HIV Transmission

D. M. Basavarajaiah •
Bhamidipati Narasimha Murthy

HIV Transmission

Statistical Modelling

Springer

D. M. Basavarajaiah
Department of Statistics and Computer Science
Veterinary Animal and Fisheries Sciences University
Bengaluru, Karnataka, India

Bhamidipati Narasimha Murthy
Department of Biostatistics
National Institute of Epidemiology, ICMR
Chennai, Tamil Nadu, India

ISBN 978-981-15-0150-0 ISBN 978-981-15-0151-7 (eBook)
https://doi.org/10.1007/978-981-15-0151-7

This Springer imprint is published by the registered company Springer Nature Singapore Pte Ltd.
The registered company address is: 152 Beach Road, #21-01/04 Gateway East, Singapore 189721, Singapore

This book is dedicated to all HIV-infected children.

Preface

HIV is a scourge. Research of almost 35 years into human immunodeficiency virus (HIV) has conceivably precipitated more questions than answers. It is widely understood that unprotected sexual intercourse, intrauterine device (IUD), and mother to child transmission (MTCT) are the main modes of HIV transmission. It's been more than three decades at global level it is an addressable issue, that has played a significant role of HIV prevention program at national and global level. Due to the paucity of enquiry-based study, the policy makers were unable to implement new scientific and innovative eradicated programs of HIV MTCT. In this propinquity of the research gap, the HIV model-based study will help to elucidate observed patterns of HIV vertical transmission rate at global scenario. However, the modelling techniques are routinely used to estimate national and global trends of the number of infants infected through HIV- MTCT. Such type of fitted models depend on the input data sets from individual antiretroviral therapy (ART) centers. The present study intervention has demonstrated different statistical and mathematical models based on the primary and secondary HIV life data sets collected from thrust area (high prevalence state). The collected HIV massive data sets were demonstrated with various mathematical and statistical models. These fitted models produce an insight analytical algorithms to prove HIV transmission rate at greater accuracy and easily substitute HIV transmission with prior and posterior probabilities (both peripartum and postnatal) for estimation of maximum likelihood (MLE's) of HIV transmission rate and algebraic bifurcations (forward/backward). Intervention of maternal infections (either incident or prevention), timing of infection, comorbidity, and clinical history have been utilized for the determination of HIV transmission rate (based on HIV MTCT infection rate). Since the fitted mathematical and statistical models would clarify the full implications of the research findings and global population dynamism of the vertical transmission (MTCT), building of this few cited mathematical models has been used extensively over the past decades to examine the epidemic of HIV and acquired immunodeficiency syndrome (AIDS) at global level. As per the normative results of the HIV vertical transmission, these fitted models will serve as an important analytical algorithms to recognize the inherent limitations of massive HIV data sets; impart scientific evidence for researchers, clinicians, and public health administrators etc. In this present book, a several important practical and statistical implications and deep illustrations are discussed, which seem to be simple yet complex, that need to be addressed and examined while analyzing HIV MTCT massive data sets. For example, HIV itself is a life-threatening deadly disease. However, too many questions arose from HIV life data sets, and the researchers/statisticians/clinicians are facing several pitfalls for the simulation and reduction of HIV massive data sets while carrying tricky situations of hypothesis testing and decision-making problems at larger population level. Majority of the chapters tailored in this book, which can attempt to demonstrate various techniques of building mathematical and statistical models while analyzing HIV transmission from mother to child in HIV real-life data sets. The present book consists of 13 chapters. Chapter 1 describes introduction of HIV transmission, brief review of the published and unpublished literature from 1997 to 2019, building of mathematical and statistical modelling techniques of HIV MTCT, objectives and chapterization of the book, real-life data sets, methodology, variables considered for the study, HIV serological markers, different patterns of HIV, TB co-infection among children living with HIV (CLHIVs), etc. Chapter 2 discusses the statistical modelling of HIV transmission. Chapter 3 describes the HIV vertical transmission DTSM simulation models from global and national perspectives and the validity of the model which was simulated by different varied parameters. Chapter 4 describes large data matrices, random walk model, and application of entropy in HIV mother to child transmission. This theoretical issue was formulated with suitable illustrations and various examples by using real-life HIV MTCT data sets and also fitted models that describe the different techniques of data reduction driven by the random walk free probability values. Chapter 5 deals with statistical modelling on postnatal transmission of HIV type I infection from mother to child on global perspectives and examines the applicability of different statistical models in real-life data sets of HIV mother to child transmission and antenatal care (ANCs) women. Chapter 6 gives survivability and growth model approach to CD_4 counts of people living with HIV (PLHIVs). This chapter also describes briefly and discusses the various issues of growth models and its applications towards estimation of survival rate in real-life data sets. Chapter 7 discusses predictive model approach to HIV TB co-infection in vertical transmission. Chapter 8 gives fitted Bayesian modelling approach to HIV transmission and describes Gaussian emulator approach that was used to extract the probability values of HIV transmission, models that were formulated by networking niche, and also describe frequentist and Bayesian model differences. Chapter 9 discusses HIV projection models, while Chap. 10 discusses the simulation modelling techniques of HIV/AIDS. Chapter 11 describes the genetic variants of HIV mother to child transmission and its meta-analysis, which was done for the real historical data sets, and have also extracted HIV subtype B and C *env* genes from 190 mother-infant pairs at global level. Chapter 12 deals with the statistical perspective approach to selection of sample. Chapter 13 describes the main significance of the entire book for induction of mathematical and statistical models to prove new formulated models of HIV mother to child transmission at population level. The prominence of the entire intact of the book traces salient objectives and practical applicability to learn what methods are available and most importantly when they should be applied in real life. Many illustrations accord to clarify the use of mathematical models and to substantiate what conclusions can be made at the right time. All the topics are driven purely on the HIV transmission research gaps and its mechanisms, according to the level of apprehension of the research scholars, policy makers, clinicians, and public health administrators.

Bangaluru, Karnataka, India
Chennai, Tamil Nadu, India

D. M. Basavarajaiah
Bhamidipati Narasimha Murthy

Acknowledgments

First and foremost, praises and thanks to the God, the Almighty, for his showers of blessings throughout our research work to complete the research successfully. We are grateful to all of those with whom we have had the pleasure to work with during this and other related HIV research works. This book is tailor based on research work conducted on children living with HIV (CLHIV) and ANCs between 2009 till date. We are grateful to a number of friends and colleagues who have encouraged us to start the research work, to preserve it, and finally to publish it. We would like to specially thank Prof. Rajashekaraiah, Vijaya PU College, for his technical supports for proof reading and all the officers of the National AIDS Control Organization, Government of India, for sharing very good HIV data for this research work. Finally, we would like to acknowledge with gratitude the support and love of our family –our parents who kept us going. This book would not have been possible without them. We feel immensely very proud for extending our heartiest thanks to the HIV-infected children who participated during this study period.

Contents

About the Authors

D. M. Basavarajaiah is an Associate Professor and Head of the Department of Statistics and Computer Science, Karnataka Veterinary Animal and Fisheries Sciences University (B), Hebbal, Bangalore. He holds a Ph.D from the National Institute of Epidemiology (NIE), ICMR, Chennai, affiliated to the University of Madras. His research focuses on statistical theory, statistical modelling on high dimensional datasets of agriculture, medicine, veterinary and animal sciences. He has written sixty-eight research articles and four academic books, and is serving as an editorial board member and scientific board advisor for various international journals. He is a life member of numerous academic organizations, and has received several accolades for his academic and research excellence, such as the "Chartered Scientist Award from the Science Council, United Kingdom in collaboration with the Royal Statistical Society; Best Reviewer award 2016 from TRANS STELLAR' Journal Publications and Research Consultancy ,TJPRC Ltd., (NAAS rated Journals); Fellow of the Royal Statistical Society, UK, Fellow of the Mathematical Society, UK , Bharathshikshratana and Indo-Dubai Achiever's Pacific award from the Global Society of Health and Educational Growth, New Delhi; Best Reviewer 2015, Best Scientific Board Advisor 2016 and Best Editorial Board Member award bestowed by the International Academy of Engineering Science and Technology, USA. He is an active member of the Board of Studies and Academic Council of Karnataka Veterinary Animal & Fisheries Sciences University

Bhamidipati Narasimha Murthy is a leading academic and researcher at the ICMR's National Institute of Epidemiology, in Chennai, He holds a Ph.D from the International Institute of Population Science (IIPS), affiliated to Bombay University (1985). His research focuses on mathematical statistics, operational research, clinical research, public health, demography and vital statistics, as well as mathematical modelling in the context of medical science and public health. He has written more than 100 research articles published in respected national and international journals. He also serves as an editorial board member, a reviewer and scientific board advisor for various leading international journals. He is a life member of various academic organisations and has received several accolades for his academic and research excellence, including the Prof. R. N. Srivastava gold medal award, Bharat Jyothi Award, and Best Citizen of India. He is a member of the board of studies of a number of national universities (University of Madras, Acharya Nagarjuna University &

University of Kerala) and a visiting emeritus Professor of Johns Hopkins University, Bloomberg School of Public Health, Baltimore, Maryland, and North Carolina University USA

Abbreviations

A

AZT+LMV	Zidovudine and lamivudine
AUC	Area under curve
ARVP	Antiretroviral prophylaxis
ARV	Antiretroviral
ART	Antiretroviral treatment
ARSH	Adolescent Reproductive & Sexual Health
ANNs	Artificial neural networks
ANC	Antenatal care
AIDS	Acquired immune deficiency syndrome
aHR	Adjusted hazard ratio
AFASS	Affordable, sustainable and safe
ACC	AIDS Control Centre

B

BF	Breast feeding
BCM	Back calculation method
BHQOL	Behavioural health related quality life domain

C

CSWs	Commercial sex workers
CPT	Cotrimoxazole prophylactic therapy
CMV	Cytomegalovirus
CLT	Central limit theorem
CLHIV	Children living with HIV
CHX	Chlorohexidine
CGR	Compound growth rate
CDC	Centers for Disease Control and Prevention
CD4	Cluster differential cells

D

DTSM	Disease transmission susceptible model
DHS	Demographic and Health Survey
DEE	Diseases epidemic equilibrium

DBS Dried blood spot
DBM Database management
DALY Disability adjusted life year

E

EPTB Extrapulmonary tuberculosis
EID Early infant diagnosis

G

GBD Global burden of disease

H

HIVRT HIV rapid test
HCV Hepatitis C virus
HBV Hepatitis B virus
HAART Highly active antiretroviral therapy
HIV Human immunodeficiency virus
Hz Hazard function

I

IVDU Intravenous drug users
IU Intrauterine
IP Intrapartum
IIDs In-depth interviews

K

KPM Kaplan–Meir model

L

LRA Logistic regression analysis
LAC Link ART centre

M

MVA Moving average model
MTCT Mother-to-child transmission of HIV
MT Modes of transmission
MLE Maximum likelihood estimation
MAC *Mycobacterium avium* complex

N

NVP Nevirapine
NRTI Nucleoside reverse transcriptase inhibitor
NNRTI Non-nucleoside reverse transcriptase inhibitor
NACP National AIDS Control Programme
NACO National AIDS Control Organization

O

OIs	Opportunistic infections

P

PTB	Pulmonary tuberculosis
PPTCT	Prevention of parent to child Transmission of HIV
PPROM	Preterm premature rupture of membranes
PCR	Polymerase chain reaction
PLHIV	People living with HIV/AIDS
PI	Protease inhibitor
PGL	Persistent generalized lymphadenopathy
PJP	*Pneumocystis jiroveci* pneumonia
PCA	Principal component analysis (PCA)

Q

QOL	Quality of life
QALIBRA	Quality of life benefit risk assessment

R

RWM	Random walk model
ROC	Receiver operating characteristics
RNA	Ribonucleic acid
RMSE	Root mean square error

S

STD	Sexually transmitted disease
SQL	Structured Query Language
SPSS	Special package for Social Sciences

T

TB	Tuberculosis

V

VL	Viral load
VCT	Voluntary counselling and testing

W

WHO	World Health Organization
WBS	Whole Blood Specimen

Y

YLL	Years of life lost
YLD	Years lived with disability

List of Figures

List of Tables

Introduction of HIV Transmission

1

1.1 Introduction

HIV is a scourge and transmitted mainly in four ways, viz., through sexual intercourse and blood transfusion, among injecting drug users, and from mother to child (MTC) (Conner et al. 1994). However, there are individual differences in the ability to transmit and acquire HIV, which remain unexplained (Abbink et al. 2003; Adriaanse et al. 1995; Agrawal et al. 2013; Ahmed et al. 1992; Aitkhaled et al. 1998; Alary et al. 2010). HIV transmission, as a result of sexual intercourse, accounts for about three quarters of all HIV infections worldwide. HIV is therefore a sexually transmitted disease (STD); the majority of the world's infections have been acquired through intercourse between men and women (heterosexual transmission). A number of studies pertaining to HIV transmission at global level showed that the likelihood of HIV was found to be statistically in an increasing trend in poor and developing countries, with the number of sexual partners and anal receptive intercourse among gay population (Agarwala et al. 2002). As with some other sexually transmitted diseases (STDs), HIV infection can also be transmitted through blood, for example, medical transfusion of infected blood or blood products, or from the use of contaminated injection and equipments by intravenous drug users. The transmission of HIV from mother to child includes transmission during pregnancy, during delivery, and through breastfeeding. Infected children under 15 years ($\leq$ 15 years) have contracted the virus by transmission from their mothers; their number reflects the prevalence in women of childbearing age (Ayaya et al. 2013). The schematic HIV mother to child transmission (MTCT) flow diagram and their risk factors are presented in Fig. 1.1. Different modes of HIV transmission were previously studied by Akaike et al. (1971), Akpa et al. (2010), Alary et al. (2010), Anderson et al. (1986), Andrea et al. (2008), Anon et al. (1999), Arya et al. (1998), Avert et al. (2008), Ayaya et al. (2013).

D. M. Basavarajaiah, B. Narasimha Murthy, *HIV Transmission*,
https://doi.org/10.1007/978-981-15-0151-7_1

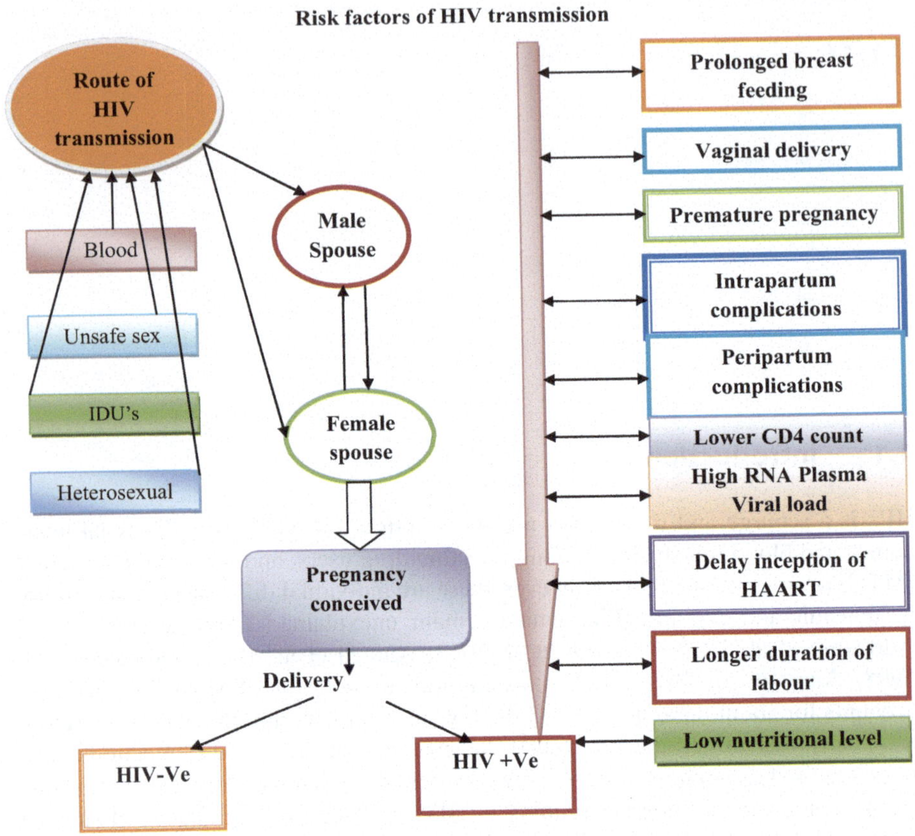

Fig. 1.1 Flow diagram of HIV—mother to child transmission (MTCT)

In the absence of any intervention, an "HIV"-positive woman has a 30–45% chance of transmitting the virus to her baby (Vajpayee et al. 2001). Approximately 5–10% of infants are infected during pregnancy, 10–20% are infected during childbirth, and 10–20% are infected through breastfeeding (BF). However, with an effective "HIV" treatment and a managed delivery, the risk of mother to child transmission (MTCT) can be greatly reduced (Shapiro et al. 2010). Transmission rates fell from 20% in India and South Asia in 2016 to <5% in 2008, as a result of the introduction of opt-out HIV testing in antenatal care (ANC), more extensive use of ARV drugs during pregnancy and delivery, Caesarean section for delivery, and formula feeding of the baby (Kapoor et al. 2004). Currently, the risk of "MTCT" in India, for women who have been diagnosed and who receive the right advise and comprehensive treatment, is <1% with transmission rates for babies of women on combination therapy and a RNA plasma viral load (VL) of <50 copies/ml at 0.10% (Creek et al. 2010). Transmission of HIV type II is less than transmission of type I. Mothers with type II are likely to have a lower viral load (VL) and slower disease progression (Kapoor et al. 2004). Between 0 and 4% of women with untreated HIV type II pass on their infections (Creek et al. 2010). HIV positive women who wish to become pregnant may be advised to choose to conceive at a time when viral load (VL) is likely to be low or easily controlled by antiretroviral (ARV) drugs. The National AIDS Control Organization (NACO) prevention of parent to child transmission (PPTCT) guidelines on managing "HIV" infection in pregnant women suggests some actions "HIV" positive women can take when preparing to conceive, including taking folic acid; avoiding transmission to their male partner, especially if she is uninfected; and aiming to delay conception until any opportunistic infections (OIs) have been treated or prophylaxis is no longer required (Taha et al. 2016). It should be stressed, however, that all HIV-positive women retain the right to make their own choices about fertility and childbirth, regardless of their health, and should be able to expect support from their physician and healthcare workers in this regard (Taha et al. 2016; Anderson et al. 1986; Andrea et al. 2008; Anon et al. 1999; Arya and Hart 1998; Avert et al. 2008; Ayaya et al. 2013). Moreover, HIV can be readily detected in the placentas of HIV positive women. The mother's viral load (VL) is a key to determine whether transmission happens during pregnancy, childbirth, or breastfeeding. The most essential preventive measure during pregnancy is the appropriate use of HIV treatment, as discussed later in this section. While transmission is most likely to take place in the third trimester (at which point viral suppression is most crucial), high viral load (VL >150,000 copies per ml) at any time in pregnancy raises the risk of transmission (Chasela et al. 2010). A recent Indian study compared women who transmitted despite having a VL (<5000 copies/ml) at the time of delivery with women who did not transmit. A higher proportion of those who transmitted had a VL (50,000 copies/ml) at 14th, 28th and 32nd weeks of pregnancy. Global data sets also show that the longer period of highly active antiretroviral treatment (HAART) use during pregnancy is associated with lower risks of "HIV" transmission. Transmission can sometimes occur before treatment is begun or before VL suppression is achieved. Treatment interruption during pregnancy including during the first trimester has also recently been associated with an increased risk of transmission. The mother's VL is likely to be exceptionally high if she has recently acquired HIV herself and so has primary HIV infection during her pregnancy (Chasela et al. 2010). In a study which specifically investigated in utero transmission, mothers with recent infection had more than twice the risk of passing on "HIV" than other mothers. One of the studies reported in New York City, USA, involved a mother who was thought to have acquired HIV during or just before her pregnancy. Illness during pregnancy has also been associated with in utero transmission. Explanations for these include temporary rises in HIV VL, increased immune activation and increased CD_4 during illness and infections, etc. In all previous studies at global level, the most important determinant of HIV transmission is the mother's VL (measured in blood around the time of delivery). For example, a large Indian-based study found that in comparison with women who had a plasma VL (< 50 copies/ml) at the time of delivery, mothers with a VL (<1000 copies/ml) had nine times the odds of transmitting HIV. If the VL (<10,000 copies/ml) had 11 times the odds of transmitting HIV and VL (>10,000 copies/ml) had 49 times the odds of transmitting HIV, while transmission is rare in mothers with undetectable VL (<50 copies/ml), it does occasionally occur. Unsurprisingly, women who do not take ARV have a higher risk of transmission. But this factor remains significant even after the impact of viral load has been taken into account. Moreover, treatment interruption during increased risk of transmission has been associated with a greatly increased risk of transmission, perhaps because they can lead to viral load rebound near the times of delivery (Csete Joanne et al. 2009). Viral load in genital and cervical secretions is also important, independent of viral load in blood (Ekouevi et al. 1985). There are clear links between herpes infections, genital ulcer disease, and raised viral load in genital secretions (Gage et al. 2006). Each of these has been associated with increased risks of "HIV" transmission. More generally, and as during pregnancy, any infection which causes inflammation of the placenta membranes surrounding the fetus will increase the risk of HIV transmission. Prolonged membrane rupture prior to delivery is a risk factor. In a large meta-analysis, for each extra hour of membrane rupture, the transmission risk increased by 2.0%. This applied whether the baby was delivered vaginally or by Caesarean section. When twins are delivered vaginally, the first-born twin spends a longer time in the birth canal than the second twin. This may account for the higher infection rate for first-born twins observed in some studies. Infants born prematurely have a higher transmission risk. In earlier studies, before effective "ARV" treatment was widely used, the effect was observed in infants born at less than 37 weeks. In the current context, it is only observed in infants born very prematurely. More specifically, bacterial vaginosis, sexually transmitted infections, and other conditions which cause inflammation of the placenta and membranes surroundings the fetus are associated with an increased risk of HIV transmission (Borkowf et al. 2015; Anon et al. 1999). Malaria can infect the placenta and is associated with increased transmission risk in some but not all studies. Tuberculosis (TB) during pregnancy is also associated with transmission. While TB has the effect of raising viral load, this doesn't account for all the increased risk. Cytomegalovirus (CMV) is a virus from the family of herpes viruses that many adults have without causing any problems. It may also be transmitted from mother to child during pregnancy or childbirth. Infants who acquire "CMV" in this way have an increased risk of acquiring "HIV" too. Some but not all studies have found that infant's girls are somewhat more likely to acquire HIV than boys. Moreover a meta-analysis report clearly states that, only including infants who were breastfed, found no gender and miscarriage for HIV-infected male infants. The use of recreational or illegal drugs during pregnancy has been linked with an increased transmission risk in a number of Indian and global studies. After controlling for other factors, substance use during pregnancy more than doubled the HIV transmission risk. However the biological relationship between drug use and "mother to child transmission (MTCT)" is not fully understood. A large proportion of mother to child transmission (MTCT) events occur during delivery as the infant passes through the birth canal and is exposed to maternal blood and genital secretions. Moreover, HIV transmission during delivery is known to occur because tests for HIV's genetic material on some infants only become positive between 14 and 28 days of birth, suggesting that they were infected at delivery. The first evidence that HIV could be transmitted via breast milk was a case report of child of previously healthy women who was delivered by a Caesarean section. Because of blood loss from the operations, the mother was given a blood transfusion after the delivery. The baby was breastfed for 6 weeks. Later, it was discovered that a unit of transfused blood had been contaminated with HIV. The mother and her infant were subsequently found to have both become infected. Moreover, HIV transmission after childbirth is known to occur because some infants test negative for HIV RNA 1 month after birth, but test positive later on. Since if the nipples are cracked or bleeding, blood may transmit the virus too. The BF and HIV global study, which analyzed data sets from 4085 infants in different African studies, found that between 24 and 42% of infants breastfed by an HIV-positive mother acquired HIV (Anon et al. 1999; Abello et al. 2002a, b; Agarwala et al. 2002; Agrawal et al. 1998; Agrawal et al. 2003; Ahuja et al. 1993; Aitkhaled et al. 1998; Akaike et al. 1971). In the absence of any interventions to reduce the risks of infection, BF is thought to account for between one third and one half of the mother to child transmissions. However in practice, the proportion population which is due to BF will vary between different populations, because the proportions of women who take "HIV" treatment and who BF vary. In Indian context, guidelines recommend that "HIV"-positive women should refrain from "BF" and should use formula feed. In much resource-limited settings, the lack of access to clean water means that the risks of MTCT through breast milk must be weighed against the risks of infant's malnutrition, infections, and mortality posed by formula feeding. The World Health Organization recommends an "either-or" approach based on available resources. HIV-positive mothers with infants who are not known to be HIV positive should either, viz., avoid BF altogether or BF with accompanying prophylactic ARV to lower the risk of HIV transmission. Should ARV drug not be available, BF may still be recommended to HIV-positive mothers. The longer the period for which an infant is BF, the greater the risk of HIV transmission. A meta-analysis of nine major studies of MTCT in HIV transmission is nearly constant throughout the period of BF. Consequently, a longer duration of BF is associated with a greater cumulative risk of transmission. A higher viral load (VL) in BF is associated with higher risk of transmission. The virus is present in lower concentration than in blood, but there is a close correlation between viral loads in blood and BF. Viral loads are highest in the first 2 weeks after childbirth. Consequently, providing ARV to the mother, the infants or birth during the BF period can significantly ($p = 0.001$) reduce the risks of HIV transmission through BF ARV taken by the mother reduce the viral load (VL) in BF but are also consumed by the infant and provide prophylaxis against infection. In African countries, a number of strategies have been investigated, including continuing maternal therapy for a few weeks after delivery and continuing maternal therapy throughout the period of BF providing prophylactic therapy to the infant throughout the period of BF. Depending on the strategy, transmission rates can be as low as 0 to 3.0%. Further, the details are given in the HIV treatment directory. Women who themselves acquire HIV after giving birth are at an elevated risks of passing on their infections due to the raised viral load (VL) in breast milk soon after infection. When the baby's only food resource is BF, the risk of infection is lower than if he or she also consumes other liquids or solids. While this seems counterintuitive, it has been observed in a number of studies. For example, a large Zimbabwean study found that mixed feeding resulted in a fourfold greater risks of HIV transmission at 6 months and threefold greater risks at 18 months. The reason for the increased risks is still not fully understood. It shows that food and water are seen by the infant gut immune system as foreign and immunological cells are recruited to fight the foreign antigens. This brings infectious BF in closer proximity to target CD_4 cells and macrophages. BF stimulates no such immunological mobilization, so that even with infectious BF, the exclusively BF infant is less likely to get infected. Because of the increased risks associated with mixed feeding, BF mothers have sometimes been advised to make a rapid switch to solid at an early stage. However viral load in BF has been observed to be considerably higher following rapid weaning than it had been beforehand. This suggests that if mothers do return to BF following weaning, the transmission risk will be greater than it was before, and many studies have found that male infants are at higher risk than female infants. This may be due to cultural differences in feeding practices, and mastitis, breast abscesses, and bleeding nipples can lead to inflammation, increasing viral levels in BF and hence transmission risks. Moreover milk becomes contaminated with blood, this also carries HIV. Should BF women develop these conditions, they are advised to avoid feeding from the affected breast until the problem clears up. In global scenario, as in developed countries, where a safe infant feeding alternatives are available (and free for women in needs), women with HIV are strongly advised against BF their babies, regardless of maternal therapy, VL, or diseases status. From birth, exclusive feeding with infant formula milk is recommended. Indian guidance has been reviewed in the light data showing the protective effect of HAART during breastfeeding. As per the PMTCT guidelines, the risk of mother to child transmission through exclusive breastfeeding from a woman who is on HAART and has a consistently undetectable HIV viral load and is likely to be low but *emphasize* that this risk has not yet been quantified. Therefore, avoidance of BF is still the best and safest option in India to prevent MTCT of HIV. In order to support women formula feed, advised to counsel and feedback recommended practical and financial measures to enable those who are poor on resources should be able to access formula milk and appropriate equipment. This includes specific measures for women subject to immigration control. Whereas an HIV positive mother's decision to BF has in the past been treated as a child protection issue., while not recommending that HIV-positive women BF, says that women who do so "should be supported to exclusively BF as safely, and for a short period as possible. This will involve:

(i) Monthly assessments of maternal viral load, side effects, and infant's HIV status.
(ii) Continuation of maternal HAART until 1 week after cessation of BF.
(iii) No mixed feeding, except in the weaning period.
(iv) Cessation of "BF" as early as possible and no later than 6 months.
(v) Education around factors that increase transmission risks.
(vi) Resources to enable switching to alternative feeding method.

The decision to avoid BF may be a very difficult one. The NACO guidelines of PMTCT recognize that in some cultural beliefs in certain communities where BF is the cultural norms, this decision may be particularly difficult, because a women's decision not to "BF" may be viewed negatively, and women's concern about this decision should be recognized and discussed in the forthcoming chapters. In specific circumstances, BF may need to be considered, for example, if women will not be remaining in India but is likely to return to a country where formula feeding is not a viable or safe option (Creek et al. 2010; Chasela et al. 2010; Chen et al. 2012; Conner et al. 1994; Creek et al. 2010; Ekouevi et al. 1985; Gage et al. 2006).

1.2 WHO Transmission Through BF Makes the Following Recommendation

The most appropriate infant feeding option for an HIV-infected mother continues to depend on her individual circumstances, including her health status and local situation, but should take greater consideration of the health services available and the counseling and support she is likely to receive. Exclusive BF is recommended for infants born to HIV-infected women for the first 6 months of life, unless replacement feeding is acceptable, feasible, affordable, sustainable, and safe (AFASS) as it usually is in India. When replacement feeding is acceptable, feasible, affordable, sustainable, and safe, avoidance of all BF by HIV-infected women is recommended. While BF will continue to carry risk of transmission, this will be reduced by the following:

The women and child being on HAART.

The woman BF exclusively. In African settings, there is evidence that mixed feeding results in a higher transmission risks than BF alone. It is suggested that mixed feeding may have exposed babies to both allergens, causing inflammation and damage to gut mucosal barriers, and HIV, which in turn led to a higher infection rate.

Minimizing the duration of "BF," switching to formula feeding if before 6 months or solid food if after 6 months.

Ensuring the woman is given early, skilled help with positioning and attachment of the baby at the breast to avoid problems such as cracked nipple and inflammatory or bacterial conditions (such as mastitis).

Treating promptly any inflammation of the mucous membranes such as oral thrush in baby mouth (Fig. 1.2, Table 1.1).

In Indian context, Caesarean birth rate is 49.0%, which is well above the national average of approximately 26.0%. This may be related to several factors. First, the majority of the group was multiparous, accounting for two thirds of the women who underwent Caesarean. Many of these women chose to undergo a repeat Caesarean,

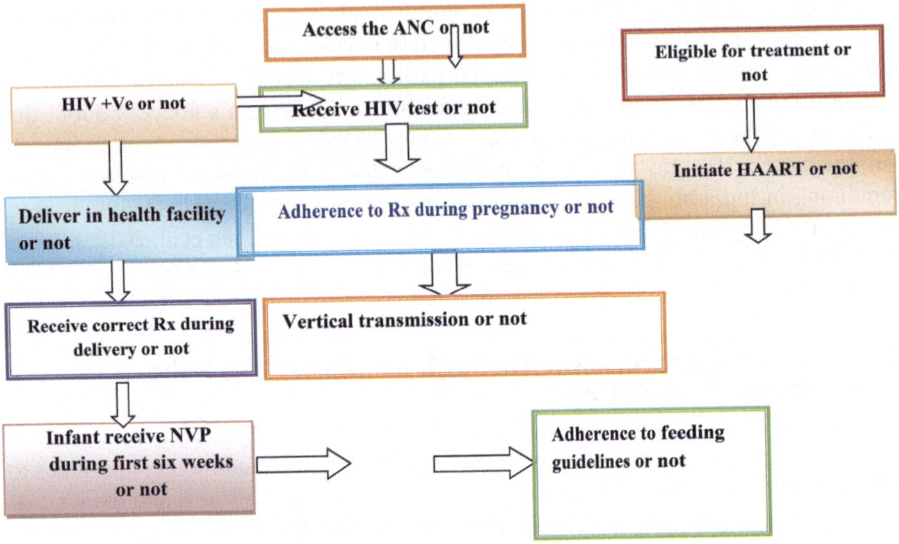

Fig. 1.2 Flow diagram of ANCs (antenatal care) for HAART treatment

Table 1.1 Estimated risk of HIV MTCT

Timing	Transmission rate
During pregnancy	5–10%
During labor and delivery	10–15%
During breastfeeding	5–20%
Overall without breastfeeding	15–25%
Overall with breastfeeding to 6 months	20–35%
Overall with breastfeeding 18–24 months	30–45%

Rates vary because of differences in population characteristics such as maternal CD_4+ cell counts, RNA viral load, and duration of breastfeeding

similar to HIV-negative women in India. Second, some "HIV"-positive women choose to undergo an elective Caesarean regardless of previous delivery status or viral load (VL). A large proportion of women in this study originate from resource-poor countries where different strategies are employed, such as Caesarean birth to prevent mother to child transmission (MTCT). Many citation describes the preterm birth rate was 16.0%, which is double the average preterm birth rate in India of 10.0%. This increased preterm birth rate has been observed in other studies of "HIV"-positive women on HAART. In previous work done (Basavarajaiah et al. 2013), the preterm delivery rate in a cohort of "HIV"-positive women was similar to the Canadian study. Possible reasons for abnormal liver function tests or preeclampsia or spontaneous preterm labor, these factors could also be a contributor to the high Caesarean birth rate observed in this intervention. More research is urgently required to further explore these relationships. Preterm premature rupture of the membrane (PPROM) in optimally managed HIV-positive women poses a clinical dilemma for management when weighing the risk of prematurity over the risk of MTCT. Our study findings (forthcoming section) clearly demonstrate that PPROM in a small number of preterm patients who were ruptured for greater than the 4-hour recommendation without a case of mother to child transmission (MTCT). Overall though, the median lengths of time of rupture for both the preterm and term patients were similar. More studies with a larger number of optimally managed patients with PPROM are required to further explore these complex issues [28–30]. Traditionally, the use of invasive procedure during labor in "HIV"-positive women has been discouraged because of the potential for increasing MTCT. In this intervention, AROM was employed for labor induction and during the active phase of labor in 46 women without increasing the likelihood of vertical transmission. There are many possible reasons for this, including an increase in the proportion of women among HIV-positive persons, changing immigration patterns, and better long-term management of HIV resulting in better overall health and an increased desire for childbearing. Since the introduction of HAART in 1998, there has been a steady decline in antenatal monotherapy use in Ontario, with an increasing acceptance of and adherence to HAART regimens. This also may have resulted in an increasing number of women who met inclusion criteria of antenatal HAART use and low VL over time. Given the number of cases from 2004 to 2014, the number for 2016 is projected to differ (Basavarajaiah et al. 2013).

1.3 CD_4 Cell Count Approach to HIV Transmission

In the HIV biological indicator, CD_4 cell counts were used to guide decision about when star HIV treatment. However, we now know that all PLHIVs with HIV benefit from HIV treatment and that it is better to start treatment sooner rather than later. Overwhelmingly CD_4 are white blood cells that play an important role in the immune system. CD_4 cell counts give an indication of the healing of HIV-infected person's immune system. This is body's natural defense system against pathogens-germs such as bacteria and virus that cause infections and illness. CD_4 cell count is the measurement of the number of blood cells in a cubic millimeter of blood (a very small blood sample). It is not a count of all the CD_4 cells in the PLHIVs. A higher number indicates a stronger immune system. The following describes in relation to CD_4 count.

(i) The CD_4 count of a person who does not have HIV can be anything between 500 μ/dL and 1500 μ/dL.
(ii) PLHIVs who have a CD_4 count over 500 μ/dL are usually in pretty good health.
(iii) PLHIVs who have a CD_4 count <200 μ/dL are significantly at risk of developing serious illness. While HIV treatment is recommended for all people living with HIV, it is especially important for people with low CD_4 counts.

If you have chosen not to start HIV treatment for the moment and then keep an eye on PLHIV, CD_4 count will help the clinician to assess how safe it is to continue without treatment. For example, if your CD_4 cell count is 200 μ/dL or less, PLHIV ANCs are at risk of developing some serious illness and infections. The physician should recommend to start treatment urgently, without delay. If the CD_4 cell count is low, physician should also offer additional drugs to try to prevent these infections, known as prophylaxis.

You should take prophylaxis whether or not you take HIV treatment. For example, you may need cotrimoxazole to prevent pneumocystis pneumonia (PCP) until PLHIV's CD_4 cell count rises above 200 μ/dL. If PLHIVs had lower CD_4 cell count, then you may take some additional tests, for example, screening of tuberculosis. If you have chosen not to take HIV treatment for the moment, PLHIV's CD_4 count will be monitored periodically once in 3 months. If it has already dropped (<250–500 μ/dL), it will be checked more often.

1.4 RNA Plasma Viral Load Approach to HIV Transmission

Once the PLHIV takes HIV treatment and viral load starts to fall, CD_4 count is likely to increase gradually. The rate at which this happens can vary a lot between individuals. During the first months of taking course of treatment, CD_4 count will continue to be monitored regularly. Nonetheless, when PLHIV takes HIV treatment, viral load is a more important indicator of the health and effectiveness of the treatment than CD_4 cell count. After a while, physician may suggest checking CD_4 cell count less often. The patients have an undetectable viral load, and when CD_4 count is over 200 μ/dL, CD_4 count will normally be checked once a year. The PLHIVs had an undetectable viral load and a CD_4 cell count over 300 μ/dL for at least a year, and then CD_4 cell counts are not needed so long as PLHIV viral load remains undetectable.

1.5 Periodic Variation of ANC CD_4 Counts

CD_4 cell counts can vary a lot between people. PLHIV's own CD_4 cell counts may go up and down in response to different factors such as exercise, lack of sleep, smoking, etc. But these factors don't seem to make any difference to how well-being of the immune system can fight against infections. Rather than attaching too much significance to an individual test result, it makes good sense to monitor any trend in changes to PLHIV CD_4 cell counts over time. It is best to have PLHIV CD_4 count measured at the same clinic and at roughly the same time of day wherever possible. If PLHIVs another infection, such as the flu or an outbreak of herpes, talks to about clinic or ART center whether it is best to delay PLHIV CD_4 counts until they had feeling better.

1.6 CD_4 Percentage of ANCs (μ/dL)

In addition to using a test to count the number of CD_4 cells, physician sometimes measures the proportion of all white blood cells that are CD_4 cells. This is called CD_4 cell percentage. Although it is not recommended that CD_4 percentage are used as general indicator of health of an adult's immune system, there can be situation where it is a useful measurement. For example, if PLHIV's CD_4 percentage is very different to PLHIV CD_4 count, it might be a sign of another health problems or HIV-associated complications. One circumstance when the physician might measure CD_4 cell percentage could be if there is a big variation in CD_4 cell count between one test and the next follow-up.

1.7 ANC Viral Load and Sexual Transmission (Copies per mL)

If ANCs have a high viral load in her blood, then she might also have a high viral load in other body fluids, including her vaginal fluid. In the first few weeks after contracting HIV viral load is usually extremely high. ANCs with high VL are more infectious and can pass on HIV more easily. On the other hand, if HIV in the blood is undetectable, it is likely to be undetectable in vaginal fluids or rectum as well. Having an undetectable VL means that the risk of HIV being passed on is extremely low. In 2014, a large scientific trials found that HIV treatment reduces the risk of passing on HIV to a regular heterosexual partner by 96%. The only reason it was not 100% is that one person in the trial did acquire HIV, but this happened just a few days before or after their partner started treatment. In 2015, a study found that no HIV transmission took place in 16,400 occasions of sex between gay men and 28,000 between heterosexual where the HIV-positive partner had a VL <200 copies per mL.

A lot of people with HIV see the reduction of infections and relief from anxiety about transmission as very important benefits of HIV treatment. PLHIV may wish to take VL and likely infectious in to consideration when thinking about safer sex. If ANC PLHIV women want to stop using condoms, it is important to wait 6 months after first undetectable VL test, to be sure that treatment is working; it is also important to discuss this issue carefully with PLHIV partners and ensure they are also comfortable with the decision. Explaining what an undetectable VL means may reduce HIV-negative partner anxiety about HIV transmission, but this information may be new to them. When HIV treatment and an undetectable VL will protect the partner from HIV, they do not protect them from other STIs (sexually transmitted infections). Also, in some countries, condom less sex without disclosing sex, is a criminal offense, regardless of the likelihood of HIV transmission. The ANCs are using HIV treatment in order to prevent sexual transmission; it is recommended to have it checked more often than might otherwise be the case. This is to check that PLHIV viral load is still undetectable. The PLHIVs are not currently taking HIV treatment, and looking at VL and CD_4 cell count can help predict the risk of becoming ill because of HIV in the future. While CD_4 count is the main indicator

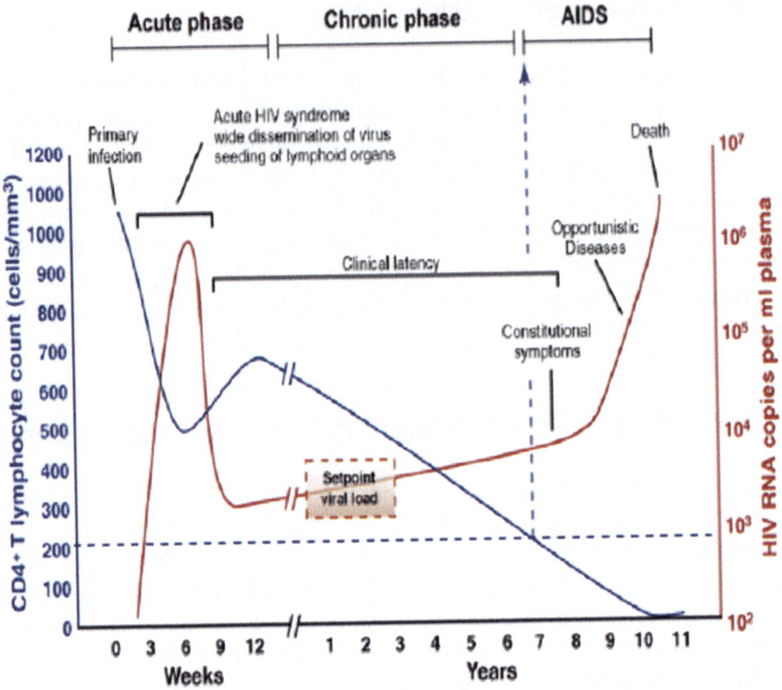

Fig. 1.3 Historical phenomena of CD_4 count and RNA plasma viral load in PLHIVs

Table 1.2 Mean CD_4 Count of ANC HIV MTCT

Status	CD_4 count Mean $\pm$ SD	P-value
Transmitter	258.55 $\pm$ 32.55	$\leq$0.0001
Non-transmitter infant survived	654 $\pm$ 16.85	$\leq$0.0001
Transmitter infant non-survived	156.88 $\pm$ 69.85	$\leq$0.0001

Recent statistical techniques in clinical research

for the physician that will be used to help monitor the health of the immune system, VL testing can also provide important information. Among PLHIV with the same CD_4 cell counts, research has shown that those with a higher VL tend to develop symptoms more quickly than those with a VL. In addition, among PLHIV with the same VL, those with lower CD_4 cell counts tend to become ill more quickly (Fig. 1.3, Tables 1.2 and 1.3).

Table 1.3 Identifying HIV-exposed infants at high risk of MTCT

Maternal factors	Infant factors
Viral load >1000 cpm from 28-week gestation	Born before 37-week gestational age
Initiated ART	Birth weight < 2500 gm regardless of GA
Defaulted ART for ≥1 month at any stage during pregnancy	Abandoned newborns/ orphans
Likely NNRTI resistance (failed 1st- or second-line ART at any stage or on second or third line during pregnancy)	Any sick HIV-exposed newborn
Diagnosed as new HIV infection from 28-week gestation or in labor/immediate postpartum	–
Diagnosed with TB/syphilis during pregnancy or immediate postnatal period clinical signs of chorioamnionitis	-

1.8 Salient Features of HIV MTCT Prevention Strategies Practiced at Global Level

Antiretroviral prophylaxis (ARP) for prevention of MTCT of HIV involves giving an ARV drugs to the mother starting at 28 weeks of gestational age, again to the mother during labor and delivery, and to her baby immediately after its birth. The drug reduces the risk of transmission of HIV to the baby. It is different from ART given to the mother to treat her own HIV infection, depending on her eligibility criteria. If an HIV-positive mother prefers and insists to deliver her baby at home, the current ARP drug that can be made available to her is nevirapine (NVP). When you know that an HIV-infected woman is near to giving birth at home, if you are authorized and trained to do so, you should give her a single dose of nevirapine (200 mg) to take when true labor starts. It is better if you make the diagnosis of true labor and administer the drug by physician. Also, the baby should receive a single dose of NVP within 3 days of being born. You should give this drug directly based on the baby's weight.

For those who decide to give birth in a health center or hospital, three types of ARP drugs are needed to be taken by the laboring mother as prophylaxis (AZT + NVP + LMV). The woman and her husband have to know that the three ARP drugs administered during labor provide better protection for the baby. Additionally, the baby will be given two drugs (AZT + LMV) for 1–4 weeks. Therefore; you have to encourage HIV-positive women to given birth in health centers or hospitals. The ARP drugs reduce the risk of MTCT of HIV to the baby, but they don't treat the mothers' HIV infection and don't improve her health. In some cases, the pregnant women can start ART drug treatment for her HIV infection before she gives birth. Therefore, you should try to encourage all HIV-infected pregnant women to go to the nearest health center to check if they can start ART that will also protect babies.

1.9 Routine HIV Testing During Pregnancy

It is advisable to carry out HIV testing on all pregnant women. The test is voluntary, and, after receiving pretest information, the woman has the right to refuse testing. The World Health Organization and the NACO promote a policy provider-initiated HIV testing and counseling. This means that when trained to do so, you should offer and provide HIV testing and counseling routinely as part of the maternal and child health services. You should not wait for the woman in these competencies, you should offer pretest education and refer the woman to the nearest health center, or you should inform her of a date for outreach testing.

1.10 Detecting of HIV Infection Using Blood Tests

HIV infection can be detected on the blood by three tests. These include the HIV rapid test (HIVRT), which is the only test which can be done in a ART center. The other two tests (the Western blot and enzyme immunoassay test) can only be done at a higher-level health facility. As it is so easy to use, the "HIVRT" is the most commonly used HIV test in India. It involves taking a very small sample of blood from the person's finger by pricking it with sterile instruments and taking a drop of blood to place onto a test kit. The principle behind all the various HIV testing kits that have been developed to screen blood is the same. The tests are highly sensitive for detecting HIV infection. They work by detecting antibodies which appear in the blood after the window period of HIV infection. The window period is the period of time between the virus entering a person's body and the appearance of detectable antibodies in the person's blood. In some cases, a person with a negative HIV test results may be infected, but the showed up because they are in the window period of infection. Testing again after 3 months from the date of infection will usually reveal an HIV-positive result.

1.11 Opt-In and Opt-Out Approach

There are two contrasting approaches to counseling pregnant women about the need for HIV testing; they are known as opt-in and opt-out approach. The opt-in and opt-out approach involves counseling a woman for about 40 minutes in a private room, to inform her about everything she wants to know, so she can agree to be tested with informed consent (i.e., opt-in and opt-out approach by the woman). Of course, at the end of the counseling session, she may refuse to have the test. Opt-in was practiced until 2006 in Ethiopia and some other countries and is still the approach in many other developing countries. Another big advantage of the opt-out approach is that HIV testing becomes a normal procedure for everyone.

The normalization of HIV testing helps to overcome fear of taking the test, so in the future, it becomes just like any other routine test for any disease, and information about HIV testing can be presented in the National AIDS Control Organization (NACO/WHO) guidelines, which also helps the community by discussing the aspect of focused ANCs and referring to the HIV test as a normal part of the routine visits. Finally, it is less time-consuming for health workers, as it does not involve a long pretest counseling with each woman.

1.12 Counseling Woman Who Refuses HIV Testing

There are some crucial points to opt-out approach that you need to understand. First the woman can refuse the test—she can opt-out. Second if the HIV test result is positive, the woman will be given posttest counseling. Third, women who opted-out (refused) will be provided with a longer session of counseling, which starts by letting them express their concerns and reasons for objections to the test, so you can address their specific questions and worries. In order to counsel opted-out effectively, you need to build trust. ***Emphasize*** that getting an early diagnosis and starting treatment or prophylaxis greatly improves the chances of survival for women who are HIV positive and their babies. Knowing her HIV status does not necessarily mean a woman's husband or partner has the right to know as well—it is her full right either to disclose her HIV status or to hide it. However, for better outcomes of follow-up and treatment, disclosing the truth to her family has a big advantage because they can support her. Assure the woman that HIV is no longer a disease that needs to be hidden or one that people should be ashamed of. Also, it is not disease that always leads to death provided that people are diagnosed early and treatment is started early.

If a woman continues to refuse the HIV test, further counseling should be provided in subsequent ANC visits. She should be reassured that opting-out of HIV testing will not affect her access to antenatal care, labor and delivery care, postnatal care, or related services. Encourage her to reconsider testing. Do not pressure her to be tested, but let her know that if she changes her mind, an HIV test and further counseling can always be provided during a later visit. Document the reasons for her refusal in your notes as reminder to offer her HIV counseling and testing the next time. Many studies documented the reasons why woman refuses HIV testing:

(i) Fear of being found HIV positive and losing hope.
(ii) Fear of positive HIV result causing marriage disharmony and divorce.
(iii) Fear of being found HIV positive and not trusting the health professionals to keep the results private.
(iv) Fear of a positive HIV test leading to stigma and discrimination by the community.

1.13 Discussing HIV Test Posttest Counseling

If a woman has agreed to and had the HIV test, you need to know how to discuss the results with her during posttest counseling. In an adult, a positive HIV test results mean that the person is definitely infected with HIV. PLHIV may be at high risk for HIV if she has recently had unprotected sexual intercourse with a man of unknown HIV status or with a man known to be HIV positive or if her husband has another sex partner or had illegal relationship or if her husband injects illegal drugs. If such a woman tests negative the first time, she should be tested again after 3 months to confirm the original results.

1.14 Posttest Counseling for HIV Pregnant Women

In talking to a woman delivering HIV test results, you should be very sensitive to her feelings, which may include shock, anger, or denial. When she is able to take in your health education messages, make sure that she understands the importance of delivering her baby in a higher-level health facility where ARP drugs are available and safe delivery methods are practiced to prevent MTCT of HIV. She can reduce the risk of becoming ill by taking ART as prescribed and medicine to prevent OIs from developing; practicing safe sex by using a condom with her partner to protect him from HIV infection, and to ensure she doesn't get any other sexually transmitted infections (STIs) from him if he has unsafe sex with anyone else; eating enough nutrition foods, as recommended for all pregnant women regardless of HIV status; and having good personal hygiene, as recommended for everyone to prevent infections with bacteria, viruses, protozoans, and fungi, infections with parasites and insects, and skin disorders.

(i) Women partner or husband and children should be tested for HIV.
(ii) The importance of preventing HIV transmission to other and the way to do this.
(iii) The importance of referral for follow-up and ongoing HIV healthcare herself, her HIV-exposed baby, and other family members.

1.15 Posttest Counseling for HIV-Negative Women

(i) Even though the woman will be very relieved that she has tested negative, you should ensure that she understands:
(ii) How to remain HIV negative through using safe sex practices.
(iii) The need for later HIV testing if additional risk exposure occurs or if the test was done during the window period of early "HIV" infection.
(iv) Exclusive breastfeeding for her baby (i.e., just breastfeeding, no bottle-feeding or feeding of solid foods before 6 months of age).
(v) If she becomes HIV infected during pregnancy or while breastfeeding, the baby has an increased risks of MTCT.

The importance of effective family planning and birth spacing.

1.16 Additional Care for the HIV-Positive Woman During Pregnancy

Finally, we should mention that a recent study conducted in India showed that most of the study participant believed that if HIV-infected women got pregnant, their general health would deteriorate because pregnancy acerbates HIV disease progression. As mentioned above, being pregnant does not mean that the healthy condition of the woman will deteriorate. However, maternal health may deteriorate during pregnancy because of the stage of HIV. If a woman gets pregnant when she has advanced HIV, she will certainly need additional nursing and palative care that guides the service providers to give her additional care (Table 1.4).

1.17 Topical Antiseptic

A large randomized trial of intrapartum vaginal chlorhexidine washes failed to demonstrate a protective effect against vertical transmission. Although there was no protection in the group overall, chlorhexidine was associated with a significantly lower rate of infection in a subgroup of women with prolonged ruptured membranes. Several observations, including the differential inflation rate of vaginally delivered first-born twins, the protective effect of Caesarean delivery, and the association of prolonged ruptured membranes with vertical transmission, suggest that infant exposure to HIV-1 in the genital tract during delivery is an important determinant of transmission. Compared with other intervention strategies, topical microbicides have

Table 1.4 Intervention to Prevent MTCT Type I

Correlate	Model	Intervention
Maternal VL	ART of syphilis, gonorrhea, chlamydia	HAART (AZT combination)
Infant VL exposure	Postnatal antibiotic treatment of infants at risk for bacterial infections acquired intrapartum (i.e., after prolonged ruptured membrane/maternal fever)	ART (AZT)
Maternal genital VL	Group B streptococcus	Topical antiseptic (i.e., chlorhexidine)
Maternal immunocompromise	Primary active HSV hepatitis B	Caesarean section
		Passive immunotherapy of infant
Breastfeeding	Human T-cell lymphotropic virus	Breast milk alternative

VL viral load, *HSV* herpes simplex virus

the advantage of being safe and inexpensive and can be used without HIV-1 screening of pregnant women; another trial of chlorhexidine is currently underway.

1.18 Caesarean Section

Although Caesarean delivery may be associated with decreased transmission, this intervention is not one that can be easily implemented in resource-poor settings. The long-term effects of operative delivery on disease progression in HIV type I-infected mothers also need to be considered as a randomized clinical trial of Caesarean versus vaginal delivery is ongoing. As a randomized trial, the study will be able to evaluate the non-confounded risk of vaginal delivery for vertical transmission. In the future, a decision algorithm which identifies high-risk transmitters, comparable to the one used for herpes simplex virus, may be useful in determining which women should undergo delivery.

1.19 Immunoglobulin

Immunoglobulin administration in combination with vaccination has been an effective intervention in the prevention of vertical transmission of HBV. Many trial is evaluating the effectiveness of postpartum administration of HIV-1-specific immunoglobulin to infants. In HBV infection, the presence of specific immunoglobulin G in the absence of antigenemia indicates clearance of infection secondary to an effective host immune response. The presence of HIV-1-specific antibody, however, is not associated with clearance of HIV-1 infection. Thus, passive protection of the infant by HIV-1-specific immunoglobulin may be a less promising intervention.

1.20 Avoidance of Breastfeeding

While it is clear that BF transmission of HIV-1 occurs, there are limited alternatives to BF in setting where HIV-1 is most prevalent. A randomized clinical trial of BF and formula feeding. Determination of the amount and timing of BF transmission will be useful in determining safe recommendations for the feeding of HIV-1-exposed infants. If there is a substantial amount of late BF transmission, early weaning might be a practical intervention.

1.21 Vitamin A

A trial of antenatal maternal vitamin A administration is ongoing. VA is inexpensive and could probably be safely administered to all expectant mothers in population with high prevalence of HIV-1 infection, without the need for HIV screening. Although V_A has been associated with teratogenicity when administered in large

Table 1.5 Rates of mother to child transmission (MTCT) assessed at 4–8 weeks after delivery (reflecting intrauterine, intrapartum, and early postpartum infection), by peripartum antiretroviral therapy used

Authors	MTCT rate %	Age at assessment year	HAART used in peripartum period	Median CD_4 count
Dabis et al., Wiktor et al.	14.73	6	ZDV	545
Guay et al. (1999)	11.92	6	NVP	461
Moodley et al.	10.72	4	ZDV + 3TC	405
The Petra Study Team (2002)	8.10	6	ZDV + 3TC	475
The Petra Study Team (2002)	6.48	4	ZDV + NVP	370
Dabis et al.	4.53	4	ZDV + 3TC + NVP	439

doses during pregnancy, supplementation with lower doses during pregnancy has not been associated with toxicity. VA has the additional benefits of decreasing childhood morbidity in infants exposed to HIV_1 (Table 1.5).

1.22 Global and National Epidemiological Trend

The epidemiology of HIV-1/AIDS dates back to early 1980s, when the first case of unusual immune deficiency was identified among gay men in the USA. There are two main types of HIV, viz., type I and type II. HIV-1 is the most common and the more virulent of the two. The infectivity of HIV-1 is lower than HIV-2 and it occurs predominantly in Asian countries. Dual infection with HIV-1 and HIV-2 can occur, and it has been suggested that HIV-2 may confer some protection against HIV-1. Based on UNAIDS estimates of December 2000, there are 36.10 million people living with HIV-1/AIDS in the world. The majority (34.7 million) are adults in their reproductive age (15–49 years), of which 16.4 million are women. Currently, over 1.4 million children under 15 years of age are infected with HIV-1. During the year 2000, 5.3 million people were newly infected with HIV-1, and three million deaths occurred from HIV-1/AIDS. In India, there are an estimated 2.1 million people living with HIV (PLHIV), with national adult HIV prevalence of 0.27% in 2011. Of these, women constitute 39% of all PLHIV, while children less than 15 years of age constitute 7% of all infections. As of March 2015, 0.1 million HIV-positive children had been registered under the antiretroviral therapy (ART) program, and 38,579 are receiving free HAART. There has been a significant scale-up of HIV counseling and testing, prevention of parent to child transmission (PPTCT), and ART services across the country over the last 5 years. Between 2004 and 2015, the number of pregnant women tested annually under the prevention of parent to child transmission (PPTCT) program increased from 0.8 million to 8.83 million, and reach of the services has expanded to the rural areas to a large extent [5]. Concurrently, there has also been a significant decentralization and scale-up of the ART services, with 7.34 lakh people living with HIV (PLHIV) receiving free ART across the country through 409 ART centers and 860 link ART centers (LAC).

Mother to child transmission of HIV is a major route of HIV infection in children. However, out of an estimated 27 million pregnancies in a year, only about 52.7% attend health services for skilled care during childbirth in India. Of those who availed health services, 8.83 million ANCs received HIV counseling and testing during March 2015, out of which 12,551 pregnant women were detected to be HIV positive. To enhance this coverage, a joint directive from the National AIDS Control Program (NACP) and the National Rural Health Mission (NRHM) regarding convergence of the two program components was issued in July 2010, explicitly stating that universal HIV screening should be included as an integral component of routine ANC checkup. There are about 33.2 million human immunodeficiency virus (HIV)-infected people in the world, of which about 22.5 million are in sub-Saharan Africa. Of adult infections, 40% are in women and 15% in individuals of 15 to 25 years of age. Prenatal infection has resulted in large number of children being born with HIV. In 2006, the National AIDS Control Organization (NACO) of India reported an estimate of 4.58 million people living with HIV/AIDS in the country[2]. The HIV seroprevalence among pregnant women has been reported to be between 0.5 and 3.3% in various parts of the country. However, recent trends suggest that the incidence of HIV infection in women seeking antenatal care may be as high as 6%, and India can expect 75,000 HIV-infected neonates to be born every year. India has the second highest number of HIV-infected individuals. Of these, approximately 2.02 million are children. These children face some of the most tragic consequences of HIV infection: being orphaned, replacing a bread winner, nursing sick and dying parents, and struggling for survival in the streets. Mother to child transmission is the largest source of HIV infection in children below 15 years of age. The transmission of HIV from mother to child can take place within the uterus, during birth, or through breastfeeding. This vertical transmission can be drastically reduced by following prevention of parent to child transmission (PPTCT) guidelines. The measures taken for prevention of parent to child transmission of HIV comprise of: primary prevention among prospective parents through education and counseling, prevention of pregnancy among HIV-positive women, testing of HIV status of all pregnant women, provision of antiretroviral drugs to HIV-positive mothers, and replacement feeding for infants.

1.23 Global Trend

Those countries that are having and implementing good programs on prevention of mother to child transmission (MTCT) of HIV, such as the USA and Western Europe, have been able to reduce the number of children with vertically transmitted infection to less than 1%. Without intervention, the risk of transmission is 25–45%. India integrated the program on prevention of mother to child transmission along with antenatal care and immunization activities long before, but it has not been effective. The main obstacles to their implementation in India are found to be lack of infrastructure and cost (CDC 2018). Only few places have adequate antenatal services with voluntary counseling. Even in places where such facilities exist, due to existing customs and beliefs, many fail to avail the resources available. There is shortage of trained counselors which result in awareness deficit among the needy population. Majority of the deliveries take place outside the hospitals which exposes the baby at high risk of acquiring infection from mother. The cost involved in antiretroviral treatment and stigmatization of HIV-positive individuals are other important contributing factors which limit the uptake of testing, treatment, and infant feeding modifications. Karnataka, still being a developing state, with vast population, diverse social and cultural groups, and limited health facilities and with an illiterate population of around 30%, is vulnerable for many health-related problems especially HIV and AIDS. Prevention is the only solution to remain away from HIV, and it can be achieved through knowledge about its transmission and prevention aspects.

1.24 Economic and Demographic Impact at National Level

The disease transmission of HIV-1 through mother to child-transmission (HIV MTCT) is expected to place enormous economic burden on national "GDP" and on healthcare facilities. Globally, in some places in Africa, Europe, and America, "AIDS" has become the leading cause of death among adults. AIDS kill people in their prime and productive years. In addition to this, HIV pandemic has already resulted in the death of over one million children. Even for those children who escape perinatal infection, survival rates will decrease because of the loss of one or both parents due to AIDS. Overall, infant and child mortality rates have exceeded previous projections by as much as 30%. Life expectancy, which had been increasing in most of these countries, is now declining in many of them. Though, as a result of medical advances, since 1931, the Indian life expectancy has more than doubled from 26.5 to 60.6 years and the IMR has decreased from 174 to 95, the country faces enormous public health problems including a high prevalence of diarrhea diseases, tuberculosis (TB), and AIDS. AIDS also poses a threat to economic growth in many countries, which are already in distress. The World Bank estimates an annual slowing in growth of income per capita by an average of 0.6% per country in the ten worst affected countries. The negative impact of AIDS on households, productive enterprises, and countries stems partly from the high cost of treatment, which diverts resources from productive investments. There is two-way relationships between HIV and economy. HIV results in high morbidity and mortality among young adults, thereby reducing the quantity and quality of labor available to produce gross national product (GNP). A declining GNP has a negative impact on other social indicators, e.g., life expectancy, access to education, future income, and capacity for the care of dependents. There are also structural changes within households brought about by the dissolution of families. Other variables include depletion of the labor force, adverse impact on productive and social sectors, declining health services, shrinking revenues, and loss of military strength. The end results can be social and political unrest, destitution, and socioeconomic disintegration, which can lead to further spread of HIV infection.

1.25 Statistical Implications

The statistical modelling is an essential tool for understanding of disease progression and its relationships with social, biological, and environmental mechanisms that influence the spread of HIV/AIDS (Lih-ing et al. 2009; May et al. 1998; Lallemant et al. 2004; Guay et al. 1999; Diallo et al. 2010; Conner et al. 1994), fitted modelling has examined by the magnitude of the AIDS epidemic and statistical techniques for estimating key aspects of the disease progression. According to Fusaro et al., the model can attempt to discover the underlying structure of a process from observed data in the presence of variability. Several standard models have been developed for HIV epidemic. Thus, the statistical models are essential tool for clinicians and policymakers for understanding the spread of HIV/AIDS and its progression in state and country. AIDS epidemiology is interdisciplinary, and it calls for coordinated scientific effort across a wide range of disciplines. To this end, there shall be an effective mechanism to share the data and to answer the following crucial questions:

(i) How does HIV transmission vary with time after infection and with disease stage?
(ii) Which is responsible for the large variation in incubation time?
(iii) What are the co-factors affecting infectivity on MTCT?
(iv) What is the time between infection and transmission?
(v) Will current trends in the spread of the HIV continue?
(vi) Can we explain the past rate of growth of the endemic?
(vii) Can we predict the future size of the endemic precisely?

It is to be noted that information on HIV/AIDS is surrounded by sensitive, social, legal, and ethical issues. Researchers attempting to answer the above questions do not have access to the important elements of raw data. Identifying the sources and availability of such data itself is the beginning. Bio-statisticians have to evaluate the available data sources and develop estimation and projection methods based on such data. Issues that are essential to the understanding and management of the disease have generated numerous statistical challenges. Some of these are as follows:

(i) Estimation of incubation distribution.
(ii) Estimation of infection rate on modern projectile mathematical and statistical models.
(iii) Designing of new epidemiological and genetic model for determination of HIV transmission.

(iv) Choosing proper infection density.
(v) Projection of the course of the endemic.
(vi) Dealing with confidentiality and analysis of incomplete data.
(vii) Inadequacy of data on HIV/AIDS for assessing the size and progression of endemic.

The statistical models have played an important role in understanding HIV infection and its manifestation of AIDS. Statistical ideas and methods enter naturally in these studies in view of the considerable amount of uncertainty in disease phenomenon. Further, data from AIDS studies have many new features, which need development of special types of statistical tools and methodology. In this context, the present thesis tries to fill the gap with the following rationale and objectives.

1.26 Review of Literature Survey

In this section, the attempt has been made to review the relevant literature linking to statistical, mathematical, and epidemiological models on HIV transmission from mother to child (MTCT). This is done particularly from the point of view of assimilating the usability and applicability of the models that have taken place in India and global level. The purpose of the review of literature is to focus analytical research gap derived from modelling techniques, those models which are bearing on HIV transmission from mother to child (MTCT), especially in the context of national and global level. From the published or unpublished research, it appears that attempts have been made during the past two decades to study the impact of modelling on "HIV MTCT" by leading bio-statistician, demographer, and economists. The modelling works that have been developed on HIV transmission from mother to child have been grouped into four categories, namely:

(i) Theoretical statistical modelling (without applications).
(ii) Mathematical modelling (parsimonious and full-blown modelling).
(iii) Statistical modelling (with applications).

Busenberg et al. discussed a variety of diseases that transmit both horizontally and vertically and gave a comprehensive survey of the formulation and the mathematical analysis of compartmental models that also incorporate vertical transmission. Tomas et al. fitted CD_4 T lymphocyte count dynamics mathematical model on antenatal care (ANCs), and study concludes that fitted dynamic models can able to incorporate a feedback mechanism regulating the production of T lymphocytes and simulates the dynamics of CD_4 cells, and also he found that CD_4 cells were good prognostic indicator of HIV infection, the fitted model was used to simulate various therapeutic interventions such as chemotherapy and active and passive immunization. Timaeus et al. fitted disease transmission simulation model, and it was fitted for utilizing population-based data, which divided the female population into two groups, those who are HIV-free and those with HIV. The model was developed in such a way that it would feed into the conventional orphan hood simulation method. Three crucial variables introduced in the model are as follows: *F* (undefined but mathematically related to *F (a,y)* which is the age-specific ratio of fertility of seropositive to seronegative women who gave birth *a* years ago at age *y*); *h*, the proportion of seropositive mothers who transmit the virus to their children prenatally; and *P* the seroprevalence rate for women seen at ANC's clinics. The model was showed to be diseases and endemic equilibrium status (R0 < 1 and R0 > 1). Aalen et al. fitted Markov chain model to know the AIDS and HIV diagnosis. The fitted model comprises of ten states. Three of the states refer to HIV infection before AIDS, but before diagnosis. Three additional states refer to these stages of HIV infection but with diagnosis. One state refers to HIV infection with diagnosis and treatment. The remaining three states refer to AIDS (without diagnosis and with diagnosis and treatment). Fitted model is more reliable for estimation of disease progression rate. Stover et al. (2000) opined that simulation modelling played a major role in increasing our understanding of the dynamics of the epidemic and in demonstrating how much we still need to learn. Its impact on policies and programs has been limited. The need for better translation of modelling findings to policy action will be even greater in the future. Nagelkerke et al. (2002) fitted dynamic compartmental simulation model for Botswana and India, developed to identify the best strategies for preventing spread of HIV/AIDS. Mother to child transmission program could reduce the HIV transmission to infants but would have no impact on the epidemic itself. In the long run, interventions targeting sexual transmission would be even more effective in reducing the number of HIV-infected children than mother to child transmission programs. Antiretroviral therapy would prevent transmission in the short term, but eventually its effects would wane because of the development of drug resistance. Vieira et al. (2003) discussed the development of an operational model that can be used to evaluate intervention options for the prevention of MTCT of HIV. The problem was approached by defining suitable pregnancy risk groups, prevention options, and the required model outputs to evaluate different intervention strategies. The method chosen to approach the problem was a discrete-event, three-phase simulation, built in Visual Basic, with a stochastic semi-Markov structure the same study put forth by Celine Maria et al. and Chasela et al. (2009). Simulation model takes individual pregnant women through each stage of their pregnancy, labor, and birth. Different intervention strategies were modelled at any time, including short-course antiretroviral drugs and cessation of breastfeeding (BF). The model was demonstrated with various MTCT parameters (Botswana data sets). The MTCT rate was geometrically progressed in Botswana, one of the highest HIV infection rates in the world reported by Low-Beeri et al. (1997). Rauner et al. (2005) fitted discrete-event simulation model that evaluates the relative benefits of two potentially affordable interventions aimed at preventing mother to child transmission of HIV, namely, antiretroviral treatment at childbirth and bottle-feeding strategies. The model uses rural Tanzanian data and compares different treatment policies. Study results demonstrated that strategic guidelines about breastfeeding (BF) are highly dependent on the assumed infant mortality due to bottle-feeding, the efficacy of antiretroviral treatment at childbirth, and the maternal health stage. The cost of averted infections, though low by Western standards, may represent significant obstacles to policy implementation in developing countries. Martin et al. (2010) and Shapiro et al. (2010) fitted semi-Markov chain mathematical simulation models to know the progression of HIV infection and HAART treatment effects. As per the resulted findings of the fitted model, the reproduction number will give an idea for HIV treatment procedures, disease progression, and possible therapeutic protocol. Further, Akpa et al. (2010) studied mathematical modelling for human immunodeficiency virus (HIV) transmission epidemics. The mathematical models are specialized by stochastic differential equations that were solved by the use of moment-generating functions (MGF). Models based on mother to child transmission (MTCT) (age group 0–5 years), heterosexual transmission (age group 15 and more years), and combined case (incorporating all groups and the two modes of transmission) were developed, and the expectations and variances of susceptible **(S)** persons, infected **(I)** persons, and AIDS cases were found in the model findings. The ***S1*** ***(t)*** susceptible model produced a constant expectation and increased quotient of variance. It was shown that the mother to child transmission and heterosexual models were special cases of the combined models. Lounes et al. (1986) developed a non-linear compartmental model for the HIV detection in Cuba with different types of detection, some random and other non-random variables. The fitted models analytically derived a different reproduction numbers and use the data from the Cuban HIV/AIDS epidemic during 1986–2008 to fit the model. The reproduction numbers for each time period were also computed from the sets of values of the parameters. He found that random screening will be most important as a mean of surveillance, since there will always be an epidemic random screening that exceeds one. Moreover, local asymptotic and stability for DEF could be achieved if random screening was sufficiently effective and importance of education for the known infections exceeds unity (due to inefficient detection by random screening or lack of behavior change by the known infectious), the endemic equilibrium was always unstable, and it was possible that the number of infectious would increase without equlibrium boundary , if the initial infective population sizes are very large and outside the domain of attraction of the disease-free equilibrium (DFE). On the other hand, if it is less than one, then either the DFE or the endemic equilibrium was globally asymptotically stable, leading to a more manageable epidemic for public health purposes, even if the diseases is not eradicated. Srinivasrao (2009) fitted higher-order differential mathematical models by using Range and Kutta method for predicting the HIV MTCT rate, the resulted model was found to have more approximation to the real value, fitted models served as a tool for understanding the epidemiology of human immunodeficiency virus and AIDS, and also he concluded that initial ARV therapy including nevirapine (NVP) or efavirenz (EFV) is effective in patients with an advanced HIV-1 infection. Lower baseline CD_4 cell count and high RNA plasma viral load (micro/dL) are more associated with the occurrences of opportunistic infections (OIs) and mother to child transmission (MTCT) rate. Roeger et al. concluded that tuberculosis (TB) is the leading cause of death among individuals infected with the human immunodeficiency virus (HIV). The study depicted that the joint dynamics of HIV and TB is formidable mathematical challenges, due to the fact that the models of transmission are quite distinct. Furthermore, although there is overlap in the populations at risk of HIV and TB infections, the magnitude of the proportion of individuals at risk of both diseases is not known. The analytical based study derived a highly simplified deterministic model that incorporate-rates the joint dynamics of TB and HIV, a model that is quite hard to analyze. Study computed various independent reproductive numbers for TB (R_1) and HIV (R_2) and the overall reproductive number for the system, $R = \max \{R_1, R_2\}$. The focus of model fitting is naturally (given the highly simplified nature of the framework) on the qualitative analytics. Further, he found that if R1 < 1, then the disease-free equilibrium was seen locally asymptotically stable. Tuberculosis is only equilibrium and found to be locally asymptotically stable if $R_1 > 1$ and $R_2 < 1$. However, the symmetric condition, $R_1 < 1$ and $R_2 > 1$, does not necessarily guarantee the stability of the HIV-only equilibrium EH, and it is possible that TB can co-exist with HIV, when R2 > 1. In other words, in the case when $R_1 < 1$ and $R_2 > 1$ (or when $R_1 > 1$ and $R_2 > 1$), present study will able to find a stable HIV/TB co-existence equilibrium. Moreover, the results showed that the prevalence level of TB was seen increased trend with $R_2 > 1$ under certain conditions. Johnson et al. described a mathematical model of HIV incidence in children, and HIV survival rate has been created by using South African data source. The model describes the size of the population under the age of 15 at monthly intervals, starting in the middle of 1985. Estimates of the 1985 population profile, non-AIDS mortality rates, and annual numbers of births to mothers who are HIV positive and HIV negative were extracted from the ASSA. So that, the fitted model will allow estimation of vertical transmission from mothers, who seroconvert after their antenatal HIV screening visits. The model will allow for building two modes of HIV transmission in children under the age of 15, transmission from infected mothers at or before birth (*intrapartum* or *intrauterine* transmission) and transmission from infected mothers after birth, as a result of breastfeeding (BF). In the absence of PMTCT, women who are HIV seropositive at the time of their first antenatal screening visit are assumed to have an average probability of transmitting the virus at delivery equal to 0.20, with the probability varying according to the mother's CD_4 counts. A higher transmission probability applies, if the mother becomes infected prior to delivery and seroconverts after her first antenatal visit. In the absence of PMTCT, women who were HIV seropositive at delivery were assumed to have a constant HIV transmission probability per month of breastfeeding (BF). If the woman acquires HIV while breastfeeding (BF), a higher transmission probability was assumed to apply during the acute phase that follows HIV acquisition. Based on the 1998 South African Demographic and Health Survey (DHS), it was assumed that 86.70% of undiagnosed HIV-positive mothers breastfeed and the median duration of breastfeeding was 18 months. Assumptions about access to PMTCT and uptake were based on District Health Information System data collected from 2004 to 2009 and from earlier surveys. The HIV transmission probability at birth was assumed to reduce by 40%, if the mother receives single-dose nevirapine during labor and by 65% if the mother receives three doses. Mohammed et al. (2012), Swaminathan et al. (2004), and Springer et al. (2004) fitted non-linear mathematical model on the spread of HIV/AIDS in a varied size of population with a constant recruitment of susceptibles. The results showed that the basic reproductive number $R_0 < 1$ corresponds to a disease-free equilibrium, indicating that the disease was under control. The diseases become endemic if R0 > 1, and thus the disease remains in the population. Pinkerton et al. (2012) fitted several mathematical modelling on studies based on the concept of "HIV MTCT" rates. The extended transmission rate approximately was found to be 51.6% of new infections in the USA which is due to the transmission risk behaviors of ANCs who were unaware of their infection, including 10.90% due to PLHIVs in the acute phase of HIV infection. Findings from this study suggested that significant reductions ($p < 0.001$) in HIV incidence likely requires a combination of increased antibody testing, enhanced early detection of acute HIV infection, appropriate medical care and antiretroviral medicine adherence counseling, and behavioral risk reduction interventions. Ayaya et al. (2013) developed a patient level (Monte Carlo) model of HIV progression among untreated children <5 years of age, using the cost-effectiveness of preventing AIDS complication model framework. The model postulated with opportunistic infections (OIs) and mortality risks from the International Epidemiology Database to Evaluate AIDS (IeDEA). The data was validated from the suitable tool for fitting the model by varying WITS-derived CD_4 percent data, comparing the corresponding model-generated survival curves to empirical survival curves from Idea, and identifying best-fitting parameter sets as those with a root-mean square error (RMSE) <0.01. Model-generated survival curves for children aged 0–60 months were compared, again using RMSE, to UNAIDS data from >1300 untreated, HIV-infected African children. The resulted model determined that the survival curves fit Idea data well; modelled and observed survival at 16 months of age were 91.2% and 91.1%, respectively. RMSE varied widely with variations in CD_4 percent parameters; the best-fitting parameter set (RMSE = 0.00423) resulted when CD_4 percent was 45% at birth and declined by 6% per month (ages 0–3 months) and 0.3% per month (ages >3 months). The CEPAC-Pediatric model performed well in internal validation analyses. Increases in modelled mortality risks required to match UNAIDS data highlight the importance of pre-enrollment mortality in many pediatric cohort studies. Nguefacket al. (2014), Goldman Emiley et al. (2007), and Vieira et al. (2003) developed a stochastic simulation model to estimate the number of new HIV infections in children and the MTCT rate (perinatal and postnatal rates) based on the level of the observed uptake of PMTCT programs over the different steps of the PMTCT CASCADE at the national level in Cameroon. A discrete-event computer simulation-based approach with a stochastic structure was proposed to generate a cohort of pregnant women followed up in several states (the different steps of the PMTCT cascade) during pregnancy until delivery (perinatal transmission) and optionally until complete weaning (postnatal transmission). Thomas et al. (2007a, b) discuss transition probabilities from one state to another, derived from published data sources at the national level in Cameroon reporting on the prevalence of HIV, access to antenatal care, coverage of HIV testing, number of women who are aware of their HIV status, coverage of CD_4 cell assessment, and live birth rates. After simulation, HIV transmission rates depended on the timing of the infection (before or during pregnancy or during breastfeeding), maternal CD_4 count, type of PMTCT treatment, and type and duration of breastfeeding. Borkowf et al. (2015) fitted Markova semi-structured simulation model (0.1,1). The fitted model parameters included the annual number of HIV-infected pregnant women, the number of perinatally infected infants, the proportion of infants exposed to antiretroviral drugs during the prenatal and intrapartum period, and the estimated mother to child transmission rate in the absence of preventive interventions. As per the resulted model, the cumulative transmission MTCT rate was 7.68%. The fitted model is best fit for HIV large data set of MTCT, and it would be serving as a tool for clinician, policymaker, and researchers for implementation of new program. Nedelman et al. fitted statistical projection models (logistic regression, exponential smoothing model) and its application to AIDS. Study revealed that, the models based study on transmission mechanisms of AIDS can able to help the medical and scientific fields to understand and anticipate its progression rate. Since, AIDS is expected to place enormous demand on healthcare facilities and implementations of care, support, and treatment program by policymakers, there is pressing need to develop flexible and understandable prediction models that also can be served as an integral part of long-range scientific research program. Timaeus et al. developed a specific model of HIV/AIDS and explained on age patterns of mortality rate of ANCs. Parameters were derived using modelled life tables that have different age patterns of HIV mother to child transmission. The model life tables were used for linking indices of survivorship over different age ranges, and also he studied age patterns of HIV-MTCT from the available data. As per his computerized model, ANCs with low demographic profile were more prone to transmission of HIV from mother to child. Timaeus et al. fitted double hit exponential smoothing statistical modelling on disease progression of MTCT and mortality in sub-Saharan Africa; the model was assessed using data from national surveys and censuses. While he pointed out that the spread of HIV infection was not the only reason for the slowdown in mortality decline in Africa, the results showed clear split between those countries where one would expect significant HIV mortality by the time the data were collected and those where one would not. Springer et al. continued the same investigation further and explored using in-depth analysis of few countries of HIV mother to child transmission. Simwa et al. study dealt with a deterministic model for HIV epidemic with three stages of disease progression among infected patients. It was assumed that the patient once infected experiences disease progression up to full-blown AIDS. Using two systems of ordinary differential equations that were coupled through a delay in one of the systems, a compartmental model for the dynamics of the HIV/AIDS epidemic was constructed. The transmission of the disease was considered to be only through heterosexual contact and vertically from an infected mother to her unborn child. Numerical integration of the equations was used for simulating the stage-specific epidemic curves, given the demographic and epidemiological parameters of the model. Simulation models were noted that all the three stage-specific prevalence rate curves also satisfied the equilibrium condition. Vieaira et al. studied mother to child transmission (MTCT) of HIV which was the most significant source of HIV infection in children below the age of 15 years. The study discussed the development of an operational model that can be used to evaluate intervention options for the prevention of MTCT of HIV. The problem was approached by defining suitable pregnancy risk groups, prevention options, and the required model outputs to evaluate different intervention strategies. The method chosen to approach the problem was a discrete-event, three-phase simulation, built in Visual Basic, with a stochastic semi-Markov structure statistical model. The developed model takes individual ANCs through each stage of their pregnancy, labor, and birth. Different intervention strategies were modelled at any time, including short-course antiretroviral drugs and cessation of breastfeeding. The model was demonstrated with data from Botswana, which had one of the highest HIV infection rates in the world. Depaoliet et al. studied factors associated with ANC's expressed willingness to accept voluntary counseling and HIV testing (VCT). A cross-sectional interview survey of 500 pregnant women, complemented by focus group discussions, was conducted in the Kilimanjaro region of Tanzania. Constructs derived from the health belief model explained 41.70% of women willingness to accept VCT. Perceived high personal susceptibility to HIV/AIDS, barriers related to confidentiality and partner involvement, self-efficacy regarding alternative feeding methods, and religion were all shown to be associated with willingness to accept VCT. The women acceptance of VCT seems to depend upon their perceiving that VCT and alternative feeding strategies provide clear benefits, primarily for the child. Whether a positive attitude to VCT and alternative feeding strategies are transformed into actual behavior depends on a set of complicated decisions in which several potential psychological consequences were assessed. Sharing the diagnosis with partners may not have the intended effect, if there is a lack of sensitivity to the women fear of blame and rejection. Gage et al. risk of MTCT can be reduced through the complementary approaches of ARV prophylaxis for the mother, with or without prophylaxis to the infant, implementation of safe delivery practices, and use of safe alternatives to breastfeeding. ARV prophylaxis followed by exclusive breastfeeding may also reduce the risk of vertical transmission when breastfeeding is limited to the first 6 months. In low-income countries, significant difficulties exist in implementing these strategies due to constraints in accessing, affording, and using voluntary counseling and testing services, reproductive health, and maternal and child health services with integrated PMTCT interventions. Montanez et al. studied universal HIV testing impact through logistic regression model. The new HIV cases would decline from 7.0 per thousand to 0.10 per thousand over 50 years, if universal testing and treatment were implemented. Study suggests that providing antiretroviral therapy infected with HIV would stop the HIV epidemic. Naresh et al. developed a model of transmission of HIV into population of varying size with vertical transmission and other demographical and epidemiological factors. Study found that an increase in the rate of vertical transmission leads to an increase in the population of infective which in turn increases the pre-AIDS and AIDS population, Thus, they concluded that the vertical spread of the disease would be controlled by the way of promoting effective treatment. Akpa et al. studied HIV MTCT statistical models; study suggests that the models would aid researchers in applying them to better understand and control the incidence and distribution of the disease in their countries. Dalva et al. estimated the risk of vertical HIV transmission and assess the associated factors and missed opportunities for prevention in a cohort of HIV+ ANCs (1995–2001) treated in Brazil, with follow-up of their children until 2005. Three data sources were compared: Information System on Reportable Diseases (SINAN), Information System on HIV+ ANCs and Exposed Children (SISGHIV), and patient clinical charts. The overall risk of vertical HIV transmission was 27.8%. The MTCT rate was 40.80% in the group without prophylaxis and 1% in the group with adequate prophylaxis, i.e., 97.5% reduction in transmission risk. Year of delivery, consultation with a specialist, and no history of injecting drug use were factors associated with adequate use of antiretroviral therapy. The study showed an important reduction in the risk of vertical transmission in ANCs, who received adequate HAART, besides identifying missed opportunities for prevention. Charlotte et al. estimate rates of perinatal mother to child transmission of HIV, and HIV assays are scheduled at multiple points in time. Still infection status for some infants at some time points is often unknown, particularly when interim analyses are conducted. Logistic regression and Cox proportional hazard regression are commonly used to estimate covariate-adjusted transmission rates, but their methods for handling missing data may be inadequate. Here, we propose using censored multinomial regression models to estimate cumulative and conditional rates of HIV transmission. Through simulation, we show that the proposed methods perform better than standard logistic models in terms of bias, mean squared error, coverage probability, and power, under a range of treatment effect and visit process scenarios. WHO mentioned in their report that exclusive breastfeeding (EBF) breastfeeding with no other food or drink, not even water was the ideal mode of infant feeding for the first 6 months of life. For optimal growth, development, and health, infants should be exclusively breastfed for their first 6 months and should then receive nutritionally adequate and safe complementary foods, while breastfeeding continues up to 24 months or beyond. With the onset of the HIV/AIDS epidemic, however, and the recognition that HIV-infected mothers can transmit HIV to their infants through breastfeeding, specific recommendations apply to infants born to HIV-infected mothers. The overall aim of these recommendations was to achieve the ultimate goal of increasing child survival while reducing HIV infection in infants and young children, respectively. Diallo et al. (2010) fitted dynamics and threshold of a simple epidemiological model; examples of HIV/AIDS in Mali, as per his study epidemiological models for infectious diseases in the sexually active population presents a crucial period; the spread of the influx or recruitment susceptible and also he assumed that the recruitment of susceptible was done among the juvenile group. The study concluded that the dynamic system model cleary demonstrates the disease spread and to know the dynamic behavior of the HIV system. Fitted model can allow algebraic treatment and provide the survival rate for controlling the dynamic system. Chibwesha et al. describe weighted regression model to examine the effect of duration of antenatal HAART on perinatal HIV infection. As per the model results, mean gestational age at first antenatal visit was 21 weeks (SD $\pm$ 6), median CD_4+ cell count was 231 cells per micro liter (interquartile range 164–329), and median duration of antenatal HAART was 13 weeks (IQR 8–19). Fifty nine (3.3%) infants were HIV infected. Duration of antenatal HAART was the most important predictor of perinatal HIV transmission. Compared with women initiating HAART at least 13 weeks before delivery, women on HAART $\leq$4 weeks had 5.5-fold increased odds of HIV transmission (CI 95% 2.6 to 11.7). Low rates of mother to child HIV transmission can be achieved within programmatic settings in Africa. Maximal effectiveness of prevention of mother to child transmission programs is achieved by initiating HAART at least 13 weeks before mother delivery. Studied mother to child HIV transmission through logistic regression model, the major source of HIV infection among children under the age of 15 years. Emily et al. (2013) fitted univariate descriptive statistical models at Naivasha District Hospital. A total of 113 mother-infant pairs were enrolled, and 99 (87.70%) mothers and 85 (92%) infants received antiretroviral drugs. Although 79 (85.60%) infants were breastfed, only 63 (55.80%) were exclusively breastfed for 6 months. About 100 (88.50%) infants had HIV deoxyribonucleic acid polymerase chain reaction testing at 6 weeks, and 84 (80.80%) had follow-up HIV antibody testing at 18 months. MTCT rate was 2.70% at 6 weeks and 4.40% between 6 weeks and 18 months. HIV-free survival at 18 months was 83.90%. High rates of antiretroviral drug use and low rates of MTCT are reported at 6 weeks in this population. However, MTCT rate increases substantially after 6 weeks indicating an urgent need for strategies to promote exclusive breastfeeding. Mother to child HIV transmission remains very high in Cameroon. Therefore follow-up of numerous HIV-infected infants is a critical issue in the country. Study fitted univariate logistic regression model. As per the model, it signifies that HIV biomarkers like lower CD_4 count and high plasma viral load were found to be statistically significant for HIV MTCT in Cameroon. The fitted model concludes that the lack of adherence, high plasma viral load, and lower CD_4 count can be able to increased high incidence rate of MTCT. Fitted logistic regression model is to determine the level of adherence among HIV-infected pregnant women on prevention of mother to child transmission (PMTCT) antiretroviral therapy and to establish the factors that contribute to poor adherence and their relative importance, in order to suggest intervention strategies that will improve treatment adherence among this population. Fitted model predicted that the most important factors influencing adherence from the study were pregnancy-related illnesses, medication side effects, and month of pregnancy of the patients, as participants tended to adhere less as they got closer to delivery. Zekiewos et al. studied cross-sectional study that was conducted at Karnataka State, Hassan district hospital during 2013–2014. Of a total of 422 sample women, 417 ANCs were included in the study, and data were collected by using pretested structured questionnaire. Binary and multiple logistic regression models were fitted to identify factors associated with KAP toward PMTCT. A total of 417 pregnant women responded to the questionnaire, yielding a response rate of 98.8%, among which, 78.2% knew that the risk of MTCT of HIV can be prevented, 69.92% responded that ART should be started as soon as the status is known, and 64% of the respondents had good knowledge (greater than average score) on PMTCT. Majority, 98.30% of the respondents had good attitude, and 90.40%

respondents were practiced PMTCT of HIV. About 90.40% of mothers were tested for HIV during current pregnancy, and 93.90% shared test results to their husbands/partners. Awareness creation activities on HIV/AIDS in general and prevention of MTCT in particular through distribution of ICE/BCC materials, mass medias, and maternal and child health service units should be strengthened. Gilbert et al. (2015) fitted inferences on relative failure rates in stratified mark-specific proportional hazard statistical models with missing marks, with application to human immunodeficiency virus vaccine efficacy trials. The study developed hypothesis testing procedures for the stratified mark-specific proportional hazard models in the presence of missing marks. The motivating application was preventive human immunodeficiency virus (HIV) vaccine efficacy trials, where the serological markers are the genetic distance of an infecting HIV sequence to an HIV sequence represented inside the vaccine. The test statistics were constructed on the basis of two-stage efficient estimators, which utilize auxiliary predictors of the missing marks. The asymptotic properties and finite sample performance of the testing procedures were investigated, demonstrating double robustness and effectiveness of the predictive auxiliaries to recover efficiency. The new techniques of statistical model can help to conduct HIV-RV144 vaccine trials and MTCT incidence on prospective basis. Thamattor et al. (2015) worked on multilevel model of the predictors of HIV prevalence among pregnant women enrolled in annual HIV sentinel surveillance in four states in southern India. As per the resulting fitted model, the average ANC HIV prevalence from 2004 to 2007 in the 24 integrated biological and behavioral assessment (IBBA) districts ranged from 0.25 to 3.25%. HIV positivity was significantly higher among ANC women with age $\geq$ 25 years; illiterate (AOR 1.62; 95% CI 1.13 to 1.62) or with occupations like driver/helper/industry/factory worker/hotel staff (AOR 1.59; 95% CI 1.0 to 1.05) and percentage women marrying under 18 years were significantly associated with ANC HIV positivity (AOR 1.02; 95% CI 1.00 to 1.04). Illiteracy of the woman, higher HIV prevalence among female sex workers (FSWs), and early marriage were associated with HIV positivity among pregnant women in southern India. In addition to targeted HIV preventive intervention among FSWs, studying and changing the behavior of FSW clients and addressing structural drivers of the epidemic might indirectly help reduce HIV infection among women in southern India. Nani et al. conducted a prospective observational study at ten human immunodeficiency virus (HIV) and treatment centers in Dar es Salaam, Tanzania. Multivariate log normal regression (Chen et al. 2012; Marazzi et al. 2011) model was used to investigate the association between ARV use and adverse birth outcomes among HIV-negative HIV-exposed infants. Study findings demonstrate an increased risk of adverse birth outcomes associated with the use of highly active antiretroviral therapy during pregnancy. Further studies are needed to investigate the underlying mechanisms and identify the safest ARV regimens for use during pregnancy. Fentaw et al. (2014) studied mother to child transmission of HIV (MTCT) which is the major source of HIV infection among children under the age of 15 years. Bayesian logistic regression, Kaplan-Meier method, and Cox proportional hazards model are applied to know the estimation rate of HIV MTCT, and the same model was adopted by Fowler et al. (2015) and Berhanu et al. (2009); within prevention programs, package of services including HIV counseling and testing, provision of prophylactic antiretroviral (ARV) drugs for mothers and babies, safe delivery practices, and infant feeding counseling is being given. Considering the prevailing high level of HIV infection rate among MTCT clients, re-organization of the PMTCT services especially raising the level of awareness of MTCT/PMTCT among pregnant women is important to prevent the babies from HIV infection. Basavarajaiah et al. (2013) studied pediatrician HIV epidemic in India using statistical models. A statistical model of HIV incidence among CLHIV survival rate has been created by using CMIS data sources. The model predicted the size of the population on monthly intervals, non-AIDS mortality rates, and annual numbers of births to mothers who are HIV positive and HIV negative that were obtained from the ASSA model. Since, the rate of vertical transmission of HIV was dependent on the maternal CD_4 counts, and uptake of HAART relative to short course of ARV prophylaxis also depends on the pregnant women CD_4 counts. The review of relevant published and unpublished literature on modelling of HIV transmission from mother to child was presented here, and the above literature suggests that there was fewer number of published literature cited to know the incidence of MTCT, and it was found that there is a paucity of literature on formulation of modelling to know the HIV transmission from mother to child (MTCT). The desired epidemiological goals can't be expected to be achieved with only one specific program, e.g., HIV HAART comprehensive support treatment program. The review also indicated that the socioeconomic variables, behavioral changes, and risk factors were already existing in a society; it was equally important to derive/determine the impact of modelling of HIV transmission from mother to child (MTCT). Thus, in the present state of knowledge of HIV transmission from mother to child, there appears to be no unique model which can determine and realize specific epidemiological goals. However, the modelling of HIV transmission from mother to child (MTCT) along with socioeconomic factors, behavioral changes, and selected risk factors can be expected to provide better understanding of complex phenomena of HIV transmission from mother to child (MTCT). Such a study on modelling will be of special significance in populations where there is limited literature on modelling to study the HIV MTCT. At population level where the HIV transmission from mother to child is relatively moderate or where there is limited use of HAART, any study of modelling of HIV transmission from mother to child and the association of socioeconomic factors, behavioral changes, and risk factors will be of great help to the public and public health administrators at larger extent. This book describes outcome of the building and application of selected mathematical and statistical models on HIV transmission from mother to child (MTCT) which is made possible by the availability of data on HIV comprehensive treatment program and HIV transmission from mother to child (MTCT); the models were fitted by utilizing primary and secondary data source of NACO and Karnataka State AIDS Control Society during 2009–2018. This book attempts to examine the development of HIV modelling and validate the fitted models with real-life HIV data sets collected in the high prevalence states of India, for example, Karnataka, Andhra Pradesh,

Manipur, Maharashtra, and Uttar Pradesh. The fitted model will help to examine the impact of HIV transmission from mother to child and its OIs and co-infection tuberculosis (TB).

1.27 Objectives of the Book

The objectives of the reference book that were tailored based on the results of mathematical and statistical modelling on simulated and real data sets are:

(i) To provide a brief introduction and background of modelling on HIV from MTCT, literature survey on both mathematical and statistical modelling, and estimation of transmission parameters of MTCT. It also includes modelling on both simulated and real-life HIV data sets to examine the impact of mother to child transmission.

(ii) To describe the real-life databases including patients, study design, and input and output parameters pertaining to state AIDS control center (SAC) HAART data sets.

(iii) To examine by developing the disease transmission simulation model—an Indian- and global-based perspectives. In this chapter, we studied the fraction of newborn infected with HIV and to examine the validity of the model.

(iv) To study the modelling of large data matrix, random walk model, and application of entropy in HIV MTCT theoretical model and examine the reduction of high-dimensional large HIV data sets, computed the probability of HIV MTCT on theoretical basis.

(v) To develop statistical modelling on postnatal transmission of HIV type I infection from mother to child and examine the genetic model, whether routine breastfeeding (BF) associated with HAART, and also to develop an epidemiological and genetic model of HIV biomarkers like RNA plasma viral load and CD_4 count. Specifically examined whether lower maternal viral load and CD_4 count was statistically significant for increase in HIV MTCT.

(vi) To develop survivability and growth models on CD_4 count of PLHIVs to determine the rate of survivability with proportion of survival growth among those who started highly active antiretroviral therapy (HAART) at lower CD_4 counts with high RNA plasma viral load (VL).

(vii) To study the association between HIV and tuberculosis (TB) in vertical transmission through predictive modelling approach by considering CD_4 counts, RNA plasma viral load, and delay in inception of highly active antiretroviral therapy (HAART) for HIV-infected mother.

(viii) To formulate Bayesian statistical model approach to HIV/AIDS on global perspectives.

(ix) To summarize the modelling research, propose recommendations, and discuss various implications of HIV future research.

1.28 Organization of Book

This book is divided into 11 chapters in which **Chap. 1** describes introduction of HIV transmission, brief review of the published and unpublished literature from 1997 to 2019, building of mathematical and statistical modelling techniques of HIV mother to child transmission (MTCT), objectives, and chapterization of the book and discusses the real-life data sets, methodology, variables considered for the study, HIV serological markers, different patterns of HIV-TB co-infection among children living with HIV (CLHIVs), etc. **Chapter 2** discusses the statistical modelling of HIV transmission. **Chapter 3** describes the HIV vertical transmission DTSM simulation models—global and national prospective; the validity of the model was simulated by different varied parameters. **Chapter 4** describes large data matrices; random walk model, and application of entropy in HIV mother to child transmission. This theoretical issue was formulated with suitable illustrations and various examples by using the real-life HIV mother to child transmission (MTCT) data sets, and also fitted models describe the different techniques of data reduction derived by the random walk free probability values. **Chapter 5** deals with statistical modelling on postnatal transmission of HIV type I infection from mother to child on global perspectives and examines the applicability of different statistical models in real-life data sets of HIV mother to child transmission and antenatal care (ANCs). **Chapter 6** gives survivability and growth model approach to CD_4 counts of people living with HIV (PLHIVs). This chapter describes briefly and discusses various issues of growth models and its applications toward estimation of survival rate in real-life data sets. **Chapter 7** discusses predictive model approach to HIV-TB co-infection in vertical transmission. **Chapter 8** fitted Bayesian modelling approach to HIV transmission, Gaussian emulator approach was used to extract the probability values of HIV transmission, the models were formulated by networking NICHE, and also frequentist and Bayesian model differences were described briefly. **Chapter 9** discusses HIV projection models, and **Chapter 10** discusses simulation modelling techniques of HIV/AIDS. **Chapter 11** discusses meta-analysis of genetic variants of HIV mother to child transmission and also describes the genetic variants of HIV mother to child transmission; meta-analysis was done for the real historical data sets, and also we have extracted HIV subtype B and C *env* genes from 190 mothers' infant pairs at global level. **Chapter 12** deals with the statistical perspective approach to selection of sample, and finally, Chap. 13 describes the main significance of the entire book for induction of mathematical and statistical models to prove new formulated models of HIV mother to child transmission at population level.

1.29 Description of Study Area

India has the third largest HIV epidemic in the world. In 2018, HIV prevalence among adults (aged 15–49) was an estimated to be 0.20%. This figure is small compared to most other middle-income countries, but because of India's huge population (1.30 billion people), this equates to 2.1 million people living with

HIV. Overall, India's HIV epidemic is slowing down. Between 2010 and 2017, new infections declined by 27%, and AIDS-related deaths more than halved, falling 56%. However, in 2017, new infections increased to 88,000 from 80,000, and AIDS-related deaths increased to 69,000 from 62,000. In 2017, 79% of people living with HIV were aware of their status, of which 56% were on ART. The proportion of people on highly active antiretroviral therapy (HAART) who are virologically suppressed is not reported. The HIV epidemic in India is driven by sexual transmission, which accounted for 86.0% of new infections in 2017–2018. The three states with the highest HIV prevalence, Manipur, Mizoram, and Nagaland, are in the east of the country. The epidemic is concentrated among key affected populations; however the vulnerabilities that drive the epidemic vary in different parts of the country. A key driver is unprotected sex among key populations and their clients, partners, and spouses. However, injecting drug use in the north and northeast of the country is also pushing HIV prevalence up. Key population groups have been priorities in the national AIDS response since its inception in 1992. Both the sex worker and men who have sex with men population groups have experienced a recent decline in HIV prevalence.

1.29.1 Subgroup Analysis Study Site

Karnataka State provenance was purposively selected for the research study because more ethnic group of population migrated from adjacent states of Andhra Pradesh, Tamil Nadu, and Red Corridor of Chennai and also from other countries of Nepal, Burma, and Afghanistan. First ART center for HIV comprehensive care support center was initiated during 2004 at Bowring and Lady Curzon Government Hospital, Bengaluru. More ANCs were registered for comprehensive HAART treatment in selected area (Figs. 1.4 and 1.5).

1.30 Methods of Model Formulation: Source of Secondary HIV Data Set

A cohort retrospective data was collected yearly from ART centers in Bangalore City. HIV HAART follow-up data at different intervals were collected from ART registers. The data pertaining to demographic features of ANCs, viz., risk factors of HIV MTCT; gravid status; clinical parameters like type of regimen, WHO staging, opportunistic infections (OIs), etc.; laboratory parameters; CD_4 cell count (micro/dL); viral load(micro/dL); transmission rate; timing of transmission; mechanisms and risk factors of transmission; breastfeeding types and methods of feeding; duration of feeding; secondary prevention strategy; tertiary strategies; HAART type of therapy (I line or II line); duration of therapy; drug toxicity; WHO clinical stages; and different modes of delivery, were considered for the study. The collected data was analyzed by using Matlab-10.50 and SPSS-16.50 version software.

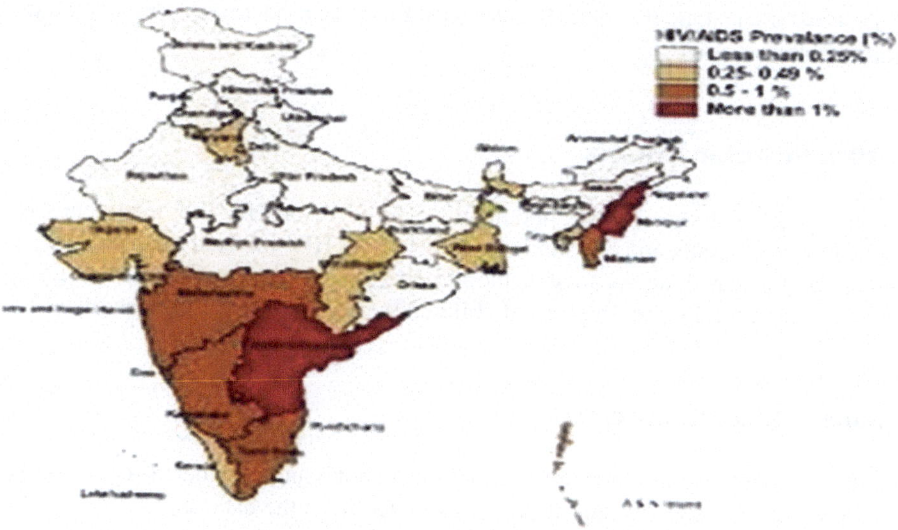

Fig. 1.4 Indian AIDS epidemic—2016 (reproduced from NACO report, 2019)

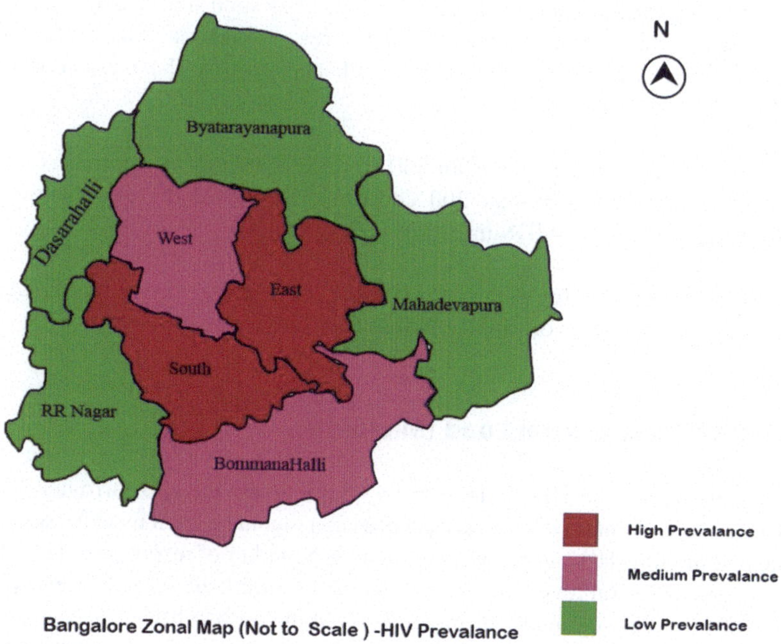

Fig. 1.5 Map showing prevalence of HIV in Bangalore City

Different statistical, mathematical, and epidemiological models were fitted to test the null hypothesis.

1.30.1 Inclusion Criteria

A retrospective study of ANC population, who were on HAART treatment over 18 years of age group, and children who were born to HIV-infected mothers between the (a) age group 6 weeks to <18 months irrespective of sex and (b) age group between >18 months and 16 years of children were considered for the study.

1.30.2 Exclusion Criteria

Highly sick and mentally disordered ANCs were not being considered for the study, and any incomplete/discrepant data was excluded from the data sets.

1.31 CD_4 Cell Count (Micro/dL)

The terms "CD_4 cell" and "T cell" both refer to the same type of cell and are often interchangeable. CD_4 cells or T cells are a type of white blood cells that play a major role in protecting the human body from infection. They send signal to active immune response, when they detect "intrudes" like virus or bacteria. Once a person is infected with HIV, the virus begins to attack and destroy the CD_4 cells of the PLHIVs.

(i) A normal CD_4 count ranges from 500 to 1200 cells/mm^3 in adults.
(ii) A CD_4 count of fewer than 200 cells/mm^3 is one of the qualifications for diagnosis of stage III AIDS infection.

ART is recommended for everyone with HIV, but the urgency to start HAART is greater in people with low or rapidly falling CD_4 cell count.

1.31.1 RNA Plasma Viral Load (Micro/dl)

The CD_4 cell counts and HIV RNA plasma viral load are the two surrogate markers of HAART response and HIV disease progression that have been used for decades to manage and monitor HIV infection. Viral load is a marker of response to HAART. A patient's pre-ART viral level and the magnitude of viral load decline after inception of HAART provide prognostic information about the probability of disease progression. The key goal of HAART is to achieve and maintain viral load suppression. The present aforesaid variable is discussed in Chaps. 5, 6, 7, and 8.

Table 1.6 Approved HAART Drugs for PLHIVs

WHO clinical stage Adults	**WHO clinical stage**
Approved for adult	Approved for pediatric population
Zidovudine +lamivudine	Zidovudine+lamivudine
Zidovudine+lamivudine+nevirapine	Stavudine+lamivudine
Stavudine+lamivudine+nevirapine	–
Abacavir+lamivudine	
Zidovudine+abacavir+lamivudine	
Lamivudine+tenofovir	
Lamivudine+tenofovir+efavirenz	
Tenofovir+emtricitabine	
Tenofovir+emtricitabine+efavirenz	
Ritonavir+lopinavir	
Amprenavir+ritonavir	
HIV infected adults and adolescents (including pregnant women	–
	–
Clinical stages I and II	–
	Start ART if CD_4 < 350 cells/mm3
Clinical stages I and II	–
	Start ART irrespective of CD_4 count
For HIV-TB co-infected patients with HIV-TB co-infection (PTB/EPTB)	Start ART irrespective of CD_4 count and type of TB (start ATT first, initiate ART as early as possible between 2 weeks and 2 months when TB treatment is tolerated)
For HIV and HBV, HCV co-infected patients	
Without evidence of chronic active hepatitis without documented evidence of chronic active hepatitis	Start ART if CD_4 count <350 cells/mm3 start ART irrespective of CD_4 count

1.31.2 Highly Active Antiviral Therapy (HAART)

Antiretroviral therapy (ART) is a treatment of PLHIVs or pregnant women with immunodeficiency virus (HIV) using anti-HIV drugs. The standard treatment consists of a combination of NRTIs and NNRTIs with boosted protease inhibitors (PIs) often called as "highly active antiretroviral therapy" or HAART that suppress HIV replications (Table 1.6).

1.31.3 WHO Clinical Stages

The following stages were identified by WHO with presenting complaints received from people living with HIV (PLHIVs) and children living with HIV (CLHIVs):

Primary Infection and Asymptomatic Acute Retroviral Syndrome

Clinical stage (i): Asymptomatic and persistent generalized lymphadenopathy (PGL).

Clinical stage (ii): Moderate unexplained weight loss, recurrent respiratory tract infections, herpes zoster, angular chalets, recurrent oral ulceration, popular pruritic eruptions, seborrheic dermatitis, fungal nail infections of finger, etc.

Clinical stage (iii): Severe weight loss (>10% of presumed or measured body weight), unexplained chronic diarrhea for longer than 1 month, unexplained persistent fever, oral candidiasis, oral hairy leukoplakia, pulmonary tuberculosis diagnosed in last 2 years, severe presumed bacterial infections, and acute necrotizing ulcerative stomatitis.

Clinical stage (iv): Wasting syndrome, pneumocystis pneumonia, recurrent severe or radiological bacterial pneumonia, chronic herpes simplex infection, esophageal candidiasis, extrapulmonary TB, Kaposi sarcoma and toxoplasmosis, HIV-encephalopathy (Table 1.7).

1.32 HIV-Opportunistic Infections (OIs)

People with healthy immune system can be exposed to certain virus, bacteria, or parasites and have no reaction to them, but PLHIVs can face serious health threats from what are known as "opportunistic infections" (OIs). These infections are called "opportunistic," because they take advantage of HIV-infected immune system and they can cause devastating illness. OIs are signs of a declining immune system. Most life-threatening OIs occur when HIV-infected PLHIV's CD_4 count is below 200 cells/mm^3. OIs are the most common cause of death for PLHIVs (CDC report, 1998). The following most common OIs observed in PLHIVs or CLHIVs are:

1.32.1 Candidiasis of Bronchi, Trachea, Esophagus, or Lungs

Candidiasis is a fungal infection due to any type of *Candida* (a type of yeast). When it affects the mouth, it is commonly called thrush. Signs and symptoms include white patches on the tongue or other areas of the mouth and throat. There are many kinds of fungus that live in the human body. One type is called candida. It's a type of yeast that normally lives in small amounts in place like your mouth and belly or on your skin without causing any problems. But when the environment is right, the yeast can multiply and grow out of control.

Table 1.7 Overview of WHO clinical stages of adult and children

Stage	Adults and adolescents	Children
(i)	Asymptomatic persistent generalized lymphadenopathy	Asymptomatic persistent generalized lymphadenopathy
(ii)	Moderate unexplained weight loss (<10% of presumed)	Unexplained persistent hepatosplenomegaly
	Recurrent respiratory tract infections (sinusitis, tonsillitis, otitis media, pharyngitis)	Recurrent or chronic upper respiratory tract infections (otitis media, otorrhea, sinusitis, tonsillitis)
	Herpes zoster	Herpes zoster
	Angular cheilitis	Lineal gingival erythema
	Recurrent oral ulceration	Recurrent oral ulceration
	Papular pruritic eruption	Papular pruritic eruption
	Fungal nail infections	Fungal nail infections
	Seborrhoeic dermatitis	Extensive wart virus infection
		Extensive molluscum contagiosum
		Unexplained persistent parotid enlargement
(iii)	Unexplained severe weight loss (>10% of presumed or measured body weight)	Unexplained moderate malnutrition not adequately responding to standard therapy
	Unexplained chronic diarrhea for longer than 1 month	Unexplained persistent diarrhea (14 days or more)
	Unexplained persistent fever (intermittent or constant for longer than 1 month)	Unexplained persistent fever (above 37.5 °C, intermittent or constant, for longer than 1 month)
	Persistent oral candidiasis	Persistent oral candidiasis (after first 6 weeks of life)
	Oral hairy leukoplakia	Oral hairy leukoplakia
	Pulmonary tuberculosis	Lymph node tuberculosis
	Severe bacterial infections (such as pneumonia, emphysema, pyomyositis, bone or joint infection, meningitis, bacteremia)	Pulmonary tuberculosis
	Acute necrotizing ulcerative stomatitis, gingivitis, or periodontitis	Unexplained anemia
	Unexplained anemia	Neutropenia
	Neutropenia	Thrombocytopenia
	Thrombocytopenia	Severe recurrent bacterial pneumonia
		Acute necrotizing ulcerative gingivitis or periodontitis
		Symptomatic lymphoid interstitial pneumonitis
		Chronic HIV-associated lung disease, including bronchiectasis
(iv)	HIV wasting syndrome	Unexplained severe wasting, stunting, or severe malnutrition not responding to standard therapy
	Pneumocystis (jirovecii) pneumonia	Pneumocystis (jirovecii) pneumonia

(continued)

Table 1.7 (continued)

Stage	Adults and adolescents	Children
	Recurrent severe bacterial pneumonia	Recurrent severe bacterial infections (such as empyema, pyomyositis, bone or joint infection, meningitis, but excluding pneumonia)
	Chronic herpes simplex infection (orolabial, genital, or anorectal of more than 1 month's duration or visceral at any site)	Chronic herpes simplex infection (orolabial or cutaneous of more than 1 month's duration or visceral at any site)
	Esophageal candidiasis (or candidiasis of trachea, bronchi, or lungs)	
	Extrapulmonary tuberculosis	
	Kaposi sarcoma	Esophageal candidiasis (or candidiasis of trachea, bronchi, or lungs)
	Cytomegalovirus infection (retinitis or infection of other organs)	Extrapulmonary tuberculosis
	Central nervous system toxoplasmosis	
		Kaposi sarcoma
	HIV encephalopathy	
	Extrapulmonary cryptococcosis, including meningitis	Cytomegalovirus infection (retinitis or infection of other organs with onset at age more than 1 month)
	Disseminated nontuberculous mycobacterial infection	
	Progressive multifocal leukoencephalopathy	Central nervous system toxoplasmosis (after the neonatal period)
		HIV encephalopathy
	Chronic cryptosporidiosis	
		Extrapulmonary cryptococcosis, including meningitis
(v)	Chronic isosporiasis	Disseminated nontuberculous mycobacterial infection
	Disseminated mycosis (extrapulmonary histoplasmosis, coccidioidomycosis)	Progressive multifocal leukoencephalopathy
	Lymphoma (cerebral or B-cell non-Hodgkin)	Chronic cryptosporidiosis (with diarrhea)
	Symptomatic HIV-associated nephropathy or cardiomyopathy	Chronic isosporiasis
	Recurrent septicemia (including nontyphoidal salmonella)	Disseminated endemic mycosis (extrapulmonary histoplasmosis, coccidioidomycosis, penicilliosis)
	Invasive cervical carcinoma	Cerebral or B-cell non-Hodgkin lymphoma
	Atypical disseminated leishmaniasis	HIV-associated nephropathy or cardiomyopathy

1.32.2 Oral Thrush

When the *Candida* yeast spread in the mouth and throat, it can cause an infection called thrush; it's most common in PLHIV, the elderly, and PLHIV with weakened systems (adults). As per the literature, the prevalence was 16.25%, also more likely to get ANCs are treated for cancer take medication like corticosteroids and wide-spectrum antibiotics wear dentures, have diabetes. The following symptoms include white or yellow patches on the tongue, lips, gums, roof of mouth, and inner cheeks, redness or soreness in the mouth and throat, cracking at the corners of the mouth, and pain when swallowing; if it spreads to the throat, thrush is treated with antifungal medicines like nystatin, clotrimazole, and fluconazole. Rinsing the mouth with chlorhexidine (CHX) mouthwash may help prevent infections in PLHIVs.

1.32.3 Invasive Cervical Cancer

Cervical cancer is mostly caused by the human papilloma virus or HPV. An HPV vaccine may reduce the risk of cervical cancer. Symptoms of cervical cancer can include painful sex, vaginal bleeding, and white discharge that are seen in ANCs. The uterine cervix is the lowest portion of a woman's uterus (womb), connecting the uterus with the vagina. Cervical cancer occurs when the cells of the cervix grow abnormally and invade other tissues of the cervix and may have spread to other parts of the body (metastasis), most notably the lungs, liver, bladder, vagina, and rectum.

Most women PLHIV diagnosed with precancerous changes in the cervix are in their 20s and 30s, but the average age of women when they are diagnosed with cervical cancer is the mid 50s. This difference in the age at which precancerous changes are most frequently diagnosed and the age at which cancer is diagnosed highlights the slow progression of this disease and the reason why it can be prevented if adequate steps are taken from the caretakers.

1.32.4 Coccidioidomycosis

It is a systemic mycosis that affects humans and wide range of animals. It is caused by the soil-dwelling dimorphic fungus *Coccidioides immitis*. The disease is acquired by inhalation of infective arthroconidia that live in the soils, where the fungus grows as saprophyte, presenting filamentous growth. The infection is usually benign and resolves spontaneously; however, a small proportion of infected individuals develop progressive, potentially lethal infection that can affect not only the lungs but other organs through hematogenous dissemination. Coccidioidomycosis manifests in one of three clinical forms; the primary pulmonary form, the progressive pulmonary forms, or the disseminated forms were found in the PLHIVs.

1.32.5 Progressive Forms

The progressive pulmonary coccidioidomycosis is generally chronic and develops after the first infection, the symptoms of which do not resolve after 2 months. The progressive pulmonary coccidioidomycosis might present as follows, viz., nodular or cavitary lesions, sometimes as an incidental radiological findings, cavitary lung disease with fibrosis, and military pulmonary dissemination, with nonspecific clinical and radiological manifestations. Due to its chronic progression, progressive pulmonary coccidioidomycosis constitutes an important differential diagnosis with PTB of HIV-infected patient.

1.32.6 Disseminated Coccidioidomycosis

In approximately 0.2% of the patients with primary pulmonary coccidioidomycosis, the lesions disseminate predominantly to the skin, the central nervous system, and osteoarticular system. The presence of mediastinal or paratracheal lymphadenomegaly is indicative of dissemination. The disseminated form generally progresses in an acute manner, reaching various organs or systems, rapidly leading to death when diagnosis and treatment are not timely. However, the disseminated form might progress in a protracted form, disseminating to various organs, presenting periods of remission and recurrence, despite antifungal treatment. The most common disseminated lesions are seen on the skin, in the central nervous system, in bones, in joints, and in the genitourinary system. The skin is the site that is most commonly affected by lesions, second only to the lungs, the face being predominantly affected. The lesions are generally papules or warts; however, they can present as plaques, superficial abscesses, pustules, and granulomatous lesions.

1.32.7 Cryptococcosis

Cryptococcosis is a disease caused by fungi from the genus *Cryptococcus* that infect humans and animals usually by inhalation of the fungus, which results in lung infection that may spread to the brain, causing meningoencephalitis. The disease was first termed "BusseBuschke disease" after the two individuals who first identified the fungus in 1894–1895. Cryptococcosis is found worldwide, the predominant way the disease is spread through inhalation of fungi that is associated with many bird species, especially old pigeon feces and bat guano. *Cryptococcus* species is found in bird feces (*C. neoformans*) throughout the world, but usually the bird themselves are not infected or sick. Human and animals usually get the infection from inhaling dust contaminated with bird feces, but human do not transmit cryptococcosis to other individual or animals. However, *C. gattii* is type of *Cryptococcus* that is acquired by inhalation of airborne plant material. Until a few years ago, almost all *C. gattii* infections were associated with plants found in tropical and subtropical climates. This has changed since an outbreak has occurred in the Pacific Northwest.

In general, the people infected with *C. neoformans* usually have some defect in cell-mediated immunity (especially HIV/AIDS patients). However, *C. gattii* usually infects immunocompetent individuals but can infect immunocompromised people. Cryptococcosis is rarely transmitted directly into the skin and by organ transplants.

1.32.8 Cytomegalovirus (CMV)

Cytomegalovirus (CMV) disease is a viral infection that can affect one part of the body, such as the eyes, or it can spread throughout the body. Before the availability of effective HIV therapy (commonly called HAART), it was common for people with HIV/AIDS to develop CMV. Today we greatly applause HAART; cases of CMV disease in HIV-positive people in India and overseas population are relatively rare. PLHIVs whose CD_4 counts are <50 cells/mm^3 are most at risk for developing this disease. Fortunately, treatment for CMV has improved dramatically in recent years. CMV is a serious infection caused by a virus called cytomegalovirus (CMV). This virus is related to the herpes viruses that cause chicken pox and mononucleosis (mono). CMV is one of a number of infections that can develop in PLHIVs, called OIs. The OIs (Opportunistic Infection) only occur if immune system unique weakened and body becomes vulnerable to infection that would not otherwise affect. Most adults carry CMV but unaware of it because the virus doesn't make them sick. In PLHIV with severely weakened immune system, CMV can make a person feel as though they have mono. CMV can also cause serious disease in different parts of the body, most commonly the eyes.

People who have a weakened immune system, due to HIV, cancer, and long-term use of drugs that weaken the immune system, or who have received transplanted tissue are at risk of developing CMV. PLHIV most at risk of developing CMV tend to have the following features:

(i) Have a CD_4 count <50 cells/mm3.
(ii) Have a VL over 1000,000 copies/ml.
(iii) Are not taking or do not respond to HAART.
(iv) Have previously had CMV or other life-threatening infection.
(v) Have wasting syndrome due to HIV.

Common OIs among HIV-infected children were discussed in Chap. 4 by using logistic regression predictive model.

1.32.9 HIV Encephalopathy

Cognitive disorder in the setting of HIV infection was recognized a long time ago and was referred to with various names. The term AIDS dementia complex was introduced by Navia and colleagues in 1986. Human immunodeficiency virus (HIV) enters the central nervous system (CNS) early in the course of the infection and causes several important CNS conditions over the course of disease, such as HIV-encephalopathy and AIDS dementia complex. As part of the acute HIV syndrome during seroconversion, patients may experience HIV-encephalopathy. HIV-associated progressive encephalopathy (HPE) is a syndrome complex with cognitive and behavioral features seen in children.

Prior to advent of HAART, dementia was a common source of morbidity and mortality in HIV-infected patients. It was usually observed in the late stages of acquired immunodeficiency syndrome (AIDS), when CD_4 counts fall below 200 cells/ml, and was seen in up to 50% of patients prior to their death.

1.32.10 Herpes Simplex

The herpes simplex virus, also known as HSV, is an infection that causes herpes. Herpes can appear in various parts of the body, most commonly on the genital or mouth. There are two types of the herpes simplex virus:

HSV1: Primarily causes oral herpes and is generally responsible for cold sores and fever blisters around the mouth and on the face.

HSV2: Primarily causes genital herpes and is generally responsible for herpes outbreaks. The herpes simplex virus is a contagious virus that can be transmitted from person to person through direct contact. Children will often contrast HSV1 from early contact with an infected adult. They then carry the virus with them for the rest of their lives. HSV1 can be contracted from general interaction such as:

(a) Eating from the same utensils.
(b) Sharing lip balm.
(c) Kissing.

The viruses spread more quickly when an infected person is experiencing an outbreak. An estimated 67% people aged 49 or younger are seropositive for HSV1, though they may never experience an outbreak. It's also possible to get genital herpes from HSV1 if some who performed oral sex had cold sores during that time. HSV2 is contracted forms of sexual contact with a person who as HSV2. An estimated 20% of sexually active adults in India and 26% at global level are infected with HSV2 according to the CDC report. Most people get HSV1 from an infected person who is asymptomatic or does not have sores.

1.32.11 Histoplasmosis

Histoplasmosis is an infection caused by a fungus called *Histoplasma*. The fungi live in the environment, particularly in soil that contains large amounts of birds or bat droppings. In Indian context, histoplamosis mainly lives in the Eastern and Western Ghat region, especially area around the Kerala, Karnataka, Tamil Nadu, Maharashtra, Sikkim, Manipur, Meghalaya, Nagaland, etc. The fungus also lives in part of Central and South America, Africa, Asia and Australia. People can get histoplasmosis after breathing in microscopic fungal spores from the air. Although most people who breathe in the spores do not get sick, those who do may have a fever, cough, and fatigue. Many people who get histoplasmosis will get better on their own without medication, but in some people, such as those who have weakened immune system, the infection can become severe. In some people, usually those who have weakened system, histoplasmosis can develop into a long-term infection, or it can spread from the lungs to other parts of the body, such as the central nervous system (the brain and spinal cord).

1.32.12 Isosporiasis, Chronic Intestinal (Greater Than 1 Month's Duration)

This is an uncommon infection of the intestine classified by the US Center for Disease Control and Prevention as an AIDS-defining condition worldwide prevalence is variable, with infection occurring most frequently to tropical or subtropical regions with the advent of combination antiretroviral therapy, isosporiasis is considered rare among PLHIVs in the developed world. However, occasional outbreaks have been reported in recent years, generally due to returning travelers or migrants from tropical regions. Isosporiasis is caused by *Cystoisospora belli* (*C. belli*) and intestinal parasites closely related to *Toxoplasma gondii* (*T. gondii*) and *Cryptosporidium*. Humans are the only known hosts for *C. belli*, the disease of which is spread through food or water that has been contaminated with feces from infected humans. Transmission through oral-anal sex is also possible. Symptoms can last for weeks and include crampy abdominal pain and profuse watery diarrhea accomplished by weakness and low-grade fever. For immunocompromised individuals, these symptoms can progress to dehydration, malnutrition, or cachexia which is often asymptomatic. The clinical presentation is distinguishable from cryptosporidiosis and requires microscopic examination of the patient's stool sample to confirm the diagnosis.

1.32.13 Kaposi Sarcoma

All forms of Kaposi sarcoma are caused by a type of herpes virus, *Kaposi sarcoma herpes virus* (KSHV). Most people with KSHV do not develop Kaposi sarcoma unless their immune system is suppressed. The incidence of Kaposi sarcoma increased 20-fold during the spread of HIV in the early 1990s, and this type of cancer is still seen most often in people with stage HIV, as well as in people taking suppressant medications. Kaposi sarcoma is a multicentric vascular tumor, meaning that it involves blood vessels and affects soft tissue in multiple areas of the body; it originates in the endothelial cells that line blood and lymphatic vessels, causing these to grow at faster rate and to survive for longer than normal. People with Kaposi sarcoma do not always present sign or symptoms of the cancer. In many people, however, asymptomatic skin lesions indicate the disease. Kaposi sarcoma often presents as marks of the skin with the following characteristic: brown, purple, pink, or red blemishes called macules.

Different types tend to have clinical presentation; HIV-associated Kaposi sarcoma is more aggressive than others and usually produces multiple lesions, often on the face and trunk. Internal tumors are also common.

Classic or Mediterranean Kaposi sarcoma normally results in a small number of lesions, usually on the skin of the lower limb and particularly on the ankles and soles of the feet. The skin lesions are slowly growing when compared with other forms. This type rarely occurs as an internal tumor. Endemic Kaposi sarcoma tends to affect younger people under 40 years of age, including children. Some forms appear identical to classic Kaposi, and others affect the system and internal organs. Immunosuppressive treatment-related Kaposi sarcoma can appear more suddenly. It is often confined to the skin but not always. Suspected lesions of Kaposi sarcoma on the skin can be confirmed by laboratory examination of a sample, typically by punch biopsy. If internal tumors are suspected or are considered likely, such as in patients with HIV infection or AIDS or other immunosuppression, tests may include, viz., CT or X-ray scan of the chest and abdomen, bronchoscopy, and gastrointestinal endoscopy. Treatment aspects will be varied from the cases. Some of the treatment options for KS are common to other types of cancer, such as:

Local therapy.
Radiation therapy.
Chemotherapy.
Immunotherapy.

Unlike almost all other cancer, treatment for KS focuses on maintaining the health of the immune system. This typically involves targeting HIVs or immunosuppressant drug use. HAART is a combination of anti-HIV drug that are more effective in treating KS alongside chemotherapy than treatments that only make use of chemotherapy.

1.32.14 Lymphoma

It is cancer that begins in infection-fighting cells of the immune system called lymphocytes. These cells are in the lymph nodes, spleen, thymus, bone marrow, and other parts of the body. When the patient had lymphoma, lymphocytes change and grow out of control. There are two main types of lymphoma: (a) non-Hodgkin (most people with lymphoma have this type) and (b) Hodgkin.

Non-Hodgkin and Hodgkin lymphoma involve different types of lymphocyte cells. Every type of lymphoma grows at a different rate and responds differently to treatment.

Lymphoma is very treatable, and the outlook can vary depending on the type of lymphoma and its stage. Lymphoma is different from leukemia. Each of these cancers starts in different type cell:

(a) Lymphoma starts in infection-fighting lymphocytes.
(b) Leukemia in blood-forming cells inside the bone marrow.

1.32.15 *Mycobacterium avium* Complex (MAC)

It is a group of bacteria-related tuberculosis. These germs are very common in food, water, and soils. Almost everyone has them in their bodies. PLHIV get easily infected from MAC because of weakened immune system. MAC usually causes problems after HIV becomes AIDS and CD_4 cell count is <50 micro/dL,. MAC by starting ART early not allow PLHIV CD_4 count to get low, If CD_4 count is very low <50, PLHIVs absolutely get MAC; the infection can be treated, but PLHIV need to take MAC drug for a long time, until CD_4 count relatively increases in response to ART. Symptoms. If MAC goes all over the body, the patient may have high fever or chill, night sweats, belly pain, diarrhea, weight loss, fatigue, swollen glands, fewer red blood cells (anemia), etc. Other serious symptoms have been noted, viz., blood infection, hepatitis, and pneumonia. Many other infections can cause the same symptoms as MAC. Getting the right diagnosis will help the healthcare workers treat it. In addition to physical exam, the physician may order lab tests to find MAC bacteria in patient blood, urine, sputum, bone marrow, and tissue.

1.32.16 Tuberculosis (TB)

Tuberculosis is a contagious disease that can spread from person to person. TB is caused by bacteria called *Mycobacterium tuberculosis*. The TB bacteria spread in the air. TB usually affects the lungs. But TB-causing bacteria can attack any part of the body, including the kidneys, spine, or brain. If not treated, TB causes death. A person with TB disease of the lungs or throat can spread droplets of TB bacteria in the air, particularity when they cough or sneeze. People who breathe in the TB bacteria can get TB. Once in the body, TB can be inactive or active. Inactive TB is called latent TB. Active TB is called TB disease. In the advent of HIV and TB called HIV-TB co-infection. latent TB is more likely to advance to TB disease in people with HIV than in people without HIV. TB disease may also cause HIV to worsen. Treatment with HIV medicines is called ART. ART protects the immune system and prevents HIV infection from advancing to AIDS. In people with HIV/TB co-infection, ART reduces chances that latent TB will advance to TB disease. Worldwide, TB is one of the leading causes of death among people with HIV. In the USA where HIV medicine is widely used, fewer people with HIV get TB than in many other countries. But TB still affects many people with HIV in the USA, especially those born outside the USA. All people with HIV should get tested for

TB infection, preferably at the time of HIV diagnosis. If test results show that a person has latent TB, additional testing is needed. More testing will determine whether the person has TB diseases.

1.32.17 *Pneumocystis carinii* Pneumonia (PCP)

PCP is a life threatening lung infection that can affect people with weakened immune system, such as those infected with HIV, the virus that causes AIDS. More than three quarters of all people with HIV disease will develop PCP if they do not receive treatment to prevent it. PCP is caused by tiny parasites. In addition to the lungs, the parasite can infect the eyes, ears, skin, liver, and other organs. The organism probably infects most people during childhood, but it usually does not cause illness in healthy people. Because the parasite remains in the body for life, it can cause disease at any time if the immune system becomes severely damaged, as in HIV infection, or is suppressed by drugs. PLHIVs are particularly prone to PCP when their CD_4 T-cell levels fall <200. CD_4 T cells are important immune system cells targeted by HIV. The respiratory symptoms of PCP include a dry cough, chest tightness, and difficulty breathing. People with this infection can experience fever, fatigue, and weight loss for weeks or even months before having any respiratory symptoms. If a person with PCP is not treated, the infection can seriously impair the lung's ability to transport oxygen from inhaled air in the blood, which can lead to death. People with respiratory symptoms usually undergo a chest X-ray to determine if signs of pneumonia are present. It can be diagnosed by detecting the organism in sputum or in fluid removed from the lung by bronchoscopy, a procedure in which a tiny tube is threaded through the patient's airways. Rarely, the physician may have to surgically remove a sample of lung tissue for further examination.

1.32.18 Pneumonia (Recurrent)

Pneumonia is an infection in one or both lungs. It can be caused by bacteria, viruses, or fungi. Bacterial pneumonia is the most common types in adults. Pneumonia causes inflammation in the air sacs in affected lungs, which were called alveoli. The alveoli fill with fluid or pus, making it difficult to breathe. Pneumonia symptoms can be mild to life-threatening. The most common symptoms of pneumonia can include coughing that may produce phlegm (mucus); fever, sweating, and chills; shortness of breath; and chest pain, and other symptoms can vary according to the cause and severity of the infection, as well as the age and general health of the individuals. Viral pneumonia may start with flu-like symptoms, such as wheezing. A high fever may occur after 12–36 hours. Bacterial pneumonia may cause a fever as high as 105 F along with profuse sweating, bluish lips and nails, and confusion. The symptoms by age are children under 5 years of age have fast breathing; infants may vomit, lack energy, or have trouble drinking or eating; older people may have a lower than normal body temperature, and PLHIVs were more affected by this infection.

1.32.19 Progressive Multifocal Leukoencephalopathy

PML is a demyelinating disease of the central nervous system (CNS) characterized by widespread lesions due to infection of oligodendrocytes by JC virus, which is a human polyomavirus (formerly known as papovavirus). It is a small non-enveloped double-stranded DNA virus that was identified as the etiological agent in 1967 and was named JC virus in 1971 after John Cunningham from whom it was isolated. It occurs almost exclusively in immunosuppressed individuals, e.g., patients with AIDS, hematological and lymphoreticular malignancies, and autorheumatological disease or those having undergone organ transplantation. PML has also been reported in patients receiving immunotherapy with monoclonal antibodies and various other immunosuppressants, including prednisone, cyclophosphamide, methotrexate, cyclosporine, etc. PML is associated with both HIV1 and HIV2; infection accounts for almost 85% of the total cases, and its prevalence in this population is around 4–5%.

1.32.20 *Salmonella* Septicemia (Recurrent)

A life-threatening *Salmonella* infection that has been spread to the bloodstream. Salmonella septicemia can be caused by any of the *Salmonella* bacteria, which are found in contaminated food and water. The infection is systemic and affects virtually every organ system. The most common symptom is fever that comes and goes in PLHIV; recurrent *Salmonella* septicemia is an AIDS-defining condition. *Salmonella* transmission usually occurs through fecal oral route. Animal can become infected through contaminated feed or water or close contact with an infected host. The bacteria can then be passed to human through tainted meat or animal products that have not been thoroughly cooked (145–160 F). Even after treatment, humans can remain infectious for months after recovery. Proper hygiene is recommended particularly for those with CD_4 counts under 200 cells/ml. In addition to the diarrhea, vomiting, and abdominal cramping commonly associated with salmonellosis, the symptoms can include high fever, swelling, flushed skin, increased heart rate, confusion, hyperventilation, and high BP.

1.32.21 Toxoplasmosis of Brain

Toxoplasmosis is the leading cause of focal central nervous system diseases in AIDS. CNS toxoplasmosis in HIV-infected patients is usually a complication of the late phase of the disease. Typically, lesions are found in the brain, and their effects dominate the clinical presentation. Rarely, intraspinal lesions need to be considered on the differential diagnosis of myelopathy. The *Protoplasm gondii* is found ubiquitously, and antibodies to the organisms can be identified in 30% of all humans. The rate varies greatly from population and has a widely reported prevalence from 6 to 90%. In most cases, the infection is asymptotic. However, in immunocompromised patients, infection can become established. Cerebral toxoplasmosis is found in 10–34% of autopsies on patients with HIV/AIDS. The infection most likely occurs once the CD_4 count has dropped below 200 cells/mm3. In immunocompetent patients, acute encephalitis is extremely rare. Even in the immunocompromised, symptoms are typically vague and indolent. Development of new neurological symptoms in these patients should raise high suspicion of cerebral toxoplasmosis.

1.32.22 AIDS (Acquired Immunodeficiency Syndrome)

AIDS as a term has also been used to describe the various clinical syndromes, specific OIs, or malignancies that occur with HIV infection and signal those in whom advanced HIV infections have occurred. It is a disease of the immune system due to infection with HIV. HIV destroys the CD_4 T lymphocytes (CD_4 cells) of the immune system, leaving the body vulnerable to life-threatening infections and cancers. Acquired immunodeficiency syndrome (AIDS) is the most advanced stage of HIV infection. To be diagnosed with AIDS, a person with HIV must have an AIDS-defining condition or have a CD_4 count less than 200 cells/mm^3 (regardless of whether the person has an AIDS-defining condition).

1.32.23 Modes of Delivery: Infected Pregnant Women

Mode of delivery is the important parameter of MTCT; many authors reported that the prevalence of HIV MTCT significantly impacts on mode of delivery.

1.32.24 Mechanisms and Risk Factors of HIV Transmission

Knowing the mechanism and risk factors of MTCT is important for the design of interventions. Risk factor for vertical transmission of HIV-1 is divided into maternal, obstetrical, and neonatal. Maternal factors are known to be positively correlated with transmission rate and elevated viral load, symptomatic HIV disease, sexual intercourse during pregnancy, and low CD_4 count at the time of inception of HAART in pregnant women. Obstetrical factors are prolonged rupture of membrane, placental inflammation, and vaginal delivery. Neonatal factors include first-born twin, prematurity, low birth weight, etc.

1.32.25 Late Pregnancy and Intrapartum Transmission

It is one of the possible mechanisms of HIV transmission in the intrapartum period, which could be due to materno-fetal transfusion due to uterine contradictions in labor. Babies born through elective Caesarean section mode of delivery have a lower chance of MTCT, probably because the mothers avoid materno-fetal transfusion by not going into labor. The order of merit of delivery was recorded in the present study.

1.32.26 Breastfeeding

Breastfeeding is a common practice in developing countries. In India, breastfeeding is generally recommended because it provides appropriate nutritional value, passively conveys protection against some microorganisms including respiratory and gastrointestinal pathogens, and is more economical and promotes child spacing.

Children who breastfed for a longer duration grow better and have fewer episode of neonatal and childhood morbidity such as fever, acute diarrhea, and upper respiratory infections than those who are not breastfed. On the other hand, breastfeeding causes late postpartum transmission of HIV depending on the duration and other underlying risk of HIV.

1.33 Timing of HIV MTCT to Infant Non-BF Population

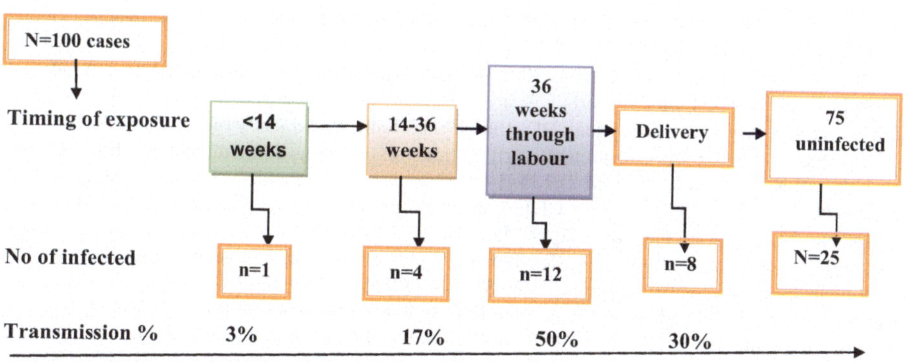

1.33.1 Interventions

There is an urgent need for effective interventions to reduce the spread of HIV-1. The HIV epidemic among children in Indian context is a very challenging issue, and caring for HIV type I-infected children is costly for families and health system.

There is a definite need for intervention to reduce the spread of HIV-1 in general and MTCT. In order to reduce the incidence, several measures are necessary to correlate different types of interventions. In this section, we have assessed the primary level, i.e., any programs implemented by NACO to prevent new infection by targeting the general population among ANCs.

1.33.2 Rates of Transmission

In India, MTCT rates in untreated non-breastfeeding populations ranged from 10% to 28%, whereas 25–38% were found in breastfeeding populations in resource-poor settings (UNAIDS report, 2009).

1.34 Confidentiality

Collected data was maintained in safe locker, and 100% confidentiality has been maintained at all times. The written consent was obtained from patient caretaker for photography and nontextual virtual data.

References

Abbink TE, Berkhout B et al (2003) A novel long distance base-pairing interaction in human immune deficiency virus type 1 RNA occludes the gag start codon. J Biol Chem 278:11601–11611

Abello J, Pardalos PM, Resende MG (2002a) Handbook of massive data sets. Kluwer Academic Publishers, Norwell, pp 201–221

Abello J, Pardalos PM, Resende MG (2002b) Handbook of massive datasets. Kluwer Academic Publishers, Norwell, pp 296–301

Adriaanse AH, Kollee LA, Muytjens HL et al (1995) Randomized study of vaginal chlorhexidine disinfection during labor to prevent vertical transmission of group streptococci. Eur J Obstet Gynecol Reprod Biol 61(Suppl 2):135–141

Agarwala BD et al (2002) On two ODE models for HIV/AIDS development in Canada and a logistic SEIR model. Far East J Appl Math (Suppl 1):25–70

Agrawal J, Gehrke J, Gunopulos L, Raghaven P (1998) Automatic subspace clustering of high dimensional data for data mining. ACM SIGMOD Rec 27(Suppl 2):94–105

Agrawal VK et al (2003) HIV and infant feeding. Indian J Clin Pract 24(Suppl 4):354–356

Agrawal VK et al (2013) HIV and infant feeding. Indian J Clin Pract 24(4):354–356

Ahmed F, Clemens J, Rao M et al (1992) Community-based evaluation of the effect of breast-feeding on the risk of microbiologically confirmed or clinically presumptive shigellosis Bangladeshi children. J Pediatr 90:406–411

Ahuja RK, Magnanti TL, Orlin JB (1993) Network flows: theory, algorithm, and applications. J Undergrad Math 32:125–136

Aitkhaled M, Lyall EG, Stains C et al (1998) Intrapartum mucosal exposure to human immunodeficiency virus type 1 (HIV-1) of infants born to HIV-1-infected mothers correlates with maternal plasma virus burden. J Infect Dis 177(Suppl 1):1097–1098

Akaike H et al (1971) A new look at the statistical model identification. IEEE Trans Autom Control 19:716–723

Akpa OM, Oyejola BA et al (2010) Modelling the transmission dynamics of HIV/AIDS epidemics: an introduction and a review. J Infect Dev Ctries 4(10):597–608

Alary M, Jayachandran AA, Lowndes CM et al (2010) Ecological analysis of the association between high risk population parameters and HIV prevalence among pregnant women enrolled in sentinel surveillance in four southern India states. Sex Transm Infect 86:174–179. (PMID 22376218; *PubMed* Central PMCID: PMC3287551)

Anderson RM, Medly GF, May RM, Johnson AM (1986) A preliminary study of the transmission dynamics of the human immunodeficiency virus (HIV), the causative agent of AIDS. IMA J Math Appl Med Biol 3(Suppl 9):229–263

Andrea L, George CR, Kenneth A et al (2008) Antiretroviral drugs for preventing mother-to-child transmission of HIV in sub- Saharan Africa: balancing efficacy and infant toxicity. JAIDS 22:2359–2369

Anon et al (1999) The mode of delivery and the risk of vertical transmission of human immunodeficiency virus type 1. N Engl J Med 340:977–987

Arya OP, Hart CA (1998) Regional epidemiology of viral STI (HIV/AIDS). Sex Transm Infect AIDS Tropics 3:12–20

Arya OP et al (1998) Regional epidemiology of viral STI (HIV/AIDS). Sex Transm Infect AIDS Tropics 43(Suppl 11):12–20

Avert et al (2008) Mother to child HIV transmission in Africa. Policy fact. HIV Treat J AIDS 13:56–63

Ayaya S, Doherty K, Leroy V, Hou T, Desmonde S, Lu Z, Noubary F (2013) Validation and calibration of a computer simulation model of pediatric HIV infection. Int J Math Comp Sci 8:110–116

Basavarajaiah DM, Chikkanarasareddy PS, Mohankumar G, Narasimha Murthy B (2013) Statistical models of postnatal transmission of HIV type I infection from mother to child–an Indian perspective. IJESIT 2(Suppl 2):588–593

Berhanu EC et al (2009) Survival analysis of time to treatment resumption for chronic HIV-1 patients interrupting Highly Active Antiretroviral Therapy (HAART). J Sex Transm Dis 52:112–118

Borkowf C, Kristen M, Little W et al (2015) Perinatal antiretroviral exposure and prevented mother-to-child HIV infections in the era of antiretroviral prophylaxis in the United States. JSM Online programme. http://www.amstat.org/meetings/jsm/2015/onlineprogram/AbstractDetails.cfm

Chasela C, Hudgens M, Jamieson D, et al (2009) Both maternal HAART and daily infant navirapine (NVP) are effective in reducing HIV-1 transmission during breastfeeding in a randomized trial in Malawi: 28 week results of the Breastfeeding, Antiretroviral and Nutrition (BAN) Study. 5thIAS conference on HIV pathogenesis, treatment and prevention; July 19–22, Cape Town, South Africa

Chasela CS, Hudgens MG, Jamieson DJ et al (2010) Maternal or infant antiretroviral drugs to reduce HIV-1 transmission. N Engl J Med 362(24):2271–2281

Chen JY, Ribaudo HJ, Souda S et al (2012) Highly active antiretroviral therapy and adverse birth outcomes among HIV-infected women in Botswana. J Infect Dis 206:1695–1705

Conner EM, Smith E et al (1994) Reduction of maternal-infant transmission of human immunodeficiencyvirustype 1 with zidovudine treatment. N Engl J Med 331:1174–1179

Creek T, Kim A, Lu L et al (2010) Hospitalization and mortality among primarily non-breastfed children during a large outbreak of diarrhea and malnutrition in Botswana. J Acquir Immune Defic Syndr 53:14–19

Diallo Q, Yagakone, Jerome et al (2010) Dynamics and threshold of simple epidemiological model; example of HIV/AIDS in mail. J Math Math Sci 24:86–91

Ekouevi D, Coffie P, Benaud B et al (1985) Antiretroviral therapy in pregnant women with advanced HIV disease and pregnancy outcomes in Abidjan, cote d'Ivoire. AIDS 22:1815–1820

Emily K et al (2013) Effectiveness of PMTCT at Naivasha District Hospital: outcomes of HIV Exposed Infants children and AIDS. Compendium of abstracts presented at the 17th ICASA. http://icsaconf2013.org

Fentaw HM, Worku A, Sahu O et al (2014) Statistical modelling and analysis of mother-to-child transmission of HIV: a case study in referral hospital and health Center of Hawassa Town, south nation nationality people, Ethiopia. Int J Data Envelop Anal Oper Res 1(3):49–52

Fowler M, Qin M, Shapiro D et al (2015) Efficacy and safety of strategies to prevent perinatal HIV transmission. In: CROI, vol 3, Seattle, pp 1897–1899

Gage et al. Percent of infants born to HIV infected mothers, who are infected. www.unaids.org.in 2006

Gilbert PB et al (2015) Inference on relative failure rates in stratified mark-specific proportional hazard models with missing marks with application to human immunodeficiency virus vaccine efficacy trail. App Statist 64:49–73

Goldman Emiley H et al (2007) The immune system of human milk: antimicrobial, anti-inflammatory and immune modulating properties. Pediatr Infect Dis J 12:664–671

Guay L, Lola et al (1999) Intrapartum and neonatal single-dosenevirapine compared with zidovudine for prevention of mother-to-child transmission of HIV-1 in Kampala,Uganda:HIVNET012 randomised trial. Lancet 354:795–802

Kapoor et al (2004) Prevention of mother to child transmission of HIV. Indian J Pediatr 71 (3):247–251

Lallemant M, Jourdain G, Le coeur S (2004) Single-dose perinatal navirapine plus standard zidovudine to prevent mother to child transmission of HIV, Thailand. N Engl J Med 351 (3):217–228

Lih-ing W, Feng RZ, Castillo-Chavez C (2009) Modelling TB and HIV co-infections. Math Biosci Eng 6(4):815–837

Lounes R, Arazoza HD, Sanchez A et al (1986) Epidemiology of HIV in Cuba, modelling detection with temporally varying parameters. Int J Math 4(1):107–117

Low-Beeri D, Stone Burner RL et al (1997) An age–and sex structured HIV epidemiological model; features and applications. Bull World Health Organ 75:312–316

Marazzi MC, Palombi L, Nielsen-Saines K et al (2011) Extended antenatal use of triple antiretroviral therapy for prevention of mother-to-child transmission of HIV-1 correlates with favorable pregnancy outcomes. AIDS 25:1611–1618

Martin DJ, Sim JG, Sole GJ, Rymer L, Shalekoff S, Van Niekerk AB et al (2010) CD_4 lymphocyte count in African patients co-infected with HIV and TB. J Acquir Immune Defic Syndr Hum Retrovirol 8:386–391

May RM, Anderson RM et al (1998) Transmission dynamic of human immunodeficiency virus (HIV). Phil Trans R Soc A 321:565–607

Mohammed I, Seidu DB et al (2012) Modelling the effect of irresponsible infective immigrants on the transmission dynamics of HIV/AIDS. Adv Appl Math Biosci 3(1):31–40

Nagelkerke NJD, Blanchard JF, Jha P et al (2002) Modelling HIV/AIDS epidemics in Botswana and India: impact of interventions to prevent transmission. Bull World Health Organ 80 (2):89–96. http://www.who.int/bulletin/archives/80(2)89.pdf

Pinkerton SD et al (2012) HIV transmission rate modelling: a primer, review, and extension. AIDS Behav 16(4):791–796

Rauner MS, Brailsford SC, Flessa S et al (2005) Use of discrete-event simulation to evaluate strategies for the prevention of mother-to-child transmission of HIV in developing countries. J Oper Res Soc 56:222–233

Shapiro RL, Hughes MD, Ogwu A (2010) Antiretroviral regimens in pregnancy and breast-feeding in Botswana. N Engl J Med 362(24):2282–2294

Springer V, Castillo-Chavez C, Songe B (2004) Dynamical models of Tuberculosis and their application. Math Biosci Eng 1:361404

Srinivasrao A (2009) Mathematical modelling on HIV. Ph.D thesis submitted to Bangalore University

Stover et al (2000) Influence of mathematical modelling of HIV and AIDS on policies and programs in the developing world. Sex Transm Dis 27(10):572–578

Swaminathan S et al (2004) Tuberculosis in HIV-infected children. Paediatr Respir Rev 5:225–230

Taha TE, Kumwenda NI, Hoover DR et al (2016) The impact of breast feeding on the health of HIV-positive mothers and their children in sub-Saharan Africa. Bull World Health Organ 84:546–554

Thamattor U, Thomas T, Banandur P et al (2015) Multilevel analysis of the predictors of HIV prevalence among pregnant women enrolled in annual HIV sentinel surveillance in four states in South India. PLoS One 10(7):1–11

Thomas T, Masaba R, Ndivo R et al (2007a) Rates of diarrhea associated with early weaning among infants in Kisumu, Kenya. 14th conference on retroviruses and opportunistic infections; February 25–28, Los Angeles, CA

Thomas T, Masaba R, Ndivo R et al (2007b) Prevention of mother-to-child transmission of HIV-1 among breastfeeding mothers using HAART: The Kisumu Breastfeeding study, Kisumu, Kenya, 2003–2007. 15th conference on retroviruses and opportunistic infections; February 3–6, Boston, MA

Vajpayee N, Kanswal S, Seth P, Wig N (2001) Spectrum of opportunistic infection and profile of cd4 counts among AIDS patients in north India. Infection 31:336–340

Vieira TI, Harper RP, Shahani AK, De Senna V (2003) Mother-to-child transmission of HIV: a simulation-based approach for the evaluation of intervention strategies. J Oper Res Soc 54 (7):713–722

Waema R, Olowofeso OE et al (2005) Mathematical modelling for human immunodeficiency virus (HIV) transmission using generating function approach. Kragujevac J Sci 27(115):130

Statistical Modeling of HIV Transmission 2

2.1 History of Modelling of HIV Transmission

Epidemic modelling is an exciting, active, and rapidly expanding field. Models based on transmission mechanisms of AIDS virus can help medical and scientific community to understand and anticipate its spread. Since AIDS is expected to place enormous demand on healthcare facilities, there is a pressing need to develop flexible prediction models. These are an integral part of long-range scientific research and are equivalent to the hypotheses to be tested. Modelling has been in use for a long time (Chasela et al. 2010; Creek et al. 2009; Dabis et al. 2000; Duff et al. 2010a, b, c) (have extensively reviewed epidemic models. They discuss the choke among alternative. Intervention strategies play a crucial role in quantifying uncertainties of "AIDS" projection. In developing a model, one creates a logical structure to organize existing information into a framework and suggest what new data that must be collected. Thus, models provide insight into the systems even when data are lacking. Hence statistical models are essential for understanding AIDS and the relation between social and biological mechanisms that influence its spread (Dietz et al. 1993; Duff et al. 2010a, b, c).

2.2 Deterministic Theory of HIV Epidemics

Incidence of HIV seroprevalence and AIDS counts is a large-scale phenomenon. The variability due to large number of susceptible and infective in such a phenomenon has to be reduced. We assume that, for a given number of susceptible and infectives and for given rates of contact, infection, and removals, certain definite numbers of new HIV and AIDS cases will result during a specified period. To begin with we outline a deterministic approach as developed by (Duff et al. 2010a, b, c; El Khatib et al. 2011; Fasoranbaku et al. 2015; Gourlay et al. 2013)

D. M. Basavarajaiah, B. Narasimha Murthy, *HIV Transmission*,
https://doi.org/10.1007/978-981-15-0151-7_2

2.3 Rationality of the Good Model

As there is generally a conflict between convenient simplicity and realistic complexity, it is essential to strike a balance between the two. Demographic transition life datasets are essential in model building for accurate assessment of "AIDS" because population change can be rapid, particularly in developing countries like India and Southeast Asia (Gilbert et al. 2010; Igwegbe et al. 2010; Kasenga et al. 2009; Kunihira et al. 2010; Kourtis et al. 2006; Lewis et al. 2001).

A single model that elaborates to address all the frequentisitc characteristics of heterosexuality would contain too many variables to be solved numerically at global level (Coovadia et al. 2004; Bhatt and Buwn 2003). Instead, simplified flexible models may be developed for each stratum separately and then aggregated. These must be tested for consistency with the history of the endemic in order to predict the future projection trend. The following are a few features of a good model:

(i) Using all available HIV life data sets
(ii) Reproducibility
(iii) Data encapsulation
(iv) Easy to import data input for formulation of the model – large data sets
(v) A simple structure and easy attributable
(vi) Stated degree of validity (>95% accuracy)
(vii) Understood in principle by those who are to be guided
(viii) Realistic to meet the administrative needs of government
(ix) Policy/clinician record/ health authorities

Providing insight into the system being modeled, etc.

Also, a model should allow for assumptions about the natural history of HIV infection and the efficacy and availability of treatment for HIV infected. It should incorporate delays in reporting of AIDS diagnoses. The logical soundness of a model in the context of its application is the basis on which we must choose our model among the alternatives. The following sections present features of HIV spread in four modes of spread and propose a methodology to evaluate the number HIV infected in the respective groups.

2.4 HIV Heterosexuality (TM_1)

In Asian countries, considerable increase in "HIV" infection has been detected among sex workers and attendees of "STD" clinics. High-risk behavior is commonly noted in "STD" patients. Sexual activity typically begins in the mid-teens, reaches a peak in early adulthood, and declines thereafter with age. The factors that influence a susceptible individual to be infected are probability of choosing an infected partner, frequency of contact, number of different partners, his behavior, and HIV prevalence in the group to which he belongs. For most infectious diseases including AIDS, infection rate increases with population density.

2.5 HIV Models for Heterosexual Transmission

Lettow et al. 2011; Moses et al. 2009; Morgan et al. 2010; Mepham et al. 2011;Naresh et al. 2011) presented two simple deterministic models to describe episodes of infection during the long incubation period by focusing on the heterogeneity in sexual activity within the heterosexual community in the UK. Models accounting for pair formation rate were also proposed (Shapiro et al. 2010; Nguyen et al. 2009). In the former, the model considers the duration of partnership and the number of contacts with same partner. An explicit formula for the number of partners during a lifetime, which is necessary to maintain the infection at an endemic level, is given. The latter discusses analytic models by considering pairing and separation rates and shows that the infection transmission depends on the contact rate in a pair and the duration of partnership. A model described by Kault et al. studies the impact of different sexual mixing patterns on the spread of HIV. Naresh et al. (2006), Oosterhoff et al. (2008), and Orie et al. (2009) present a hierarchical sequence of deliberately oversimplified models which combine the demography of a population with the epidemiologic characteristics of the heterosexual population as homogeneous, neglecting the variability in rates of acquiring sexual partners (Pai et al. 2009; Rollins et al. 2007). An exception is the "CASCADE" model, presented in the same paper, which captures heterogeneity factor and assumes the flow of infection from CSWs to young males and hence to the majority of child-bearing women. An outline of this model follows.

2.5.1 Probability of Infection

Consider a heterosexual HIV-risk population of size "N" consisting of three categories of persons:

(i) Sexually active young males (y)
(ii) Sexually active young females (x)
(iii) Commercial sex workers (z)

Categories **(i)** and **(ii)** are divided into married (m) and unmarried (u), each of which is further subdivided into susceptible (o) and infective (1), while category (c) is divided into males (Z_y) and females (Z_x) which is further split into susceptible and infective. At any time t, the number of persons in each of the above groups is denoted by using the subcategory notation as subscript, for example, Y_{uo} denotes the number of susceptible unmarried males. Let "M" denote the number of married couples. The objective is to estimate the probability of infection by computing the number of infected pairs and the number of possible pairs and taking their ratio. Assuming heterosexuality, a simple accounting of possible pairs is given by

$$\{\mathbf{A(t)} = \mathbf{Y_u.Z_x} + \mathbf{Z_u.Z_y} + \mathbf{M} \qquad (2.1)$$

In reality, heterosexuality is an intentional act and is subject to social norms, attitudes, and behavior. Also in many societies, there is no free mixing of the sexes.

Thus, the materialized number of pairs is to be computed by applying suitable discounting factors f_1 and f_2 ($0 \leq f, < 1$; $i = 1, 2$) to the first two terms on the right side of Eq. (2.1). Closeness of fi to 0 will indicate higher discounting while closeness to mean the opposite. Applying these actors and assuming faithful partnership among the married, expression (2.1) reduces to

$$\mathbf{A(t)} = (\mathbf{Y_u.Z_{x)}f_1} + (\mathbf{X_u.Z_y})\mathbf{f_2} + \mathbf{M} \tag{2.2}$$

which represents the effective number of pairs, with a reasoning that for a new infection, a pair should have precisely one infected person; the total number of infected pairs $A_1(t)$ is evaluated as a sum as follows:

$$\mathbf{A_1(t)} = [(\mathbf{Y_{uo}Z_{x1}}) + (\mathbf{Y_{ul}.Z_{xo}})]\,\mathbf{f_1} + \left[(\mathbf{X_{uo}.Z_{y1}}) + (\mathbf{X_{u1}.Z_{yo}})\right]\mathbf{f_2} + \mathbf{M_x} + \mathbf{M_y}, \tag{2.3}$$

where M_x and M_y, respectively, denote the number of married pairs in which only female and male members are infected. The proportion of infected pairs **p(t)** with only one infected member is therefore obtained by dividing $A_1(t)$ by $A(t)$. To estimate probability of HIV infection, we have to consider the rate of transmission (ø) as well as the frequency of contact per unit time (c). It is noted in literature that males and females have different transmission rates. Let these be $Ø_m$ and $Ø_f$, respectively.

Accordingly, the combinations in (2.3) are segregated into "female only" and "male only" infected groups and the rates Øf and $Ø_m$ applied. Then in turn, this probability can be applied to susceptible group ($N_1(t) = X_0 + Y_o + Z_0$) to give the expected number of new infections during the period. Thus the model is more suited to describe the infective population at large data sets.

2.6 Knowledge of Parameters

The data on the variables X, Y, Z, and M in the above model are generally available from census and other demographic records. The values of the parameters Øm, Øf, and Øp defined in previous section can be taken from the African study. The discounting factors may be computed by $f_1 = ZX/Yu$ and $f_2 = Zy/Xu$. These values of f may also be assessed by special behavioral studies.

2.7 Global Illustration

Let us consider a hypothetical heterosexual population of size $N = \mathbf{1000}$ with the following breakup: Y = **500**; X = **470**; Z = **30**.

{ You = 225, Ymo = 200} {Xuo = 250, Xmo = 170}
{ Yul = 25, Yml = 50 } { Xul = 20, Xml = 30}

T = 1 year, C = 96/year, Øm = 0.001	Zyo = 3
Øf = 0.0005	Zyl = 7
	Zxo = 5
	Zzl = 15
	f1 = 0.08
	f2 = 0.037

On using expressions (2.2) and (2.3), we get A(t) =700 and A_1(t) = 428. The proportion of infected pairs is p(t) = 0.61.The use of expression (2.4) results in the estimated probability of HIV infection, P_1(t) = 0.037, and expression (2.3) gives n_1(t) = 31.

2.8 CASCADE Linkage Model

Let N_1, Y_1, respectively, denote the total and infected number of males in a heterosexual population and N_2,Y_2 be the corresponding numbers for females. The other notations are as follows:

C_1 and C_2 denote the average number of commercial sex workers.
CSWs contacted by females and males, respectively, in unit time.

β1: Transmission probability in female – CSW contact
β2: Transmission probability in female – CSW contact
γ: Rate of acquiring AIDS
μ: Death rate from all other causes
B: Recruitment of susceptible, i.e., additions to heterosexual population per unit time. Treating the variables as continuous functions of time, the following differential equations are obtained, where prime denotes rate of change with respect to time t. However, t is suppressed for brevity. On the right side of these relations, the first term represents the addition to the quantity of interest. The other terms refer to removals due to various reasons. For example, in the expression for N_1, B represents the number of susceptible cases that were recruited, μN_1 gives the removals due to deaths from causes other than AIDS, and γY_1 refers to the number of infected males who develop AIDS (Shapiro et al. 2010). Numerical studies of cascade model reveal properties which are qualitatively similar but quantitatively different from those of other models.

The "cascade" model may explain the virus spread scenario in African countries like Nigeria. This assumes that "HIV" spreads through both male and female CSWs and ignores the changes that take place in the sizes of the two categories. Also, the model is confined to infected persons and avoids discussion on persons with AIDS. As such this model may not suit Asian countries like India where the majority of infections occur in female CSWs young male contact. Hence we propose a projection-oriented deterministic model for rapid growth of HIV spread which considers sexual contact between female CSWs and young unmarried males by noting their infection status. It also provides for a stratified heterosexual population with different mixing patterns (Chasela et al. 2010). The model centers around the four stages of HIV spread phenomenon are susceptibility, infectivity, AIDS symptoms, and death due to AIDS and determines the annual number of HIV infections and AIDS cases (Rahangdale et al. 2010; Rakoasi 2005; Ujiji et al. 2011).

2.9 The Proposed Model

As in the cascade model, the proposed model captures heterogeneity factors including variable rates in acquiring partners and considers time t as continuous since the HIV infection process is continuous. A schematic presentation of the infection process is the following:

2.9.1 The Assumptions of the Model Are as Follows

(i) There is no significant change in sexual habits or behavior during the period of projection, and no medical intervention changes the risk of infection.
(ii) Diagnosed AIDS patients are isolated and therefore no risk of infection from them.
(iii) All the infected are seropositives (the window period *ie* the time lag between infection and seroconversion is ignored since it lasts only for a couple of weeks).
(iv) Sexual contact of males other than with CSWs is negligible.
(v) Married couples have negligible extramarital relations.
(vi) Unmarried group includes widowed and divorced cases.

2.9.2 Structure and Notations

A closed heterosexual adult population in the age group of 16–49 years is considered and divided into four mutually exclusive groups, viz, CSWs (z), unmarried males (y), unmarried females (x) , and married couples (M). Each group is further divided into susceptible (S) and infectives (I). Let subscript "0" denote susceptible and "1" infective. A susceptible person does not carry "AIDS" virus but can contract it through sexual contact with an infected. An infected is not an "AIDS" case but only carries the virus and transmits it to a susceptible through sexual contact. An "AIDS" case is an infected person who has developed AIDS symptoms. Since there is no effective cure for "AIDS" yet, there is a high probability that the person will die from "AIDS." The subscript t denoting time dependence is implied throughout but suppressed for brevity. A letter along with subscript/s denotes the size of the respective groups. For example, M10 denotes number of couples in which only male partner is infected. If P_1 and P_2, respectively, denote proportion of males and females infected at the time of marriage and pair formation is independent of infection status, then four combinations arise.

The numbers in the last column may be computed by multiplying the proportion in Co1.3 by M, the total number of pairs formed. We note that new infections can occur only in combinations 3 and 4. The total size of the heterosexual population is $\mathbf{N = (X_o+Y_o+Z_0)+ (X_1+Y_1+Z_1) + 2\,[M_{10}+M_{01}+M_{00}+M_{11}]}$ which may be split into

$$\mathbf{S = (X_o + Y_o + Z_0)[2M_{00} + M_{01} + M_{10}]\,and\,I}$$
$$\mathbf{= (X_1 + Y_1 + Z_1) + [2M_{11} + M_{01} + M_{10}].Clearly, S + I = N.}$$

Entry into susceptible group: As time elapses, new persons enter sexually active group. Their number (S) can be evaluated with the following notations: Let the age of onset of sexual activity for women and men.

xc: Number of females at age (af – 1)
yc: Number of males at age (am – 1)
d: Death rate among (Xc + Yc) persons

Then $\mathbf{S = (X_c+Y_c)\,(1-d)}$, which can be taken as the recruitment rate for singles into sexually active group.

Recruitment may be computed for males and females separately. Denote them by S_m and S_n, respectively.

Two crucial parameters in the transmission of HIV used in the model are:

A: Recruitment rate of CSWs. This may be taken to be proportional to number of number of young women
B: Recruitment rate for singles into sexually active group which is equal to S.

We denote category-wise rates of removal due to death, migration, or withdrawal from sexual activity as follows:

Description	Rate
Susceptible	μ1
Infectives	μ2
CSWs without AIDS	μ3
CSWs with AIDS	μ4

Assume the following contact rates:

Group	Rate
Young males	Cm
CSWs	Cf
Partners in a pair	Cp

The transmission probabilities are denoted as follows:

Event	Probability
Male to female transmission in a pair	Øm
Female to male transmission in a pair	Øf
Transmission in a contract with an infected (for singles)	Øi

A few other rates are denoted as follows:

Event	Rate
Developing AIDS by infected individuals	γ
Deaths due to AIDS	δ
Formation of pairs	r
Infection per susceptible individual	λ
Separation of pairs	r

The assumptions stated above lead to a set of differential equations (Table 2.1) which indicate the net change in different categories (variables) during a unit time as sums of appropriate numbers.

Stratum	Expression
Developing AIDS by infected individuals	γ
Deaths due to AIDS	δ
Formation of pairs	r
Infection per susceptible individual	λ
Separation of pairs	r

An explanation of the terms in Table 2.1 is as follows: In the expressions for Y_0 and X_0, the first term, respectively, represents the rate of recruitment of males and females into sexually active group. The next two terms are additions to this group from the pairs due to death or separation of a member. The last term indicates removals of singles due to death or pair formation.In the expression for Y_1, the coefficient of Y_0 gives the rate of infection among males due to contact with CSWs, and the second term represents the number of infected males removed. In X_1, the last term represents the removals due to death or marriage. It can be noted that the 3rd term in Zo represents the number of new infections among susceptible CSWs. This number may be denoted by Zc. The first term in Z_1 gives the number of infections among susceptible CSWs. In the second term, Z_1 (NA) and Z_1 (A), respectively, denote CSWs without and with AIDS. Thus the set of equations in Table 2.1 are the

Table 2.1 Overview of combination and proportion

Sl	Combination	Proportion	Number
1	Both partners susceptible	(1−p1)(1−p2)	M00
2	Both partners infective	p1 p2	M11
3	Only female infected	p1(1−p2)	M01
4	Only male infected	P2(1−p1)	M10

deterministic computational expressions for the quantities of interest which are obtained via a few simplifying assumptions mentioned earlier.

The equations in table are in fact the set of differential equations for the deterministic approach. It is difficult to obtain explicit solutions to these equations. But for the homogeneous case (where different rates are assumed to be independent of t), one may always solve these equations numerically to assess effect of various factors on the expected numbers. If **S(t)** is very large, the deterministic approach is equivalent to working with the expected values of 1(t) and a(t). Further for the homogeneous case, one may always fit equations in Table 2.1 to real data (if available) by using various methods (Simbayi et al. 2007; Sprague et al. 2011). As an approximation we suggest adding the rates of change evaluated to the known respective initial numbers for updating the quantities of interest.

2.10 Computation of Infection Rate

In order to compute the infection rate (X (t)) per susceptible person, we note the following:

When a pair has either both susceptibles or both infectives, a new infection cannot take place, but this can occur when there is precisely one infected. If r_o and r_1, respectively, denote the rates of pair formation for susceptible and infective persons, then the rate at which male partner is susceptible and female is infective is $\mathbf{r_{01} = [r_o.Y_o.X_1/(X_o{+}X_1)]}$. Similarly $\mathbf{r_{1o} = [r_1Y_1X_o/(X_0{+}X_1)]}$. Thus, the rate of pair formation where precisely one member is infected is $\mathbf{r = (r_{ol} + r_{1o})}$. Also the sequence of events associated with a new infection are the following:

(a) Pair formation with precisely one infected (with probability r. I(t)/N(t))
(b) Sexual contact between the members of the pair (with rate Cp)
(c) Transmission of infection (with probability θ)

$$\text{Now it follows that } \boldsymbol{\lambda(t) = \theta.C_p.r.I(t)/N(t)} \tag{2.6}$$

Disease Process

The infection rate λ(t) computed using the expression 2.6 is useful in several ways, especially in determining the number HIV infected. The sequence of events (in the order of occurrence) in the HIV disease process and the corresponding numbers are shown in Table 2.2.

Table 2.2 Events in HIV disease process

Order	Event	Associated
1	Susceptibility	S1(t)
2	HIV infection	Y(t)
3	AIDS case	a(t)
4	AIDS death	D(t)

The rate of change in the number of AIDS cases during unit time is given by

$$\mathbf{a}^1(\mathbf{t}) = \mathbf{Y}(\mathbf{t}).\gamma - \mathbf{D}(\mathbf{t}) \tag{2.7}$$

$$\mathbf{a}^1(\mathbf{t}) = \sum_{i=1}^{n} \mathbf{Y}_i(\mathbf{t}_i).\gamma - \mathbf{D}(\mathbf{t}_i) \tag{2.8}$$

Where $t_i =$ rate of change in number at ith period obtained from back calculation method

$$\mathbf{a}^1(\mathbf{t}_{i=1..n}) = \sum_{i=1}^{n} \mathbf{Y}_i(\mathbf{t}_{i-1})\,(\mathbf{t}_{i-2})\ldots..(\mathbf{t}_{i-ni}).\gamma - \mathbf{D}(\mathbf{t}_i) \tag{2.9}$$

Geometric progression at n^{th} period was calculated from Eq. (2.9)

$$\mathbf{a}^1(\mathbf{t}_{i=1..n}) = \sum_{i=1}^{n} \mathbf{Y}_i(\mathbf{t}_{i-1})\,(\mathbf{t}_{i-2})\ldots..(\mathbf{t}_{i-ni}).\frac{\mathbf{1}}{\gamma} - \mathbf{D}(\mathbf{t}_i) \tag{2.10}$$

$$\mathbf{a}^1(\mathbf{t}_{i=1..n}) = \frac{\mathbf{1}}{\gamma^2}\left[\sum_{i=1}^{n} \mathbf{Y}_i(\mathbf{t}_{i-1})\,(\mathbf{t}_{i-2})\ldots..(\mathbf{t}_{i-ni}). - \mathbf{D}(\mathbf{t}_i)\right]^{1/n} \tag{2.11}$$

The total number of "AIDS" cases in any interval of time (t_1, t_2) is obtained by cumulating the different components over the interval. Alternatively, a^1 (t) can also be arrived at by back-calculation. But this pre-supposes knowledge of I (.) and F (.), which is difficult to obtain in many regions. Thus the proposed method implied in (3.2) is a handy alternative, though approximate, to back-calculation.

2.11 Assessment of the Parameters

The set of equations in Table 2.1 and Eq. (2.7) are the computing expressions which need information of 3 types: (a) characteristics related to the population under study (e.g., 142, 514., the values of the variables X_o, Y_1, Z_1), (b) features determined by past studies or experience in the form of rates and proportions (e.g., μi ($i = 1, 2, 3, 4$); θ_m, θ_f), and (c) parameters estimated through sample surveys on human sexual practices (e.g., C_p, C_m, C_f). It may be noted that the input of the types (b) and (c) may come from other similar regions, while information under (a) is to be necessarily for the region under study. The estimates of some parameters can be taken from the past studies, especially the African study (Stangl et al. 2013). A few of these are listed below:

Parameter	μ1	μ2	μ3	μ4	θm	θf	Cm	Cf	ro
Value	0.05	0.1	0.5	0.9	0.004	0.0067	120	300	0.3

Parameter	r1	Cp	r	Γ	P0	P1	d	θ	K
Value	0.1	96	0.02	0.1	0.03	0.05	0.15	0.0038	0.05

2.12 Model Discussion

In the Indian subcontinent, TM1 has been the major cause for the rapid spread of HIV infection among adults. Commercial sex dominates the causes of spread in the region. The use of "cascade" model is extended to explain HIV spread mechanism in a heterosexual population of adults where most of the spread is between young males and female sex workers. The extended cascade model which is centered around the four stages of infection, viz., susceptibility, infectivity, "AIDS" case, and death due to AIDS, determines the number of HIV and AIDS cases during an interval of time. For practical convenience, the interval can be taken as 1 year, which suits data availability.

A few simplifying assumptions result in a set of differential equations as in (Table 2.1, which evaluate rates of change in a few quantities of interest. These are useful both individually and on aggregative basis. The information gained is expected to be useful to know the extent of HIV spread in different strata and also in designing effective intervention strategies. The infection rate per susceptible person ($\lambda(t)$) is computed and used to assess the number of HIV infections. Some authors report that the probability of transmission from female to male is higher than from male to female (Turan et al. 2011). However, a few others have noted the situation to be reversing (Stangl et al. 2013). Thus there is no finality over the opinion. A significant change in sexual attitudes and habits can drastically affect the projections, particularly over a relatively long period of time. In this context it may be pointed out that a survey conducted in eight metropolitan cities of India in the year 1996 by a reputed market research organization for the Outlook Magazine (Turan et al. 2008) has recorded considerable changes in sexual behavior primarily due to awareness programs. This can result in realized numbers being lower than predicted numbers. It may be noted that the probability of nonuse of condoms does not figure in the model described. An assessed value of this parameter is 0.9. Incorporation of this probability in the computational expressions in Table 1.1 will slightly reduce the projected numbers. More importantly, the model presented here focuses on the epidemiological parameters that need to be measured accurately to predict future trends and helps to assess how the values of these parameters affect the quantities of interest. More complex models may also be formulated incorporating the variation in T, but their solution will require numerical method.

2.13 Infected Needles (TM_2)

Globally, sexuality (TM_1) is by far the most common way of passing on HIV, followed by use of needles (TM_2). We now focus on the latter briefly (Abdallah et al. 2012). Up to now 114 countries have reported TM2 spread. This is the main

Table 2.3 Percentage of new HIV infections in IVDUs during 1998–2000

Country	Percentage	Country	Percentage
Canada	49	Malaysia	76
Vietnam	66	Ukraine	78
China	70	Maldova	85
Latvia	71	Russian Federation	92

UNAIDS annual report, 2001

mode of HIV transmission for adults in Eastern Europe and Central Asia where the epidemic started only in the early 1990s. About 1 million people are living with the virus today in this region. TM_2 is the dominating mode of spread followed by heterosexuality in most parts of the world including North Africa, Middle East, South and Southeast Asia, and the Pacific Region, accounting for nearly ten million seropositives. On an average 30% of the seropositives are women. Intravenous drug users (IVDUs) form the major component of TM_2. Table 1.3 shows the percentage of HIV positive cases attributable to this component in a few selected countries (Table 2.3).

In India, as at the end of 1998, based on HIV serosurveillance data, a total of 3855 seropositives were estimated among IVDUs accounting for 4% of the total prevalence in the country (Duff et al. 2010a, b, c; Balcha et al. 2011; Turan et al. 2011; Gourlay et al. 2013). The number of AIDS cases was reported to be 645 making up 5.2% of the total of 12,389 cases registered. The state of Manipur with hardly 0.2% of country's population accounts for nearly 8% of the total seropositivity. Nagaland and the adjoining Northeastern states of India are the epicenters for seropositivity. Apart from intravenous drug use, the other component comes from use of unsterilized needles for clinical injections. Let us denote these by A and B, respectively. Some work has been reported about A, while little is known about B. The dynamics of needle infection among IDUs has been modelled by (UNAIDS 2009). An outline of this is as follows: a two-state Markov process to capture the essence of needle infection is assumed since the needle alternates between uninfected and infected states (0 and 1) according to a stochastic process.

The rate of transition to state 1 is denoted by "λ," and "μ" is the reverse rate. These rates depend on factors like frequency of drug injection. It is assumed that the circulation time of needles follows an exponential distribution with mean "T." Denoting by "Q" the probability that a needle is HIV infected at time "t" after its introduction and by the probability that a randomly selected needle is "HIV" infected, and shown that "Qo" is the probability that the needle is infected at the time of induction. Equation (2.8) implies that the longer a needle remains in use, the higher the probability that it becomes infected. Equation (2.9) indicates that the chance of encountering an infected needle at a random point in time depends on T. The use of this concept is illustrated in the model proposed later in Chap. 3 (mathematical DTSM simulation modelling).

A few basic differences in the characteristics of the components A and B are as follows:

(i) Component A is a network indulging in an intentional act which is illegal and involves confidentiality, while B is an unintentional clinical act.
(ii) Activity A is restricted to a geographical area and to a subpopulation while B is unrestricted and has its impact throughout the region.
(iii) A is age dependent involving mostly the young while B is independent of age.
(iv) The HIV infection risk is higher for A since most of the IUDs are associated with the risk of TM I also. The risk is lower under B as it involves only clinical injections. Component B has a few other features which include the following: (i) the first use of needle poses no risk. Only its reuse provides scope for new infection. (ii) Infection depends on the time interval between successive uses as HIV survives for only a few minutes in media other than blood. (iii) Proper sterilization before use eliminates risk of infection. But sterilization, though it is mandatory, may not be implemented due to negligence or ignorance. (iv) The number of infections caused depends directly on the duration of the needle in circulation and the number of reuses.
(v) If a needle is used, w times and infection takes place in the ith use, then only (w – 1) usages have the infection risk, where i = 1, 2... (w – 1).

2.14 HIV Spread Through Clinical Injections

In the light of the special features of HIV infection through needles in clinical injections, the following method is developed which estimates the annual number of infections due to needles used in clinics. The important parameters of the model are as follows:

γ: Probability of needle reuse
n: Probability of non-sterilization before reuse
w: HIV transmission rate in TM2

If a needle is used w times and infection takes place in the ith use then (w – i) further uses have the infection risk where i = 1, 2,....... (w – 1). If "X" denotes the number of times a needle is in infected state, then X may be taken to follow a right truncated Poisson distribution (truncated at (w – 1)) with parameter k, the average number of times a needle is infected. This assumption is justified since there is ample opportunity for a needle to be in infected, whereas the actual probability of infection is small. Let 4 denote the probability that a needle is in infected state at least once.

Then we have further we define the following events:-.

E1: {reuse of a needle),
E2: {non-sterilization of a needle)
E3: {transmission of infection by an infected needle}

For a new infection to take place, a needle should be in infected state followed by the occurrence of the events E_1, E_2 and E_3 in that order. The probability of this compound event is, P = .γ.n.w (assuming E_i (i = 1, 2, 3) to be independent).

If m(t) is the number of needles used in a year in clinics and hospitals in the given region, then the expected number of HIV infections is, $n_{2B}(t) = m(t).\theta.P$. Then the estimated number of HIV infections due to component.

(B) is given by :n2B (t) = m(t).θ. P

Knowledge of Parameters

One source for the value of m (t) is the drug association while the parameters γ and n are to be assessed by experts. The value of w can be taken to be 1 unless there is some information to the contrary. The choice of k will be difficult in the absence of any definite information on it and also due to complexity in collecting the relevant data which estimates k. However, the value of k depends on (i) the total circulation time of a needle in use and (ii) the expected number of reuses of a needle. In fact k and w are positively correlated. As such the value of k may be taken to be equal to (w−1)/3.

2.14.1 Remarks

In Eq. (2.3), if only the first term in the numerator sum is considered which corresponds to x = 1, then n_{2B} (t) in Eq. (2.2) provides a lower bound for the number of infections. On the other hand, if we take all the terms up to X = (w−1), Φ will be the highest, and therefore $n_{2B}(t)$ provides an upper bound. Use of n_{2B} (t) – the values of the estimator from in Eq. (2.2) will be useful for the following practical purposes:

(i) To assess the spread of HIV through TM_2
(ii) To measure the magnitude of the epidemic in the given region
(iii) To plan intervention strategies

It is possible that a particular needle in circulation is reused by the same person. The impact of this is to reduce the number of new infections due to the needle and $m_{2(b)}(t)$ as an upper bound as stated above.

An alternative expression for n_{2B} (t) is $n_{2B}(t) = m(t).(1-\Phi)$ P, where Φ (or P (X = 0)) is the complementary probability. This is simpler for computation purpose.

2.14.2 Drug Abuse

It is difficult to estimate the total number of persons "HIV" infected in a country as a whole due to TM_2 because of large variation in population characteristics, seropositivity rate, cultural characteristics, and practices with reference to needle use. Since drug abuse is illegal in many countries, it is all the more difficult to estimate the size of the “IVDU” population. A single model for the spread of “HIV” under TM_2 cannot be easily developed and applied to a large and diverse country. However, the components A and B due to drug abuse and unsterilized needles can be separately studied. A method for estimating the number of HIV infected due to component A is initiated next, but mathematical models are modeled in Chap. 3.

2.14.3 Sample Proportion Method

Let N_t be the average size of the IVDU population in a given region which is exposed to the risk of infection due to component A and r_t be the HIV prevalence rate. Then the number infected in the region is estimated by

$$\mathbf{I_t = N_t . r_t} \tag{2.12}$$

The rate r_t is obtained at the national level which is generally reported annually. If there is a delay in getting value of r_t, we may assume r_{t-1} to apply during the current year t. The exact value of N_1 is difficult to get as it is the size of an evasive subpopulation. Thus it is to be estimated. Two methods may be used for this purpose. (i) Use of sample proportion obtained from an appropriate sampling design and (ii) sample-resample method. In case of (i), the size of the IVDU population is estimated by multiplying the sample proportion p of IVDUs by the total size of the adult population (M_t) in the age group of (16–49 years). Thus

$$\mathbf{N_t(1) = p_t . M_t;} \tag{2.13}$$

where M_t may be obtained by projecting the census population. The traditional method of data collection and estimation has a major drawback since drug abuse is an illegal activity involving social stigma. Respondents are generally reluctant to give reliable answers to direct questions relating to such issues. Thus, special methods are required. We propose a sample-resample technique incorporating randomized responses at two levels. This method is on the lines of Petersen mark-recapture method which was used to estimate the size of the diabetic population (UNAIDS 2011) by tackling the problem of errors in the lists. The formal procedure is described in later part as an application of a new covariate RR method.

2.15 Blood Transfusion (TM_3)

The first instances of blood transfusion-associated HIV positive cases were documented in India, in 1987, and since then there is a rising trend of HIV infection through this mode. There is a large gap between demand and supply of blood, and it appears that not all the blood is screened for HIV before use. The gap is positive in most countries as in India.

Table 2.4 Blood samples screened for HIV in Karnataka State (1987–2016)

Year	Blood samples screened	Number HIV positive
1987	913	0
1988	2264	6
1989	25,930	32
1990	48,350	58
1991	66,830	86
1992	102,340	168
1993	76,240	863
1994	24,210	425
1995	11,590	439
1996	8880	697
1997	15,450	874
1998	15,910	1023
1999	16,710	1319
2000	20,510	1965
2001	32,156	2122
2002	40,582	1632
2003	56,331	1521
2004	63,147	1622
2005	70,856	1322
2006	85,241	1589
2007	92,144	1254
2008	93,654	1141
2009	96,587	1211
2010	112,522	1018
2011	156,321	1126
2012	178,362	894
2013	185,968	925
2014	186,221	896
2015	195,632	744
2016	198,742	632

A mushrooming of private blood banks is noted here, and the regulations governing transfusion are not strictly followed. A 5-year study based on yearly screening of about 15,000 donor blood samples (WHO 2014) reveals that the prevalence of HIV has increased over the years from 1.1 to 2.1 per 1000, and this indicates the rising seroprevalence in general population. Estimated that about 9200 haemophiliacs became infected during 1986–1992 in the USA. The following table summarizes blood screening scenario in Karnataka State (Table 2.4).

An advantage with this data is that the date of infection can be ascertained retrospectively as the date of transfusion, which is usually recorded. The following sections discuss the role of a needle and infected blood to determine the probability of infection in TM_3 and outline estimation of number HIV infected. An illustration is also provided.

2.15.1 The Model Fitting

The needle plays an important role in transfusion, being the main tool, while the effect of other components such as tube may be overlooked. Many a time the occurrence of new HIV infection depends on the infection status of the needle. In the absence of an effective needle replacement program, the same needle is reused in several transfusions either for receiving blood from donors or for transfusion or for both. Non-sterilization of needle before use causes the risk of HIV infection. The chance of transfusion through an infected needle depends both on its infection status and the time lapsed after previous use. A sterile needle may become infected when used by an infected person. But due to lapse of time before its reuse, the virus present at the tip of the needle may become inactive resulting in an uninfected state. This two-state process continues until the needle is replaced. Assume that transition of uninfected needle to the infected state occurs with a rate A and it returns to the uninfected state at A rates. These rates depend on several factors including frequency of use and HIV prevalence rate among users.

The needle infection process in TM3 is similar in many respects to that among drug users as discussed by Kaplan et al. He assumed that the duration of a needle in circulation follows an exponential distribution with mean T. Then the probability that a randomly selected needle is HIV infected,

$$D = \frac{\gamma_o + \lambda t}{1 + (\lambda + \mu)t} \tag{2.14}$$

where γ_o is the probability that a needle is infected at the time of introduction. Repeating Kaplan's assumption on distribution of needle circulation time, the probability that a randomly selected needle is HIV infected is γ, so that the probability of its being not infected is $\gamma = (1-\gamma)$. The use of γ in determining the number of new HIV infections in TM_3 is outlined later.

2.15.2 Role of Blood Units

The infection status of a blood unit directly determines the occurrence of new infection in TM3. The parameter associated with this component the proportion (p) of screening of blood units, and the 'HIV' prevalence rate (δ) among donors, bridge population and unknown transmitters. Consider a closed population which includes all the donors and recipients of blood (Dietz et al. 1993). A specified volume of blood is considered as a unit. For simplicity, supply of blood from outside the region is overlooked. The other simplifying assumptions are the following:

(i) The screening of blood is error free, i.e., all the screened units are correctly classified.

(ii) Supply of blood of a particular group and the demand for blood which matches with this group are considered.

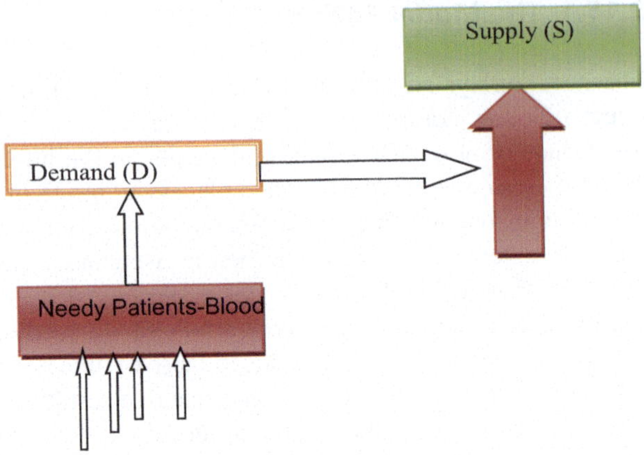

Fig. 2.1 Flow of blood for testing

Two types of donors are considered: (a) voluntary donors (Group-I) who donate blood when there is a request (especially in emergencies) and (b) professional donors (Group-II) who give blood frequently at regular intervals of time motivated by monetary reward. Experience shows that HIV prevalence is higher in Group-II. Further, not all the units will be screened for virus due to lacunae in the blood banking system, which introduces risk of infection due to non-screening (Fig. 2.1).

The blood supply is thus a mixture of units from two sources. Depending on the supply-demand relation, two cases arise:

(i) (D) for blood exceeds supply (S)
(ii) Supply exceeds demand

There is a difference in the spread of infection in the two cases. Situation as in case (ii) is unlikely in many countries. In this, since the supply is in excess of demand, mostly uncontaminated blood will be used. In case (i) all the supply will be utilized. We pursue case (i). If $S_1(t)$ and $S_2(t)$ denote the supplies from Groups 1 and 2 in year t and $h_1(t)$ and $h_2(t)$ are number of units screened out, then the effective supply S(t) will be $[(S_1(t) + S_2(t)) - (h_1(t)) + h_2(t)]$. Here D(t) is limited to S(t) as all the demand cannot be met. Then the proportion of uninfected blood transfusion is

$$D = \frac{\text{Number of transfusion not prone to new infection}}{\text{Total number of transfusion}} \tag{2.15}$$

Here the subscripts 1 and 2 indicate the groups. The proportion $(1-P_{u1})$ estimates $\acute{\alpha}$, the probability that a bottle of blood is HIV infected. The numerator on the right side of (2.13) is the sum of two components which, respectively, correspond to Group-I and Group-II, respectively. The first component has two terms: the expected number of virus-free transfusions among the screened bottles and among unscreened blood units. A similar interpretation holds for the other component. In both cases the infected bottles identified are removed from use.

2.15.3 Joint Effect of γ and $\acute{\alpha}$

The occurrence of a new HIV infection in TM_3 depends on two factors; infection status of needle and of blood. If E_l and E_2, respectively, denote the presence of HIV in needle and in blood and E_l and E_2 are the complementary events, then the following possibilities arise:

Blood Needle	Infected (E2)	Uninfected (E2)
Infected (E1)	E1 E2	E1 E2
Uninfected (E1)	E1 E2	E1 E2

It may be noted that considering both the components (needle and blood), a new infection is possible in all cases except the last (E_l E_2). Thus probability of infection is given by

$\beta = 1 - P(E1 \text{ n } E2) = 1 - P(E1).\ P(E2)$, as E1 and E2 are independent events

$$= 1 - (1-\gamma)\ (1-\acute{\alpha})$$
$$= \acute{\alpha} + \gamma(1-\acute{\alpha}) \quad (2.16)$$

The value of a can be estimated by ($1 - P_{u1}$) of Eq. (2.13), while γ can be taken from result (2.14). Hence,

$$\boldsymbol{\beta} = \acute{\alpha} + \boldsymbol{\gamma}(\mathbf{1} - \acute{\alpha}) \quad (2.17)$$

which represents the estimated infection rate under TM_3.

Note: The probability γ is a function of hospital environment. The risk of infection due to needle can be reduced by taking proper precaution. On the other hand, $\acute{\alpha}$ is a standardized rate. Infection through blood is a stochastic phenomenon, namely, the event of infection being carried through. This risk can be controlled by proper screening of blood.

2.15.3.1 Use of β

One immediate use of β as the rate of HIV incidence is to estimate the number infected under TM_3. If N(t) denotes the number of transfusions in the region during the year t, then the estimated number of HIV infections is given by

$$\mathbf{M(t) = N(t).\boldsymbol{\beta}} \quad (2.18)$$

This does not necessarily indicate the number of infected persons, since each individual may receive more than one unit of blood during the year. If θ is the average number of blood units received by an individual, then the estimated number of persons infected is

$$\mathbf{M(t) = N(t)}\ \boldsymbol{\beta}$$
$$\boldsymbol{\theta} \quad (2.19)$$

2.15.4 Cumulative Incidence

If To is the starting year and TL is the current year, then total estimated number of HIV infected persons due to TM3 during an interval of time (t_i, t_j) ; $T_o < t_j < t_j < T_L$; i = 1, 2, . . . (L−1); i, j = 1, 2,. . . ..L and i < j is given by

$$\mathbf{n_3}\left(\mathbf{t_i}, \mathbf{t_j}\right) = \sum_{\mathbf{t}=\mathbf{t_j}}^{\mathbf{t_j}} \mathbf{m(t)}$$

And if $t_i = T_o$ and $t_j = T_L$, then the estimated incidence of HIV during the period is

$$\mathbf{n_3} = \sum_{\mathbf{t}=\mathbf{T_o}}^{\mathbf{T_{ij}}} \mathbf{m(t)} \tag{2.20}$$

The component n3 will be added to the components due to other modes to give total HIV incidence. It may be noted that both n3 and n3 are the upper bounds on the number of infections as they do not account for the deaths during the period. However, knowledge of n3 will help design of blood transfusion-related interventions in the region adequately.

2.15.5 Standard Error (S.E) of m (t)

One way to evaluate this SE is to assume the HIV infection to be a continuous process following a specific probability distribution. If g(m(t)) denotes the pdf, then the expected number HIV infected during the interval (T_o, T_L) is given by

$$\mathbf{E(m)} = \mathbf{S_i m(t).g(m(t)).dtt} = \mathbf{T_o} \tag{2.21}$$

n view of the rising trend of HIV infections, m(t) may be assumed to follow a two parameter gamma distribution. With parameters λ^{-1}(scale) and φ(shape), the pdf is

$$\mathbf{g}\left(\mathbf{m(t)}/\frac{\boldsymbol{\lambda\varphi}}{\boldsymbol{\lambda}, \boldsymbol{\varphi}} = \mathbf{r}(\boldsymbol{\varphi})\left(\mathbf{m(t)}^{\boldsymbol{\varphi}-1}.\mathbf{e}^{-\boldsymbol{\lambda}\mathbf{m(t)}}; \mathbf{0} < \mathbf{m(t)} < \infty\right.\right.$$

The mean and variance of the distribution are $\mu = \varphi/\lambda$ and $a = \varphi/\lambda^2$. Thus, parameters X and φ are determined by and $\lambda = \mu/\sigma^2$ and $\varphi = \mu^2 / \varphi^2$. The parameters μ and σ^2 can be estimated from time series data for, e.g., as in (Table 2.5. The SE of the estimate of m is then given by $\sqrt{}\varphi/\lambda$.

Table 2.5 Illustration: Consider the following hypothetical setup

W(x,t) = 1,00,000	Q = 0.9
f (x,t) = 0.09 r1(t) = 2%	r2(t) = 0.1
	s(t) = 0.04

2.15.6 Estimation of Parameters

The estimation of β, the rate of infection, needs estimates of 5 parameters, viz, γ, ά, δ^1, $\delta^{2,}$ and θ. It is unlikely that all these are available from a single source. Some sources identified for this purpose are previous studies, data from clinics, and the assessment by experts. Of these the value of γ may be taken from (2.14), while ά is estimated by Eq. (2.15), the values of δ_1 and δ_2 are generally reported region-wise with $\delta_2 > \delta_1$. The value of θ, the average number of blood units given to a person, may be computed from the records kept in clinics. The proportion of blood units screened and P1 and P2 for groups 1 and 2 may assessed by the experts (Bashiru et al. 2017).

2.15.7 Practical Illustrations in Indian Context

The total demand for blood in the Karnataka State during the year 2000 was 2, 44,590 blood units. We assume that the probability of a needle being infected is $\gamma = 0.03$. The other parameters are assumed to be as follows:

Parameters	Group 1	Group 2
Proportion screened	$P1 = 0.95$	$P2 = 0.85$
HIV prevalence rate	$\delta 1 = 0.02$	$\delta 2 = 0.06$

We take $S_1(t)$, the supply of blood from voluntary donors (Group 1) to be 50,000 units, while that from professional donors (Group 2) to be S2 (t) 50,000 units. Out of these $h_1(t) = 1200$ and $h_2(t) = 5625$ ace assumed to be the removals after screening. Using result (3.1.5) we get $\acute{\alpha} = 0.007$. Now from Eq. (2.14), β is obtained as $\beta = \acute{\alpha} + \gamma\ (1-\acute{\alpha}) = 0.0368$, which is the estimated infection rate under TM3. Applying this rate for the blood demand in Karnataka and with a value of $\theta = 3$, the estimated number of HIV infected during the year 2000 is obtained as

$$m(t) = \frac{N(t)\,\beta}{\theta} = \frac{244590}{3}(0.0368) = 3008$$

Using the data for Karnataka State as in Table 3.5, the estimated parameter values are $\lambda = 0.0038$ and $p = 2.15$ with an estimated SE of 386.

Important Note In practice it is desirable to have a and γ low, if not zero. When the assessed ά and γ are serious, the control steps become critically important. Therefore it is necessary to (i) evaluate ά and γ for a given region and (ii) initiate steps to reduce ά and γ, if serious, so that infection rate β reduces. Here (i) is a statistical work, while (ii) is the responsibility of "AIDS" health planners.

2.16 Perinatal Transmission (TM_4)

Model-wise projection of HIV and AIDS cases is useful for predicting the path and interventions separately. It is likely that a few persons may be exposed to the risk from more than one mode under TM_1–TM_3 leading to overlapping of cases. But this factor is absent in TM_4. Thus, a person involved in unprotected sexual act may also be a drug abuser and a blood recipient, whereas a newborn with HIV has no other exposure (except possibility of receiving blood), since it will not survive until adulthood. Some HIV projection methods and the problem of overlap will be discussed in Chap. 2 mathematical modeling intervention (Naresh et al. 2006).

2.16.1 The Model Formation

We define a few notations as follows:

t: Unit time
X: Age of mother in years; $15 < x < 49$. (Reproductive age group)
W(x,t): Number of women aged "x" years at time t
f(x,t): Age-specific fertility rate
r1(x,t): Prevalence of HIV among women aged x at time t
q: Probability of HIV transmission from infected mother to child
B(t): Total number of births during the period (t, t+1)
Bi(t): Total number of births with HIV infection
r2(t): Infant mortality rate

Then the estimated number of births is n.
B(t) = Σ W(x,t) f(x,t) and the estimated number with HIV infection is
x = 1

$$\mathbf{B_1(t) = q \cdot \sum_{x=i}^{nk} W(x,t)\, f(x,t) \cdot r_1(x,t)}$$

2.16.2 Estimation Techniques

The probability P_2 (t) of a baby being born with HIV infection at time t can be estimated by the proportion P_2 (t) = B_1(t)/B(t). In this setting there are two practical aspects of interest: healthcare (a) for mothers and (b) for children. P_2(t) is an indicator of infection status among mothers and hence in the general population. This will help in planning healthcare for mothers. But, for (b) an adjustment for still births and infant mortality (whose effect may not be negligible) may first be made to get the net number of children with perinatal infection. In order to do this, B_1 (t) should be adjusted for still births as well as infant mortality. The former may be estimated by

$$\mathbf{S(t) = s(t).P_2(t)B(t)} \tag{2.22}$$

where s(t) is the rate of still births which can be computed from hospital records. The estimated number of deaths under age 1 among the children born with HIV is given by

$$\mathbf{D(t) = r_2(t)P_2(t)B(t)} \tag{2.23}$$

Thus, the estimated number of HIV infected due to TM_4 is obtained as

$$\mathbf{n_2\ (t) = B_1(t) - (S(t) + D(t))} \tag{2.24}$$

Region-Wise Estimation

In geographically large countries like India, perinatal infection may be estimated for different regions. Since the HIV prevalence rate $r_1(t)$ among women is likely to vary over regions (e.g., rural/urban/ metropolitan), we may use the estimation formula (2.24) region-wise and then pool the results.

2.16.3 Follow-Up

The AIDS forecasting model, which mimics the standard demographic cohort component technique, may be used for a follow-up of perinatal infections. Each group of individuals born in a given year (birth cohort) is followed from birth to death, and all necessary events are recorded over the life cycle. The following lexis diagram plots life lines of successive cohorts by age and calendar time. To obtain estimates of key variables like the number of AIDS cases in a given year t, it is necessary to combine the numbers from all cohorts at that time. Since single year cohorts are used in the model, the total number of cohorts that have to be taken into account in a given year equals the maximum number of years lived by individuals.

We obtain the following results on using expression (2.22, 2.23 and 2.24).

B1(t) = 162	D(t) = 16
P2(t) = 0.018	n2(t) = 140 infections
S(t) = 6	

2.17 National/Global Policy Implications of Modelling

The AIDS endemic has raised a number of important health policy issues. Some of these have been raised by scientific advances and others by the societal implications of AIDS. But little progress has been made in understanding and dealing with such implications. The major policy issues arising from AIDS are research priorities and directions, testing for antibodies and education, confidentiality, discrimination, and healthcare for the infected. Modelling is the best approach to identify future policy considerations. A model could give better insight into the future number of "AIDS" patients. This number is the basis for planning the healthcare system which includes educating health professionals and requirement of medical facilities. Evaluation of potential costs is also an important issue. Modelling should also take care of data requirements to know the prevalence of infected people in different population groups by suggesting special studies. Mandatory testing for HIV positivity is a sensitive issue and incurs expenditure. Another potential issue is that the models may suggest directions for research. We must focus attention on persons with high-risk behavior. Yet another policy implication is the evaluation of potential intervention strategies and points of interventions in the disease process.

2.18 Summary

Statistical modelling of HIV infection is very useful for predicting HIV positive and AIDS classes and for forecasting healthcare needs. This chapter stresses the need for modelling of AIDS and discusses a new approach. HIV spread mechanism in four modes of transmission, viz, heterosexuality, drug abuse, blood transfusion, and **perinatal** mode (TM_1–TM_4), was examined in terms of their basic attributes. A separate model was formulated in each causes of transmission to know the number of new HIV and AIDS cases geometrically progressed in the course of its spread.

References

Abdallah SW, Estomih S, Massawel S, Oluwole DM (2012) Mathematical modelling of HIV/AIDS dynamics with treatment and vertical transmission. J Appl Math 2(3):77–89. https://doi.org/10.5923/j.am.20120203.06

Balcha TT, Lecerof SS, Jeppson AR (2011) Strategic challenges of PMTCT program implementation in Ethiopia. J Int Assoc Phys AIDS Care 10(Suppl 3):187–192

Bashiru KA, Fasoranbaku OA et al (2009) Statistical modelling of mother to child and heterosexual modes of transmission of HIV/AIDS epidemic the pacific. J Sci Technol 10(Suppl 2):186–192

Bashiru KA, Fasoranbaku AO, Olukayode A, Ojurongbe TA (2017) 1stability analysis of mother-to-child transmission of hiv/aids dynamic model with treatment Anale. Seria Informatică 15 (Suppl 2):89–96

Bhat K, Buwn C (2003) Barriers to the implementation of programs for the prevention of mother-to-child transmission of HIV: a cross-sectional survey in rural and urban Uganda. AIDS Res Ther 2:10

Chasela CS, Hudgens MG, Jamieson DJ, Kayira D, Hosseinipour MC, Kourtis AP et al (2010) Maternal or infant antiretroviral drugs to reduce HIV-1 transmission. N Engl J Med 362 (24):2271–2281

Coovadia H et al (2004) Antiretroviral agents – how best to protect infants from HIV and save their mothers from AIDS. N Engl J Med 351(Suppl 3):289–292

Creek T, Ntumy R, Mazhani L, Moore J, Smith M, Han G et al (2009) Factors associated with low early uptake of a national program to prevent mother to child transmission of HIV (PMTCT): results of a survey of mothers and providers, Botswana, 2003. AIDS Behav 13:356–364

Dabis S et al (2000) Prevention of mother-to-child transmission of HIV In developing countries: recommendations for practice. The Ghent international working group on mother-To-child transmission of HIV. Health Policy Plan 15(1):34–42

Dietz K et al (1993) The estimation of the basic reproduction number for infectious diseases. Stat Methods Med Res 2:23–41

Duff P, Walter K, Wild T, Rubaale T, Okech-Ojony J (2010a) Barriers to accessing highly active antiretroviral therapy by HIV-positive women attending an antenatal clinic in a regional hospital in western Uganda. J Int AIDS Soc 13(Suppl 37):1421–1436

Duff P, Kipp W, Wild TC, Rubaale T, Okech-Ojony J (2010b) Barriers to accessing highly active antiretroviral therapy by HIV-positive women attending an antenatal clinic in a regional hospital in western Uganda. J Int AIDS Soc 13(Suppl 37):1–9

Duff P, Walter K, Wild T, Rubaale T, Okech-Ojony J (2010c) Barriers to accessing highly active antiretroviral therapy by HIV-positive women attending an antenatal clinic in a regional hospital in western Uganda. J Int AIDS Soc 13(Suppl 37):138–140

El Khatib Z, Ekstrom AM, Coovadia A, Abrams EJ, Petzold M, Katzenstein D et al (2011) Adherence and virological suppression during the first 24 weeks on antiretroviral therapy among women in Johannesburg, South Africa-A prospective cohort study. BMC Public Health 11(Suppl 88):1–13

Fasoranbaku OA, Bashiru KA, Yusuf TT (2015) Stochastic analysis of mother to child transmission of HIV/AIDS epidemic in the presence of treatment. Eur J Stat Probab 3(Suppl 5):12–23

Gilbert L, Walker L et al (2010) My biggest fear was that people would reject me once they knew my status. Stigma as experienced by patients in an HIV/AIDS clinic in Johannesburg, South Africa. Health Soc Care Community 18(Suppl 2):139–146

Gourlay A, Birdthistle I, Mburu G, Iorpenda K, Wringe A (2013) Barriers and facilitating factors to the uptake of antiretroviral drugs for prevention of mother-to-child transmission of HIV in sub-Saharan Africa: a systematic review. J Int AIDS Soc 16(Suppl 1):1611–1613

Igwegbe AO, Ugboaja JO, Nwajiaku LA (2010) Prevelance and determinants of non-adherence to antiretroviral therapy among HIV-positive pregnant women in Nnewi, Nigeria. Int J Med Med Sci 2(8):238–245

Kasenga F, Byass P, Emmelin M, Hurtig AK et al (2009) The implications of policy changes on the uptake of a PMTCT programme in rural Malawi: First three years of experience. Glob Health Action 2:1–7

Kourtis P, Lee K et al (2006) Mother-to-child transmission of HIV-1: timing and implications for prevention. Lancet Infect Dis 6(11):726–732

Kunihira NR, Nuwaha F, Mayanja R, Peterson S (2010) Barriers to use of antiretroviral drugs in Rakai District of Uganda. Afr Health Sci 10(Suppl 2):120–129

Lettow M, Bedell R, Landes M, Gawa L et al (2011) Uptake and outcomes of a prevention-of mother-to-child transmission (PMTCT) program in Zomba District, Malawi. BMC Public Health 11(Suppl 426):1859–1867

Lewis A et al (2001) Determinants of VCT uptake among pregnant women attending two ANC clinics in Addis Ababa City: unmatched case control study. Ethiop Med J 45(4):335–342

Mepham S, Zondi Z, Mbuyazi A, Mkhwanazi N, Newell ML (2011) Challenges in PMTCT antiretroviral adherence in northern KwaZulu-Natal, South Africa. AIDS Care 23(Suppl 6):741–747

Morgan MC, Masaba RO, Nyikuri M, Thomas TK (2010) Factors affecting breastfeeding cessation after discontinuation of antiretroviral therapy to prevent mother-to-child transmission of HIV. AIDS Care 22:866–873

Moses AE, Chama C, Udo SM, Omotora BA (2009) Knowledge, attitude and practice of ante-natal attendees toward prevention of mother to child transmission (PMTCT) of HIV infection in a tertiary health facility, northeast Nigeria. Internet J Third World Med 8(Suppl 1):9–11

Naresh R, Tripathi A, Omar S (2006) Modelling the spread of AIDS epidemic with vertical transmission. Appl Math Comput 178:262–272

Naresh R, Sharma D et al (2011) An HIV/AIDS model with vertical transmission and time delay. World J Model Simul 7(Suppl 3):230–240

Nguyen TA, Oosterhoff P, Pham YN, Hardon A, Wright P (2009) Health workers' views on quality of prevention of mother-to-child transmission and postnatal care for HIV-infected women and their children. Hum Resour Health 7(Suppl 39):944–947

Oosterhoff P, Hardon AP, Nguyen TA, Pham NY, Wright P (2008) Dealing with a positive result: routine HIV testing of pregnant women in Vietnam. AIDS Care 20(Suppl 6):654–659

Orie EF, Songca PP, Moodley J (2009) An audit of PMTCT services at a regional hospital in South Africa. S Afr Fam Pract 51(Suppl 6):492–495

Pai NP, Klein MB et al (2009) Improving a mother to child HIV transmission programme through health system redesign: quality improvements, protocol adjustments, and resource addition. Womens Health 5(Suppl 1):55–62

Rahangdale L, Banandur P, Sreenivas A, Turan JM, Washington R, Cohen CR (2010) Stigma as experienced by women accessing prevention of parent-to-child transmission of HIV services in Karnataka, India. AIDS Care 22(Suppl 7):836–842

Rakoasi S (2005) HIV counselling and testing of pregnant women attending antenatal clinics in Botswana. J Health Popul Nutr 1:58–65

Rollins N, Little K, Mzolo S, Horwood C, Newell ML (2007) Surveillance of mother-to-child transmission prevention programmes at immunization clinics: the case for universal screening. AIDS 21(Suppl 10):1341–1347

Shapiro RL, Hughes MD, Ogwu A et al (2010) Antiretroviral regimens in pregnancy and breast-feeding in Botswana. N Engl J Med 362(24):2282–2294

Simbayi LC, Kalichman S, Strebel A, Cloete A, Henda N, Mqeketoa A (2007) Internalized stigma, discrimination, and depression among men and women living with HIV/AIDS in Cape Town South Africa. Soc Sci Med 64(Suppl 9):1823–1831

Sprague C, Chersich MF, Black V (2011) Health system weaknesses constrain access to PMTCT and maternal HIV services in South Africa: A qualitative enquiry. AIDS Res Ther 8(Suppl 10):1–9

Stangl AL, Lloyd JK, Brady LM, Holland CE, Baral S (2013) A systematic review of interventions to reduce HIV-related stigma and discrimination from 2002 to 2013. J Int AIDS Soc 16(Suppl 3):135–142

Turan JM, Miller S, Bukusi EA, Sande J, Cohen CR et al (2008) HIV/AIDS and maternity care in Kenya: how fears of stigma and discrimination affect uptake and provision of labor and delivery services. AIDS Care 20(Suppl 8):938–945

Turan JM, Bukusi EA, Onono M, Holzemer WL, Miller S, Cohen CR (2011) HIV/AIDS stigma and refusal of HIV testing among pregnant women in rural Kenya: results from the MAMAS study. AIDS Behav 15(Suppl 6):1111–1120

Ujiji OA, Ekström AM, Ilako F, Indalo D, Wamalwa D (2011) Reasoning and deciding PMTCT-adherence during pregnancy among women living with HIV in Kenya. Cult Health Sex 13 (Suppl 7):829–840

UNAIDS and WHO (2009) Joint United Nations Programme on HIV/AIDS: AIDS epidemic update. Join United Nations Programme on HIV/AIDS and WHO, Geneva

UNAIDS Reference Group on Estimates (2011) Working paper on mother-to-child HIV transmission rates for use in spectrum. UNAIDS, Washington, DC

WHO (2014) Global guidance on criteria and processes for validation: elimination of mother-to-child transmission (EMTCT) of HIV and syphilis. WHO, Geneva

HIV Vertical Transmission DTSM Simulation Models: Global and National Perspective

3

3.1 Introduction

An epidemiology is the study of the distribution and determinants of diseases of both infectious and noninfectious nature. Originally, the term was used to refer only epidemic infectious diseases, but it is now applied more broadly to other diseases as well (Israel-Ballard et al. 2005). Mathematical modelling was used extensively in research into the epidemiology of HIV/AIDS to improve our understanding of major contributing factors in a given epidemic (Kupriyashkina et al. 2010). The goal of any modelling exercise is to extract as much information as possible from available data and provide an accurate representation of both the knowledge and uncertainty about the epidemic (Korenromp et al. 2002). A number of various models of HIV and AIDS have been derived, ranging from simple extrapolations of past curves to complex transmission models (Longini et al. 1989). A major tradition modelling of HIV/AIDS epidemics was used only for back calculation or back projection techniques, etc.. These techniques were produced statistical solutions to different convolution derivatives that relate the number of AIDS diagnoses over time to past trends in HIV infection and to the distribution of the HIV incubation period (Li et al. 1996). In the reality of past literature of HIV transmission, many mathematical models have been developed to understand how HIV infection might spread among the human population, such as a mathematical model that discussed how HIV might spread among the community of injecting drug users and mother-to-child transmission (Luo et al. 2012). The literature cited with various fitted patrimonial mathematical models through ordinary differential and partial differential equations by Thompson-iteration method for estimation of different reproduction numbers and population equilibrium analysis about the existence and their global stability criterion and also Bendixson-Dulac criteria for the local stability check (Mhawej et al. 2010). The model results found that the HIV will spread among the injecting drug users and mother-to-child transmission if and only if the basic reproduction number is larger than one $R_0 < 1$, and the diseases will appear if and only if the basic reproduction number is smaller than one. A contrasting feature of HIV syndrome in relation to other infectious

D. M. Basavarajaiah, B. Narasimha Murthy, *HIV Transmission*,
https://doi.org/10.1007/978-981-15-0151-7_3

diseases is its incubation period which is a random variable and probably the longest one (Morris et al. 1997, 2006). An HIV infective exhibits disease symptoms after completion of this period and thereafter presents in AIDS case (Markowitz et al. 2003). The levels of CD4 T lymphocyte immune cells and HIV RNA in the human body determine the progression of the infection (Chen et al. 2016). HIV spread mechanism and its manifestation to AIDS are random phenomena, and hence mathematical modelling is expected to be a better descriptor of the present global scenario for implementation policy at global level (Naresh et al. 2006). Some of the literature explained about benefits and risk of HAART treatment of ANCs with comprehensive treatment supports and various randomized trail data study was conducted at national and global level for estimation of risks and benefits of HAART as compared with zidovudine and single-dose nevirapine to prevent transmission of the HIV from PLHIV (Newell et al. 1998) The primary outcomes were HIV transmission at first week of age in the infants and maternal and infant safety (Nosova et al. 2010). The mechanism of HAART resulted in significantly lower rates of early HIV transmission than without intervention of HAART (Nordic Medical research Council's HIV therapy group 1992; Putter et al. 2002; Palella et al. 1998; Phillips et al. 1980; Porco et al. 2004). In the present chapter, we have fitted mathematical models for estimation of transmission of HIV considering with varying population size subject to vertical transmission, demographics transition, clinical parameter, epidemiological factors, etc (Perelson et al. 1997).

3.2 Model Formulation of Disease Transmission and Susceptible Model (DTSM–Model)

Model Variables Description: *N* Total population, *S* Susceptible class, *I* Infective class, *P* Pre-AIDS class, *T* Treated class, *A* AIDS class

Symbols Used for Fitting Up of Mathematical Model

π	Rate of recruitment into susceptible population
c	Average number of sexual partners per unit time
β	Sexual contact rate
δ	Rate of movement from infectious class
ε	Fraction of newborns infected with HIV who die immediately after birth
θ	Rate of newborns infected with HIV
μ	Natural mortality rate
α	Inducted death rate due to AIDS
$\sigma 1$	Fraction of δ joining the pre-AIDS class
γ	Rate of movements of pre-AIDS class individuals into AIDS class
$\sigma 2$	Fraction of δ joining treated class
v	Rate at which AIDS group get treatment
m	Fraction of γ who get treatment
k	Rate at which treated group becomes full-blown AIDS

3.3 Description of the Model

3.3.1 Model Implications

Consider a population of size $N(t)$ at time "t" with constant inflow from the susceptible class with rate πN. The population size $N(t)$ was divided into five subclasses, which are either susceptible $S(t)$ or infective $I(t)$ (also assumed to be infectious), pre-AIDS patients or $P(t)$ treated class or $T(t)$ and AIDS patients or A (t) with natural mortality rate μ in all classes, disease-induced death rate α in the AIDS patients class, and v as the rate at which AIDS patients get treatment. In the model, it is assumed that the susceptible becomes HIV infected via sexual contacts with infectives which may also lead to the birth of infected children. It was assumed that a fraction of newborn children are infected during birth and hence are directly recruited into the infective class with a rate $(1 - \varepsilon)$ θ and others die effectively at birth $(0 \leq \varepsilon \leq 1)$. It was assumed that some of the infectives join pre-AIDS class, depending on the viral counts with a rate $\sigma 1\delta$,and then proceed with a rate γ to develop full-blown AIDS. It was also assumed that some of the infectives move to join treated class with a rate $\sigma 2\delta$ and then proceed with a rate k to develop full-blown AIDS, while others with serious infection directly join the AIDS class with a rate $(1 - \sigma 1 - \sigma 2)$ δ. The interaction between susceptible and infectives was assumed to be of standard mass action type.

There are various modes of transmission of the HIV/AIDS epidemic, but two of the major modes of transmission are mother-to-child transmission and heterosexual transmission of HIV (Prud'homme et al. 1998). As the epidemics move from the group's first affected to women of reproductive age, an increasing number of infants are becoming infected with HIV through MTCT. Infants of HIV infected mothers are at great risk of becoming infected with HIV during childbirth. During 2011–2016, between 10% and 20% have become infected through biological phenomena even though many preventive steps have been taken from NACO. In this present chapter, a mathematical model of MTCT will analyze the effectiveness of disease endemic equilibrium (DEE) and diseases epidemic equilibrium (DEE) were discussed briefly (Pankavich et al. 2016) (Fig. 3.1).

The above figure that showed the disease transmission was governed by the ordinary differential equations.

$$\frac{\mathrm{ds}}{\mathrm{dt}} = \pi N - \frac{\mathrm{C}1\beta 1\mathrm{IS}}{N} - \frac{\mathrm{C}2\beta 2\mathrm{PS}}{N} - \frac{\mathrm{C}3\beta 3\mathrm{TS}}{N} - \frac{\mathrm{C}4\beta 4\mathrm{AS}}{N} - \mu\frac{\mathrm{dI}}{\mathrm{dt}}$$

$$\frac{\mathrm{dI}}{\mathrm{dt}} = \frac{\mathrm{C}1\beta 1\mathrm{IS}}{N} + \frac{\mathrm{C}2\beta 2\mathrm{PS}}{N} + \frac{\mathrm{C}3\beta 3\mathrm{TS}}{N} + \frac{\mathrm{C}4\beta 4\mathrm{AS}}{N} - (\delta + \mu)I + (I - \epsilon)\theta(I + P + A)$$

$$\frac{\mathrm{dP}}{\mathrm{dT}} = \sigma 2\delta I - (\gamma + \mu)p \tag{4.11}$$

$$\frac{\mathrm{DT}}{\mathrm{dt}} = \sigma 2\delta I + \mathrm{mrp} + \mathrm{vA} - (k + \mu)T,$$

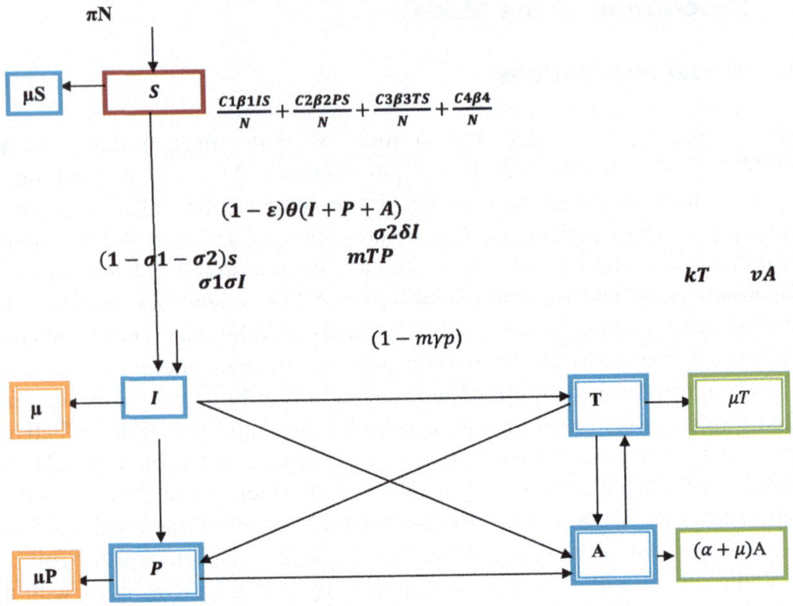

Fig. 3.1 Flow diagram of HIV mathematical model

$$\frac{\mathrm{dA}}{\mathrm{dt}} = (1 - \sigma 1 - \sigma 2)\delta I + (1 - m)\gamma p + \mathrm{kT} - (v + \alpha + \mu)A$$

The initial condition of the HIV disease was

$$\mathrm{S}(0) = \mathrm{S}_0, \mathrm{I}(0) = \mathrm{I}_0, \mathrm{P}(0) = \mathrm{P}_0, \mathrm{T}(0) = \mathrm{T}_0 \text{ and } \mathrm{A}(0) = \mathrm{A}_0$$

To simplify the above model setting, it is reasonable to assume that the AIDS women patients and those in pre-AIDS classes were isolated and sexually inactive, and hence they are not capable of producing children, i.e., $(1 - \varepsilon)\,\theta p = (1 - \delta)\,\theta A = 0$, and also they do not contribute to RNA plasma viral transmission horizontally, i.e., β_2 and $\beta_2$are taken negligible; this was reported by Naresh et al. (2006).

In view of the above assumptions, the system can now be written as follows:

$$\frac{\mathrm{ds}}{\mathrm{dt}} = \pi N - \frac{\mathrm{C1}\beta 1\mathrm{IS}}{N} - \frac{\mathrm{C3}\beta 3\mathrm{TS}}{N} - \mu k$$

$$\frac{\mathrm{dI}}{\mathrm{dt}} = \frac{\mathrm{C1}\beta 1\mathrm{IS}}{N} + \frac{\mathrm{C3}\beta 3\mathrm{TS}}{N} - (\delta + \mu)I + (1 - \varepsilon)\theta I$$

$$\frac{\mathrm{dP}}{\mathrm{dt}} = \sigma 1\delta I - (\gamma + \mu)P \tag{3.2}$$

$$\frac{dT}{dt} = \sigma 2\delta I + m\gamma p + vA - (k+\mu)T$$

$$\frac{dA}{dt} = (1-\sigma 1-\sigma 2)\delta I + (1-m)\gamma p + kT - (v+\alpha+\mu)A$$

From the Eq. 3.2, it was pointed out here that not all infected individuals take part in spreading the disease, as in the case of infected children, but they will all develop their own AIDS. However, the model can be modified to include a delay to make the infected children become adults to further spread the infection either vertically or horizontally.

The total population "N" was calculated by

$$N = S + I + P + T + A \quad \text{differentiate with respect to "t"}$$

$$\frac{dN}{dt} = \frac{dS}{dt} + \frac{dI}{dt} + \frac{dP}{dt} + \frac{dT}{dt} + \frac{dA}{dt}$$

$$\frac{dN}{dt} = \pi N - \frac{C1\beta 1IS}{N} - \frac{C3\beta 3TS}{N} - \mu S + \frac{C1\beta 1IS}{N} + \frac{C3\beta 3TS}{N} - (\delta+\mu)I + (1-\varepsilon)\theta I$$
$$+ \sigma 1\delta I - (\gamma+\mu)P + \sigma 2\delta I + m\gamma P + vA - (k+\mu)P + \sigma 2\delta I(1-m)\gamma P + kT$$
$$- (v+\alpha+\mu)A$$

Therefore

$$\frac{dN}{dt} = \pi N - \mu N - \alpha A + (1-\varepsilon)\theta I$$

Thus, we normalize the model. Without loss of generality, let $S = \frac{S}{N}, i = \frac{I}{N.}$

$$P = \frac{P}{N}, h = \frac{T}{N}, a = \frac{A}{N}$$

Therefore, the normalized system can be calculated as follows:

$$S = sN$$

$$\frac{dS}{dt} = S\frac{dN}{dt} + N\frac{dS}{dt}$$

$$\frac{dS}{dt} = \frac{1}{N}\left(\frac{dS}{dt} - S\frac{dN}{dt}\right)$$

Therefore

$$\frac{ds}{dt} = \pi - C_1\beta_1 is - C3\beta 3hs - (\pi - \alpha a + (1-\varepsilon)\theta i)\, S$$

$$i = iN$$

$$\frac{\mathrm{dI}}{\mathrm{dt}} = i\frac{\mathrm{dN}}{\mathrm{dt}} + N\frac{\mathrm{di}}{\mathrm{dt}}$$

$$\frac{\mathrm{di}}{\mathrm{dt}} = \frac{1}{N}\left[\frac{\mathrm{dI}}{\mathrm{dt}} - i\frac{\mathrm{dN}}{\mathrm{dt}}\right]$$

$$\therefore \frac{di}{dt} = C_1\beta_1\mathrm{is} + c3\beta3\mathrm{hs} + (1-\varepsilon)\theta i - (\pi + \delta - \alpha a + (1-\varepsilon)\theta i)i$$

$$P = \mathrm{PN}$$

$$\frac{\mathrm{dP}}{\mathrm{dt}} = P\frac{\mathrm{dN}}{\mathrm{dt}} + N\frac{\mathrm{dP}}{\mathrm{dt}}$$

$$\frac{\mathrm{dP}}{\mathrm{dt}} = \frac{1}{N}\left[\frac{\mathrm{dP}}{\mathrm{dt}} - P\frac{\mathrm{dN}}{\mathrm{dt}}\right]$$

$$\frac{\mathrm{dP}}{\mathrm{dt}} = \sigma_1\delta i - [\pi + \gamma - \alpha a + (1-\varepsilon)\theta i]P$$

$$H = \mathrm{Hn}$$

$$\frac{\mathrm{dT}}{\mathrm{dt}} = h\frac{\mathrm{dN}}{\mathrm{dt}} + N\frac{\mathrm{dH}}{\mathrm{dt}}$$

$$\frac{\mathrm{dh}}{\mathrm{dt}} = \frac{1}{\mathrm{dN}}\left[\frac{\mathrm{dT}}{\mathrm{dt}} - h\frac{\mathrm{dN}}{\mathrm{dt}}\right]$$

$$\frac{\mathrm{dh}}{\mathrm{dt}} = \sigma 2\delta i + \mathrm{m}\gamma\mathrm{p} + \mathrm{va} - (\pi + k - \alpha a + (1-\varepsilon)\theta i)h$$

$$A = \mathrm{aN}$$

$$\frac{\mathrm{dA}}{\mathrm{dt}} = a\frac{\mathrm{dN}}{\mathrm{dt}} + N\frac{\mathrm{da}}{\mathrm{dt}}$$

$$\frac{\mathrm{da}}{\mathrm{dt}} = \frac{1}{N}\left[\frac{\mathrm{dA}}{\mathrm{dt}} - a\frac{\mathrm{dN}}{\mathrm{dt}}\right]$$

$$\frac{\mathrm{da}}{\mathrm{dt}} = (1 - \sigma 1 - \sigma 2)\delta I + (1-m)\gamma p + kh - [\pi + v + \alpha - \alpha a + (1-\varepsilon)\theta i]a$$

Now the system of equation is as follows:

$$\frac{\mathrm{di}}{\mathrm{dt}} = C_1\beta_1 is + C_3\beta_3 hs + (1-\varepsilon)\theta i - [\pi + \delta - \alpha a + (1-\varepsilon)\theta i]i$$

$$\frac{\text{dp}}{\text{dt}} = \sigma 1\delta i - [\pi + \gamma - \alpha a + (1 - \varepsilon)\theta i]p \tag{3.3}$$

$$\frac{\text{dh}}{\text{dt}} = \sigma 2\delta i + \text{m}\gamma\text{p} + va - (\pi + k - \alpha a + (1 - \varepsilon)\theta i)h$$

$$\frac{\text{da}}{\text{dt}} = (1 - \sigma 1 - \sigma 2)\delta i + (1 - m)\gamma p + \text{kh} - [\pi + \gamma + \alpha - \alpha a + (1 - \varepsilon)\theta i]a,$$

Such that

$$s + i + p + h + a + = 1$$

3.4 Positivity of Solutions

For the model (3.3) to be epidemiologically meaningful and well posed, we need to prove that all state variables are non-negative $\forall \geq 0$.

Theorem (3.0) Let $\Omega = \{(s, i, p, h, a)\} \in \mathbb{R}+ \ : s + i + p + h + a = 1\}$, then the solution $\{s(t), i(t), p(t), h(t), a(t)\}$ of the system 3.1.3 are the $\forall \geq 0$.

P.V.T the theorem, we have to use the differential equation of the system 3.3; using the first equation, we have

$$\frac{\text{ds}}{\text{dt}} \leq \pi - \pi s$$

$$\frac{\text{ds}}{\text{dt}} + \pi s \leq \pi$$

We have derived the integrating factor $IF = e^{\pi} \int dt = e^{\pi t}$.

$$\frac{d}{\text{dt}} = (s\ e^{\pi t}) \leq \pi e^{\pi t}$$

Integrating on both the sides

$$S(t) \leq 1 + \text{Ce}^{-\pi t}$$

Applying initial condition, when $t = 0$, $s(t)\ s(0)$, $s(0) \leq 1 + C$.

$$s(t) \leq 1 + (s(o) - 1)e^{-\pi t}$$

When $t \to \infty$, $s(t) \leq 1$

Therefore

$$0 \leq s(t) \leq 1$$

Similarly, by using the second system of Eq. 3.30, we get

$$\frac{\mathrm{di}}{\mathrm{dt}} \geq -(\delta + \pi)$$

$$\mathrm{IF} = e \int (\delta + \pi)\mathrm{dt} = e^{(-\delta+\pi)t}$$

$$\frac{d}{\mathrm{dt}}\left(\mathrm{ie}^{\delta+\pi t}\right) \geq 0$$

Integrating both sides $t = 0$, $i(t) = i(o)$, $i(0) \geq 0$

$$i(t) \geq i(0)e^{(\delta+\pi)t}$$

$$t \to \infty, i(t) \geq 0$$

Therefore

$$i(t) \geq 0$$

Also in the third system of Eq. (3.3)

$$\frac{\mathrm{dp}}{p} \geq -(\pi + \gamma p)\mathrm{dt}$$

Integrating both sides, we get

$$p(t) \geq p(0)e^{-(\pi+\gamma)t}$$

Applying initial conditions at $t = 0$, $p(t) \geq p(0)$.
When $t \to \infty$, $p(t) \geq 0$.
Similarly, by using the equation of the system (4.3), we have

$$\frac{\mathrm{dh}}{\mathrm{dt}} \geq -(\pi + k)h$$

$$\frac{\mathrm{dh}}{h} \geq -(\pi + k)\mathrm{dt}$$

Integrating both sides we get

$$h(t) \geq h(o)e^{-(\pi+k)t}$$

Applying initial conditions at $t = 0$, $h(t) \geq h(0)$
When, $t \to \infty$, $h(t) \geq 0$

Finally, by using the equation of the system (3.3), we have

$$\frac{\mathrm{da}}{\mathrm{dt}} \geq (\pi + v + \alpha)a$$

$$\frac{\mathrm{da}}{a} \geq -(\pi + v + \alpha)dt$$

Integrating both sides, we get

$$a(t) \geq a(0)e^{-(\pi+\gamma+\alpha)t}$$

Applying initial condition: at $t = 0$, $a(t) \geq a(0)$
When $t \rightarrow \infty$, $a(t) \geq 0$

3.5 Stability Analysis of the Model

In this section, the result of stability analysis of the equilibrium points is presented in the discussion part. A mathematical model was fitted for induction of the HAART, for prevention of HIV progression is derived using HIV data sets and includes HIV vertical transmission. Local analysis of the unique equilibrium of this nonlinear model provides conditions for stability. Techniques are developed to determine Hopf bifurcations, and stability switching is found for the delayed HAART treatment near a double bifurcation point which was estimated. Global analysis provides conditions on the model for asymptotic stability. The biological and clinical significance of our results was discussed in the result part.

3.6 Equilibrium Points of the Model

The model 3.3 has two non-negative equilibrium points which are the disease-free equilibrium pointE_0 and endemic equilibrium E^*.

At equilibrium points

$$\frac{\mathrm{ds}}{\mathrm{dt}} = \frac{\mathrm{di}}{\mathrm{dt}} = \frac{\mathrm{dp}}{\mathrm{dt}} = \frac{\mathrm{dh}}{\mathrm{dt}} = \frac{\mathrm{da}}{\mathrm{dt}} = 0.$$

Hence, the following system of equation is solved for equilibrium points:

$$0 = \pi - C_1\beta_1 \mathrm{is} - C_3\beta_3 \mathrm{hs} - (\pi - \alpha a + (1 - \varepsilon)\theta i)s$$

$$0 = C_1\beta_1 \mathrm{is} + C_3\beta_3 \mathrm{hs} + (1 - \varepsilon)\theta i - [\pi + \delta - \alpha a + (1 - \varepsilon)\theta i]i$$

$$0 = \sigma 1\delta i - [\pi + \gamma - \alpha a + (1 - \varepsilon)\theta i]p$$

$$0 = \sigma_2\delta i + \mathrm{m}\gamma\mathrm{p} + \mathrm{va} - (\pi + k - \alpha a + (1-\varepsilon)\theta i)h$$

$$o = (1 - \sigma_1 - \sigma_2)\delta i + (1-m)\gamma p + \mathrm{kh} - [\pi + v + \alpha - \alpha a + (1-\varepsilon)\theta i]a$$

For the disease-free equilibrium $i = p = h = a = 0$, when substituted above, the system of the equation reduced to $\pi - s\pi = 0$, hence $s = 1$.

Therefore, the disease-free equilibrium E_0 is $(1, 0, 0, 0, 0)$;the linear stability of E_0 can be established by its basic reproduction number. It is determined by using next-generation method on the Eq. 3.3 in the form of matrices F and V. Let F_i be the rate of appearance of new infection in compartment be the transfer of individuals out of compartment by another means X_0be the disease-free equilibrium state

$$R_0 \text{ is the largest eigenvalue of } \left[\frac{\partial \mathrm{Fi}(x0)}{\partial(\mathrm{xi})}\right]\left[\frac{\partial \mathrm{Vi}(x0)}{\partial(\mathrm{xj})}\right] - 1 \quad (3.9)$$

3.7 Computation of the Basic Reproduction Number (R_0)

The basic reproduction number R_0 is defined as the effective number of secondary infections caused by a typical infected individual during his interred periods of infectiousness. It was obtained by taking the largest (dominant) eigenvalue (spectral radius) of

$$F = \begin{bmatrix} \pi + \sigma - (1-\varepsilon)\theta\, 0\, 0\, 0 \\ -\sigma\delta 0.\pi + \gamma\, 0\, 0 \\ 0 - -m\gamma\ \pi + k - v \\ -(1 - \sigma 1 - \sigma 2\delta\ (1-m)\gamma - k\ \pi + v + \alpha \end{bmatrix}$$

$$R_0 = \mathrm{FXV}^{-1}$$

$$R_0 = \frac{c1\beta1}{\pi + \delta - \theta + \theta\varepsilon} + \frac{C_3\beta_3(\sigma_2\pi^2 + \sigma_2\pi\alpha + \sigma_2\gamma\pi + \sigma_2\gamma\alpha + \sigma_1 m\gamma\pi + \sigma_1 m\gamma\alpha + v\pi + v\gamma + \sigma_1 v\pi)\gamma}{(\pi + \delta - \theta + \theta\varepsilon)(\pi + \gamma)(\alpha\pi + \pi k + \pi^2 + \alpha k + \gamma\pi)} \quad (3.10)$$

Thus if $R_0 > 1$,the infection triggers an epidemic; otherwise its prevalence is zero, i.e., for $R_0 < 1$. From the solution, it was found that with an increase in R_0, which can be viewed as a function of c, the number of sexual partners, the number of infectives increases which in turn increases the AIDS patient population. Thus in order to keep the spread of the disease at minimum, the number of sexual partners should be restricted accordingly.

3.8 The Endemic Equilibrium and Local Stability

The endemic equilibrium point of the model (4.3) is given by $E^* = (s, i^*, p^*, h^*, a)$; to obtain an endemic equilibrium $E^*$of this model, we set to zero each equation in the model. Then by solving the system of equations in (4.3), we express each equilibrium point in terms of $i^*$and a^*at steady state, and we get

$$\pi - C_1\beta_1\text{is} - C_3\beta_3\text{hs} - [\pi - \alpha a + \sigma_1 - \varepsilon)\theta i]s \tag{a.1}$$

$$C_1\beta_1\text{is} + C_3\beta_3\text{hs} + (1-\varepsilon)\theta i - [\pi + \delta - \alpha a + (1-\varepsilon)\theta i]i \tag{a.2}$$

$$\sigma_1\delta i - [\pi + \gamma - \alpha a + (1-\varepsilon)\theta i]p \tag{a.3}$$

$$\sigma 2\delta i + \text{m}\gamma\text{p} + \text{va} - [\pi + \text{k} - \alpha a + (1-\varepsilon)\theta i]h \tag{a.4}$$

$$(1 - \sigma_1 - \sigma_2)\delta i + (1-m)\gamma p + \text{kh} - [\pi + \text{v} + \alpha - \alpha a + (1-\varepsilon)\theta i]a \tag{a.5}$$

Adding Equation (a.1) and (a.2), we get the value of s^*

$$S^* = \frac{\pi + (1-\varepsilon)\theta^* - (\pi + \delta - \alpha a^* + (1-\varepsilon)\theta^*)i^*}{\pi - \alpha a^* + (1-\varepsilon)\theta i^*}$$

Using the Equations (a.3) and (a.4) to get the value p^*

$$p^* = \frac{\sigma_1\delta i^*}{\pi + \gamma - \alpha a^* + (1-\varepsilon)\theta i^*}$$

Soling Equation (a.4) and (a.5) to get the value of $h^* and\ a^*$, we get

$$h^* = \frac{k}{\varnothing\omega}$$

$$a^* = (1 - \sigma_1 - \sigma_2)\delta i^*\varnothing\psi + (1-m)\sigma_1\gamma\delta i\psi + k\frac{(\sigma 2\delta i\varnothing + m\gamma\sigma_1\delta i^*)}{\varnothing(\omega\psi - kv)}$$

where:

$\phi = (\pi + \gamma - \alpha a^* + (1-\varepsilon)\theta i^*)$
$\psi = (\pi + k - \alpha a^* + (1-\varepsilon)\theta i^*)$
$\omega = (\pi + v + \alpha - \alpha a^* + (1-\varepsilon)\theta i^*$ and
$k = \sigma 2\delta i^*\varnothing + m\gamma\sigma 1\delta i^* + V(1 - \sigma 1 - \sigma 2)\delta i^*\varnothing\psi + (1-m)\sigma 1\gamma\delta i^*\psi + k\frac{(\sigma 2\delta i\varnothing + m\gamma\sigma_1\delta i^*)}{\varnothing(\omega\psi - kv)}$

The value i^* is in the form of polynomial

$$i^*(A_5 i^* + A_4 i^* + A_2 i^* + A_1 i^* + A_0) = 0 \tag{3.3}$$

After some algebraic calculation, the expression can be reduced as

$$Ai^{*2} + Bi^{*} = 0 \tag{3.4}$$

where:

$A = -(\pi + k - \alpha a^{*})(\pi + \delta - \alpha a^{*})\Gamma$

$\Gamma = C_1\beta_1\pi^3 - C_1\beta_1(\alpha a^{*})2 - 2C_1\beta_1\pi v\alpha a^{*} - 2C_1\beta_1\pi\alpha^2 a^{*} + C_1\beta_1\pi k\alpha - C_1\beta_1 k\alpha a^{*} - C_1\beta_1\gamma v\alpha a^{*} + C_1\beta_1\gamma k\alpha - C_1\beta_1\gamma\alpha^2 a^{*} + C_1\beta_1\pi\gamma k - 2C_1\beta_1\pi\gamma\alpha a^{*} + C_3\beta_3\delta\pi\sigma_2\gamma + C_3\beta_3\delta\pi m\gamma\sigma 1 - C_3\beta_3\delta\gamma\alpha a^{*} + C_3\beta_3\delta\gamma\sigma_1\sigma_2\sigma + C_3\beta_3\delta m\gamma\sigma_1\alpha + C_3\beta_3\delta\gamma v - C_3\beta_3\delta\gamma\sigma_2\alpha a^{*} + C_3\beta_3\delta\sigma_2\pi^2 - C_1\beta_1 k\alpha^2 a^{*} - 2C_1\beta_1\pi k\alpha a^{*} + C_3\beta_3\delta\sigma_2\pi\alpha + C_3\beta_3\delta v\pi - C_3\beta_3\delta\sigma_1 v\pi - 2C_3\beta_3\delta\sigma_2\pi\alpha a^{*} + C_3\beta_3\delta v\alpha a^{*} - C_3\beta_3\delta v\alpha a^{*} + C_3\beta_3\delta\sigma_2\pi(\alpha a^{*})2 + C_1\beta_1\pi\gamma v + C_1\beta_1\pi\gamma\alpha - 3C_1\beta_1\pi^2\alpha a^{*} + C_1\beta_1\pi^2 k + C_1\beta_1 k(\alpha a^{*})2 + 3C_1\beta_1 k(\alpha a^{*})2 + 3C_1\beta_1\pi(\alpha a^{*})2 + C_1\beta_1\pi^2 v - C_3\beta_3\delta\sigma 2\alpha^2 a^{*}$

$B = (\pi + k - \alpha a^{*})\Lambda$

$\Lambda = -\pi^4 k + 4\pi^3\alpha a^{*} - \pi^3\alpha k - \pi^3\delta v + 4\pi^3\alpha^2 a^{*} - \pi^3\delta\alpha + 3\pi^2\delta\alpha^2 a^{*} - \pi^2\gamma v - \pi^2\delta k\alpha + 3\pi^2 k\alpha^2 a^{*} - \sigma\pi^2 v(\alpha a^{*})^2 - \sigma\pi^2\alpha(\alpha a^{*})^2 + 4\pi v(\alpha a^{*})^4 + 4\pi v(\alpha a^{*})^3 - \pi^4 v - \pi^4\alpha - \pi^4\gamma - \gamma(\alpha a^{*})^4 + k\gamma(\alpha a^{*})^4 - \alpha(\alpha a^{*})^4 + 4\pi\alpha(\alpha a^{*})^3 - \pi^4 v - \pi^4 v - \pi^4\alpha - \pi^4\gamma - \gamma(\alpha a^{*})^3 - k\gamma(\alpha a^{*})^3 - \pi^3 k\gamma + \delta k\gamma\alpha^2 a^{*} + 4\pi^3\gamma\alpha a^{*} + 2\pi\delta\gamma\alpha^2 a^{*} + \delta v(\alpha a^{*})^3 + \gamma v(\alpha a^{*})^3 + c_1\beta_1\pi^4 + 3\pi^2\gamma k\alpha a^{*} - \pi^5 + 2\pi\gamma\alpha k\alpha a^{*} + 2\pi\delta v\alpha a^{*} - \pi\gamma\alpha\delta k + 4\pi\gamma(\alpha a^{*})^3 - \alpha\delta k(\alpha a^{*})^2 - \gamma(\alpha a^{*})^4 - 3k\gamma\pi(\alpha a^{*})^2 - \pi^2\gamma\delta k + 3\pi^2\gamma\delta\alpha a^{*} - 3\pi\gamma\delta(\alpha a^{*})^2 + c_1\beta_1\pi^3\alpha + c_1\beta_1\pi^3 v + c_1\beta_1\pi^3\gamma - 3c_1\beta_1\pi^3\alpha a^{*} + 3c_1\beta_1\pi^2(\alpha a^{*})^2 + c_1\beta_1\pi^3 k - c_1\beta_1\pi(\alpha a^{*})^2 + \gamma\alpha(\alpha a^{*})^3 + 2\pi\delta k\alpha^2 a^{*} - 3\pi k\alpha(\alpha a^{*})^2 - 3\pi\delta\alpha(\alpha a^{*})^2 - 3\pi\delta v(\alpha a^{*})^2 + 3\pi^2\gamma\alpha^2 a^{*} + 3\pi^2\gamma v\alpha a^{*} - \pi^2 k\gamma\alpha - \pi^2\gamma\delta\alpha - \pi^2\gamma\delta v - 3\pi\alpha^2 a^{*} - 3\pi\gamma v - 3\pi\gamma v(\alpha a^{*})^2 - k\gamma\alpha(\alpha a^{*})^2 - \delta\gamma v(\alpha a^{*})^2 - \delta\gamma\alpha(\alpha a^{*})^2 + C_3\beta_3\delta\sigma_2\pi^3 - \sigma\pi^2\gamma(\alpha a^{*})^2 - \delta\gamma v(\alpha a^{*})^2 - \delta\gamma\alpha(\alpha a^{*})^2 + C_3\beta_3\delta m\gamma\alpha\sigma_1\pi + C_3\beta_3\delta\gamma v\pi + C_1\beta_1\pi\gamma v\alpha a^{*} - C_3\beta_3\delta v\pi\alpha a^{*} - C_3\beta_3\delta\sigma_2\pi\alpha^2 a^{*} + C_3\beta_3\delta\sigma_1 v\alpha a^{*} + C_1\beta_1\pi v(\alpha a^{*})^2 + C_1\beta_1\pi v(\alpha a^{*})^2 + C_1\beta_1\pi\alpha(\alpha a^{*})^2 - C_1\beta_1\pi\alpha^2 a^{*} + C_1\beta_1\pi^2 kv - C_3\beta_3\delta m$

3.9 Model Forward Bifurcation

The local asymptotic stability of endemic equilibrium was analyzed by using the theorem of center manifold. The linearization matrix has at least one eigenvalue with zero real part. Also, we shall describe the possibility of forward bifurcation (FB) from the non-hyperbolic equilibrium. To describe it, consider a general system of ODEs with F. This theory is convenient by changing variables. Consider $s = x_1$, $i = x_2 p = x_2$, $h = x_4$, $\alpha = x_5$. By using vector notation $X = (x_1, x_2, x_3, x_4, x_5)^T$ in the model (4.3) can be written in the form.

$\frac{dX}{dt} = F(x)$, where by $F = (x_1, x_2, x_3, x_4, x_5)^T$ as follows:

$$\frac{dx_1}{dt} = f_1 = \pi - c_1\beta_1 x_2 x_1 - c_3\beta_3 x_4 x_1 - [\pi - \alpha x_5 + (1-\varepsilon)\theta x_2]x_1$$
$$\frac{dx_2}{dt} = f_2 = \pi - c_1\beta_1 x_2 x_1 + c_3\beta_3 x_4 x_1 + x_1(1-\varepsilon)\theta x_2 - [\pi + \delta - \alpha x_5 + (1-\varepsilon)\theta x_2]x_2$$
$$\frac{dx_3}{dt} = f_3 = \sigma_1\delta\sigma_2[\pi + \delta - \alpha x_5 + (1-\varepsilon)\theta x_2]x_3 \text{ from (4.5)}$$
$$\frac{dx_4}{dt} = f_4 = \sigma_1\delta\sigma_2 + m\gamma x_3 + v x_5[\pi + k - \alpha x_5 + (1-\varepsilon)\theta x_2]x_4$$
$$\frac{dx_5}{dt} = f_5 = (1 - \sigma_1 - \sigma_2)\delta x_2 + (1-m)\gamma x_3 + k x_4 - [\pi + v + \alpha - \alpha x_5 + (1-\varepsilon)\theta x_2]x_5$$

where

$$R_0 = \frac{c_1\beta_1}{\pi+\delta-\theta+\theta\varepsilon} + \frac{c_3\beta_3(\sigma_2\pi^2+\sigma_2\pi\alpha+\pi_2\gamma\alpha+\sigma_1 m\gamma\pi+\sigma_1 m\gamma\alpha+v\pi+v\gamma+\sigma_1 v\pi)\delta}{(\pi+\delta-\theta+\theta\varepsilon)(\pi+\gamma)(\alpha\pi+\pi k+\pi^2+\alpha k+v\pi)}$$

Suppose $\beta_1 = \beta^*$ is the chosen bifurcation parameter and if we consider $R_0 = 1$ and solve for $\beta_1 = \beta^*$ it gives

$$\beta^* = \frac{(\pi+\delta-\theta+\sigma\theta)(\pi+\gamma)(\alpha\pi+\pi k+\pi^2+\alpha k+v\pi - c_3\beta_3\delta\varnothing}{c_1(\pi+\gamma)(\alpha\pi+\pi k+\pi^2+\alpha k+v\pi)} \tag{3.7}$$

where

$$\varnothing = (\sigma_2\pi^2+\sigma_2\pi\alpha+\sigma_2\gamma\pi+\sigma_1\gamma\alpha+\sigma_1 m\gamma\pi+\sigma_1 m\gamma\alpha+v\pi+v\gamma-\sigma_1 v\pi$$

The system of the transformed equation with $\beta_1 = \beta^*$ has a simple zero eigenvalue. Hence, the center manifold theory can be used to analyze the dynamic of $\frac{\mathrm{dX}}{\mathrm{dt}} = F(x) = f(f_1, f_2, f_3, f_4, f_5)T$ near $\beta_1 = \beta^*$; it can be shown that the Jacobians of $\frac{\mathrm{dX}}{\mathrm{dt}} = F(x) = F = (f_1, f_2, f_3, f_4, f_5)T$ at $\beta_1 = \beta^*$ has a right eigenvector associated with the zero eigenvalues by $w = [w_1, w_2, w_3, w_4, w_5]T$.

$$w_1 = \frac{(c_3\beta_3\mathrm{vn}(-c_1\beta_1+(1-\varepsilon)\theta+\Psi)+\alpha(\eta\varphi\Psi)-c_3\beta_3 m\upsilon\sigma_1\delta-c_3\beta_3\eta\sigma_2\delta}{c_3\beta_3 v\eta}w_2$$

$$w_3 = \frac{\sigma_1\delta}{\eta}w_2$$

$$w_4 = \frac{-(c_1\beta_1+(1-\varepsilon)\theta-\pi-\delta)}{c_3\beta_3}w_2$$

$$w_5 = \frac{-[\eta\varphi(c_1\beta_1+(1-\varepsilon)\theta-\pi-\delta]+c_3\beta_3 m\gamma\sigma_1\delta+c_3\beta_3 n\sigma_2\delta}{c_3\beta_3 v\eta}w_2$$

$$w_2 > 0$$

where

$\eta = (\pi + \gamma)$
$\varphi = (\pi + k)$
$\varpi = (\pi + v + \alpha)$
$\Psi = (c_1\beta_1 + (1 - \varepsilon)\theta - (\pi + \delta))$

The right eigenvector of $J(E_0)$ associated with the zero eigenvalues at $\beta_1 = \beta^*$ is given by

$$u = (u_1, u_2, u_3, u_4, u_5)T \text{ when } u_1 = 0$$

$$u_2 = \frac{-[\sigma_1\delta(m\gamma\varpi + (1-m)\gamma\nu) + \sigma_2\delta\varpi\eta + (1-\sigma_1-\sigma_2)\delta\eta]}{\varpi\eta\Psi}u_4$$

$$u_3 = \frac{[m\gamma\varpi + (1-m)\gamma\nu]}{\varpi\eta}u_4$$

$$u_5 = \frac{\nu}{\varpi}u_4$$

$$u_4 > u_5$$

Theorem 3 From Castillo-Chavez and Song, we considered the following general system of ordinary differential equations with a parameter such that

$$\frac{\mathrm{d}x}{\mathrm{d}t} = f(x, \varnothing), f : \mathbb{R}^n X\mathbb{R} \to \mathbb{R}^n \text{ And } f \in C^2(\mathbb{R}^n X\mathbb{R})$$

where "O" is an equilibrium point of the system that is $f(0, \varnothing) = 0$ for all and:

1. $A = D_x f(0, \varnothing) = \left(\frac{\partial f_i}{\partial x_j}(0,0)\right)$ is the linearization matrix of the system around the equilibrium 0 with evaluated at 0.
2. Zero is a simple eigenvalue of A and all other eigenvalues of A have negative real parts.
3. Matrix A has a right eigenvector ω and left eigenvector q corresponding to zero eigenvalues.
   Let f_k be the kth component of f and

$$a = \sum_{k,i,j=1}^{n} u_k\omega_i\omega_j \frac{\partial^2 f_k}{\partial_{x_i}\partial_{x_j}}(0,0) \to \tag{3.18}$$

$$b = \sum_{k,i,j=1}^{n} u_k\omega_j \frac{\partial^2 f_k}{\partial_{x_j}\partial_{\beta}}(0,0) \to \tag{3.19}$$

The local dynamics of the system around the equilibrium point is totally determined by the signs of a and b particularly; if $a > 0$ and $b > 0$, then a backward bifurcation occurs at $\varnothing = 0$:

1. $a > 0, b > 0$. When $\varnothing < 0$ with $|\varnothing|$ 1, 0 is locally asymptotically stable, there exists a positive unstable equilibrium; when $0 < \varnothing 1$, 0 is unstable, there exists a negative and locally asymptotically stable equilibrium.

2. $a < 0, b < 0$. When $\varnothing < 0$ with $|\varnothing| |1,0$ is unstable and when it is locally $0 < \varnothing 1,0$ asymptotically stable, there exists a positive unstable equilibrium.
3. $a < 0, b < 0$. When $\varnothing < 0$ with $|\varnothing| |1,0$ is unstable, there exists a locally $0 < \varnothing 1,0$ asymptotically stable negative equilibrium, when stable and positive unstable equilibrium appears.
4. $a < 0$, $b < 0$. When it changes from negative to positive, 0 changes its stability from stable to unstable. Correspondingly, a negative unstable equilibrium becomes positive and locally asymptotically stable.

3.10 Determination of Bifurcation Parameters (a and b)

From model (4.15), the associated non-zero partial derivatives of "*F*" at the disease-free equilibrium are given by

$$\frac{\partial^2 f_2}{\partial x^2{}_2} = \frac{\partial^2 f_2}{\partial x_5 \partial x_5} = \frac{\partial^2 f_3}{\partial x_2 \partial x_3} = \frac{\partial^2 f_3}{\partial x_3 \partial x_5} = \frac{\partial^2 f_4}{\partial x_2 \partial x_4} = \frac{\partial^2 f_4}{\partial x_4 \partial x_5} = \frac{\partial^2 f_5}{\partial x_2 \partial x_5} = \frac{\partial^2 f_5}{\partial x^2{}_5} = 0$$

$$\frac{\partial^2 f_2}{\partial x^2{}_2} = -2(1-\varepsilon)\theta, \frac{\partial^2 f_2}{\partial x_5 \partial x_5} = \alpha, \frac{\partial^2 f_3}{\partial x_3 \partial x_5} = -(1-\varepsilon)\theta, \frac{\partial^2 f_3}{\partial x_3 \partial x_5} = \alpha$$

$$\frac{\partial^2 f_4}{\partial x_2 \partial x_4} = -(1-\varepsilon)\theta, \frac{\partial^2 f_4}{\partial x_4 \partial x_5} = \alpha \ \frac{\partial^2 f_5}{\partial x_2 \partial x_5} = -(1-\varepsilon)\theta \ \frac{\partial^2 f_5}{\partial x^2{}_5} = 2\alpha$$

It follows from above expressions that

$$a = u_2 \sum w_i w_j \frac{\partial^2 f_2}{\partial x_i \partial x_j} + u_3 \sum w_i w_j \frac{\partial^2 f_3}{\partial x_i \partial x_j} + u_4 \sum w_i w_j \frac{\partial^2 f_3}{\partial x_i \partial x_j} + u_5 \sum w_i w_j \frac{\partial^2 f_5}{\partial x_i \partial x_j} \tag{4.2.0}$$

$$u_2\left[\alpha w_2 w_5 + 2(1-\varepsilon)\theta w^2{}_2\right] - u_3\left[\alpha w_3 w_5 + (1-\varepsilon)\theta w_2 w_3\right]$$
$$+ u_4\left[\alpha w_4 w_5 + (1-\varepsilon)\theta w_2 w_4\right] + u_5\left[2\alpha w^2{}_5 + (1-\varepsilon)\theta \, w_2 w_5\right]$$

Therefore a > 0, if

$$\left[\alpha w_3 w_5 + (1-\varepsilon) \, w_2 w_5\right] < \frac{q_1}{u_3}$$

where q_1

$$u_2\left[\alpha w_2 w_5 + 2(1-\varepsilon)\theta w^2{}_2\right] - u_3\left[\alpha w_3 w_5 + (1-\varepsilon)\theta w_2 w_3\right]$$
$$+ u_4\left[\alpha w_4 w_5 + (1-\varepsilon)\theta w_2 w_4\right] + u_5\left[2\alpha w^2{}_5 + (1-\varepsilon)\theta \, w_2 w_5\right]$$

Hence a > 0, if

$$\frac{\alpha\sigma_1\delta}{\eta}\left[\frac{\eta\varphi\Psi + c_3\beta_3 m\gamma\sigma_1\delta + c_3\beta_3\eta\sigma_2\,\delta + c_3\beta_3 v\sigma_1(1-\varepsilon)\theta}{c_3\beta_3 v\,\eta\sigma_2}\right] < \frac{\varpi\eta\ominus}{m\gamma\varpi + (1-m)\gamma v}$$

where

$$\begin{aligned}\ominus = &\frac{\alpha\Psi}{c_3\beta_3}\left(\frac{\eta\varphi\Psi + c_3\beta_3 m\gamma\sigma_1\delta + c_3\beta_3\eta\sigma_2\delta}{c_3\beta_3 v\eta}\right) + \frac{v_2\alpha}{\varpi}\\ &\times\left(\frac{\eta\varphi\psi + c_3\beta_3 m\gamma\sigma_1\delta + c_3\beta_3 m\gamma\sigma_1\delta}{c_3\beta_3 v\eta}\right)2 + \frac{(1-\varepsilon)\theta\Psi}{c_3\beta_3}\\ &+\left(\frac{\sigma_1\delta(m\gamma\varpi + (1-m)\gamma v) + \sigma_2\delta\varpi\eta + (1-\sigma_1-\sigma_2)\delta_n}{\varpi\eta\Psi}\right)\\ &+ v(1-\varepsilon)\theta\left(\frac{\eta\varphi\Psi + c_3\beta_3 m\gamma\sigma_1\delta + c_3\beta_3\eta\sigma_2\,\delta}{\varpi c_3\beta_3 v\eta}\right)\\ &+\alpha\left(\frac{\eta\varphi\Psi + c_3\beta_3 m\gamma\sigma_1\delta + c_3\beta_3\eta\sigma_2\delta}{c_3\beta_3 v\eta}\right) + 2(1-\varepsilon)\theta\end{aligned}$$

For the sign of "b," it can be shown that the associated non-vanishing partial derivatives is $\frac{\partial^2 f^2{}_2}{\partial\beta 1\partial X_2} = c_1$, so that

$$\begin{aligned}b &= u_2\sum w_i\frac{\partial^2 f_2}{\partial\beta_1\partial x_i}\\ &= u_2 w_2 c_1 - \frac{[\partial_1\delta(m\gamma\varpi + (1-m)\gamma v + \sigma_2\gamma\varpi\eta + (1-\sigma_1-\sigma_2]\delta\eta}{\varpi\eta\Psi}\end{aligned}$$

Therefore, $b< 0$, hence, we have established the following result. Since $b< 0$ and $a >0$ if the inequality satisfies, there exists a forward bifurcation (Fig. 3.2).

3.11 Global Stability of the Endemic Equilibrium

Theorem 3.12.1 If the endemic equilibrium E^*exists, then it is globally asymptotically stable provided that $R_0 > 1$.

Consider the following positive definite function about E^*:

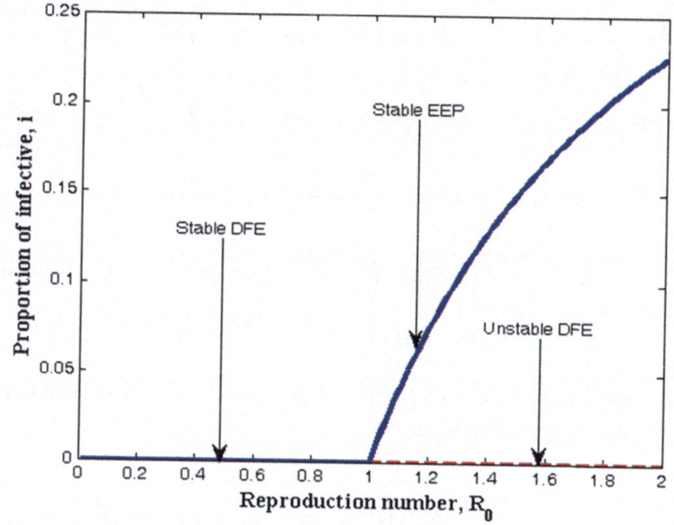

Fig. 3.2 Forward bifurcation of the model 3.3

$$V(s^*, i^*, p^*, h^*, a^*) = s\left(s - s^* - \text{slog}\frac{s^*}{s}\right) + \left(i - i^* - \text{ilog}\frac{i^*}{i}\right) + \left(p - p^* - \text{plog}\frac{p^*}{p}\right) + \left(h - h^* - \text{hlog}\frac{h^*}{h}\right) + \left(a - a^* - \text{alog}\frac{a^*}{a}\right) \tag{3.2.2}$$

By the direct calculation of the derivation of V along the solution of (3.3), it can be written as $\frac{dV}{dt} = \left(\frac{s-s^*}{s}\right)\frac{ds}{dt} + \left(\frac{i-i^*}{i}\right)\frac{di}{dt} + \left(\frac{p-p^*}{p}\right)\frac{dp}{dt} + \left(\frac{h-h^*}{h}\right)\frac{dh}{dt} + \left(\frac{a-a^*}{a}\right)\frac{da}{dt}$.

$$\frac{ds}{dt} = \pi - c_1\beta_1 \text{is} - c_3\beta_3 \text{hs} - [\pi - \alpha a + (1 - \varepsilon)\theta_i]s$$

$$\frac{di}{dt} = \pi - c_1\beta_1 \text{is} + c_3\beta_3 \text{hs} + (1 - \varepsilon)\theta_i - [\pi + \delta - \alpha a + (1 - \varepsilon)\theta_i]i$$

$$\frac{dp}{dt} = \sigma_i\delta_i - [\pi + \delta - \alpha a + (1 - \varepsilon)\theta_i]p$$

$$\frac{dh}{dt} = \sigma_2\delta_i + \text{m}\gamma\text{p} + va - [\pi + k - \alpha a + (1 - \varepsilon)\theta_i]h$$

$$\frac{da}{dt} = (1 - \sigma_1 - \sigma_2)\delta_i + (1 - m)\gamma p + \text{kh} - [\pi + v + \alpha - \alpha a + (1 - \varepsilon)\theta_i]a$$

It can now be written as

$$\frac{\mathrm{dV}}{\mathrm{dt}} = \left(\frac{s - s^*}{s}\right)[\pi - c_1\beta_1 \mathrm{is} - c_3\beta_3 \mathrm{hs} - [\pi - \alpha a + (1-\varepsilon)\theta_i]s +] + \left(\frac{i - i^*}{i}\right) c_1\beta_1 \mathrm{is}$$
$$+ c_3\beta_3 \mathrm{hs} + (1-\varepsilon)\theta_i - [\pi + \delta - \alpha a + (1-\varepsilon)\theta_i] i + \left(\frac{p - p^*}{p}\right)\sigma_i\delta_i$$
$$- [\pi + \delta - \alpha a + (1-\varepsilon)\theta_i] p + \left(\frac{h - h^*}{h}\right)\sigma_2\delta_i + m\gamma p + va$$
$$- [\pi + k - \alpha a + (1-\varepsilon)\theta_i] h + \left(\frac{a - a^*}{a}\right)(1 - \sigma_1 - \sigma_2)\delta_i + (1-m)\gamma p + \mathrm{kh}$$
$$- [\pi + v + \alpha - \alpha a + (1-\varepsilon)\theta_i] a$$

Therefore, substitute $s = s - s^*$, $i = i - i^*$, $p = p - p^*$, $h = h - h^*$ and $a = a - a^*$ After some algebraic calculation, we get

$$\frac{\mathrm{dV}}{\mathrm{dt}} = [c_1\beta_1 i^* + c_3\beta_3 h^* + \alpha a + \theta i + \varepsilon\theta i]\left(\frac{s - s^*}{s}\right)^2 + [c_1\beta_1 s + \theta + \alpha a]\left(\frac{i - i^*}{i}\right)^2$$
$$+ [\alpha a + \theta i^* + \varepsilon\theta i]\left(\frac{p - p^*}{p}\right)^2 + [\alpha a + \theta i^* + \varepsilon\theta i] + \left(\frac{h - h^*}{h}\right)^2$$
$$+ [\theta i^* + \varepsilon\theta i]\left(\frac{a - a^*}{a}\right)^2 + \theta\frac{i^{*3}}{i} + c_3\beta_3 h^*\frac{i^*}{i} + \sigma 1\delta i^*\frac{p^*}{p} + \sigma 2\delta i^*\frac{h^*}{h} + m\gamma p^*\frac{h^*}{h}$$
$$+ va\frac{h^*}{h} + \sigma 1\delta_i\frac{a^*}{a} + \gamma p^*\frac{a^*}{a} + m\gamma p\frac{a^*}{a} + kh^*\frac{a^*}{a} + 3\theta ii^* + \varepsilon\theta i^2 + 3\varepsilon\theta i^{*^2} + \pi$$
$$+ c_3\beta_3 h + \sigma 1\delta i + \sigma 2\delta i + m\gamma p + va + \alpha a^2 + 3\alpha a^{*^2} + \delta i\sigma 1\delta i + \sigma 2\delta i^* + \gamma p$$
$$+ m\gamma p^* + kh\frac{h^*}{h} + m\gamma p^*\frac{h^*}{h} + va\frac{h^*}{h} + \sigma 1\delta_i\frac{a^*}{a} + \gamma p^*\frac{a^*}{a} + m\gamma p\frac{a^*}{a} + kh^*\frac{a^*}{a}$$
$$+ 3\theta ii^* + \varepsilon\theta i^2 + 3\varepsilon\theta i^{*^2} + \pi + c_3\beta_3 h + \sigma 1\delta i + \sigma 2\delta i + m\gamma p + va + \alpha a^2$$
$$+ 3\alpha a^{*^2} + \delta i\sigma 1\delta i + \sigma 2\delta i^* + \gamma p + m\gamma p^*$$
$$+ kh[c_1\beta_1 i + c_3\beta_3 h + \pi + \alpha a^* + \theta i + \varepsilon\theta i^*]\left(\frac{h - h^*}{h}\right)^2$$
$$- [\pi + \gamma + \alpha + \theta i + \varepsilon\theta_i^*]\left(\frac{p - p^*}{p}\right)^2 - [\pi + k\alpha a^* + \theta i + \varepsilon\theta i^*]\left(\frac{h - h^*}{h}\right)^2$$
$$- [\pi + \gamma + \alpha + \theta i + \varepsilon\theta i^*]\left(\frac{a - a^*}{a}\right)^2 - \pi\frac{s^*}{s} - c_3\beta_3 h\frac{i^*}{i} - \sigma 1\delta i\frac{p^*}{p} - \sigma 2\delta i\frac{h^*}{h}$$
$$- m\gamma p\frac{h^*}{h} - 3\varepsilon\theta\frac{i^*}{i} - \alpha\frac{\alpha^{*^3}}{a} - \delta i\frac{a^*}{a} - \sigma 1\delta i^*\frac{a^*}{a} - \sigma 2\delta i^*\frac{a^*}{a} - \gamma p\frac{a^*}{a} - kh\frac{a^*}{a}$$
$$- 3\varepsilon\theta ii^* - 3\alpha aa^* - \theta i^* - 3\theta i^* - c_3\beta_3 h^* - \sigma 1\delta i^* - m\gamma p^* - \gamma a - \sigma 1\delta i$$
$$- \sigma 2\delta i - \delta i^* - \gamma p^* - m\gamma p - kh$$

Hence the sufficient condition for $\frac{dV}{dt}$ to be negative definite is that $Z - \Upsilon < 0$, where

$$\Upsilon = -[c_1\beta_1 i + c_3\beta_3 h + \pi + \alpha a^* + \theta i + \varepsilon\theta i^*]\left(\frac{s - s^*}{s}\right)^2$$
$$- [c_1\beta_1 s^* + \varepsilon\theta + \pi + \delta + \alpha a]\left(\frac{i - i^*}{i}\right)^2$$
$$- [\pi + \gamma + \alpha a^* + \theta i + \varepsilon\theta i^*]\left(\frac{p - p^*}{p}\right)^2$$
$$- [\pi + k + \alpha a^* + \theta i + \varepsilon\theta i^*]\left(\frac{h - h^*}{h}\right)^2 - [\pi + \nu + \alpha + \theta i + \varepsilon\theta i^*]$$
$$\times \left(\frac{a - a^*}{a}\right)^{-2}\pi\frac{s^*}{s} - c_3\beta_3 h\frac{i^*}{i} - \sigma 1\delta i\frac{p^*}{p} - \sigma 2\delta i\frac{h^*}{h} - m\gamma p\frac{h^*}{h} - va\frac{h^*}{h} - 3\varepsilon\theta\frac{i^*}{i}$$
$$- \alpha\frac{a^{*3}}{a} - \delta i\frac{a^*}{a} - \sigma 1\delta i^*\frac{a^*}{a} - \sigma 2\delta i^*\frac{a^*}{a} - \gamma p\frac{a^*}{a} - m\gamma p^*\frac{a^*}{a} - kh\frac{a^*}{a} - 3\varepsilon\theta i i^*$$
$$- 3\alpha a a^* - \theta i^* - 3\theta i^* - c_3\beta_3 h^* - \sigma 1\delta i^* - \sigma 2\delta i^* - m\gamma p^* - va - \sigma 1\delta i - \sigma 2\delta i$$
$$- \delta i^* - \gamma p^* - m\gamma p - kh^*$$

Therefore, the largest compact invariant set in $\left\{(s^*, i^*, p^*, h^*, a^*) \in \Omega : \frac{dV}{dt} = 0\right\}$ is the single $\{E^*\}$, where E^* is the endemic equilibrium of the normalized model system (3.3). By La Salle's invariant principle, it implies that $E^*$is globally asymptotically stable in Ω; if $Z < \Upsilon$, this completes the proof of Theorem 3.4.

3.12 The Numerical Simulations of the Model

To study the dynamical behavior of the model (3.3) numerically, the system is integrated by using Runge-Kutta method using the following set of parameter values (Table 3.1, Figs. 3.3a, 3.3b and 3.3c).

It is observed from the figures that for any initial start, the solution curve tends to equilibrium E^*. Hence, we infer that the system 3.3 may be globally stable about this endemic equilibrium point E^*. The computed values are

$$s^* = 0.6028, i^* = 0.243, p^* = 0.228, h^* = 0.0423, a^* = 0.0892$$

The results of numerical simulation are shown graphically in Figs. 3.4a. In Fig. 3.4a the distribution of proportion of population with time is shown in different classes with neither new infected children into the population nor recruitments, i.e., $\pi = 0$ and $\theta = 0$. It was seen that in the absence of vertical transmission into the community, the proportion of susceptible population decreases continuously as the population is closed, which results in an increase in proportion of infective

Table 3.1 Different parameters used for simulation

Sl. no.	Name of the parameters	Values	Name of the parameters	Value
1	θ	0.30	k	0.08
2.	ε	0.20	γ	0.90
3.	v	0.10	c_1	3.00
4.	β_1	0.40	c_3	1.00
5.	β_3	0.05	m	0.40
6.	σ_1	0.20	π	0.40
7.	σ_2	0.01	δ	0.60
8.	–	–	α	1.00

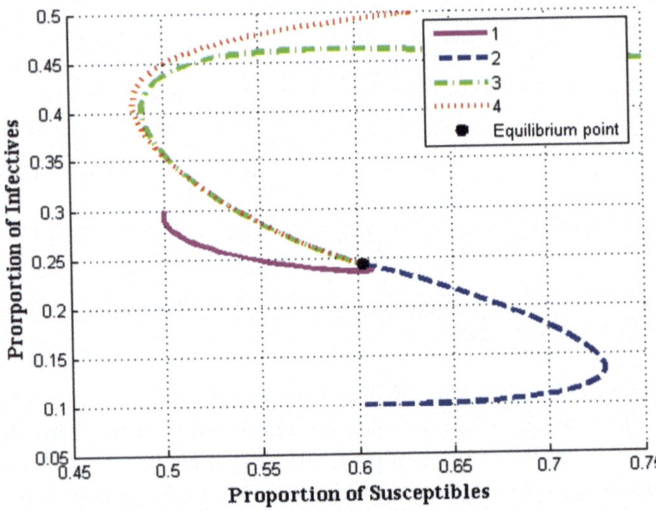

Fig. 3.3a Endemic equilibrium of proportion of infectives with susceptibles

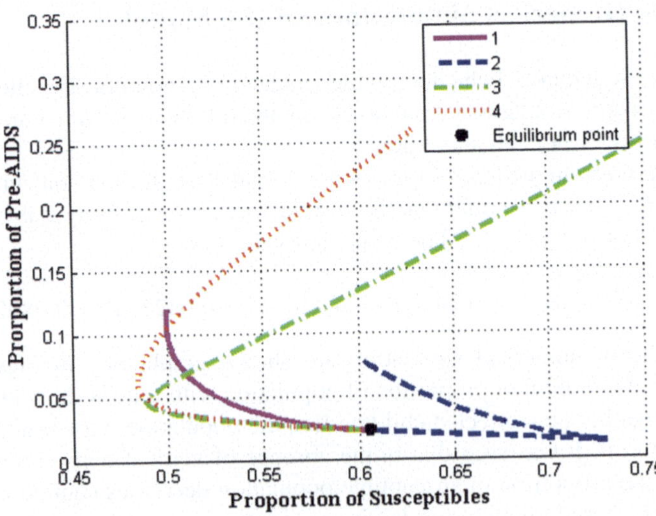

Fig. 3.3b Endemic equilibrium of proportion of pre-AIDS population

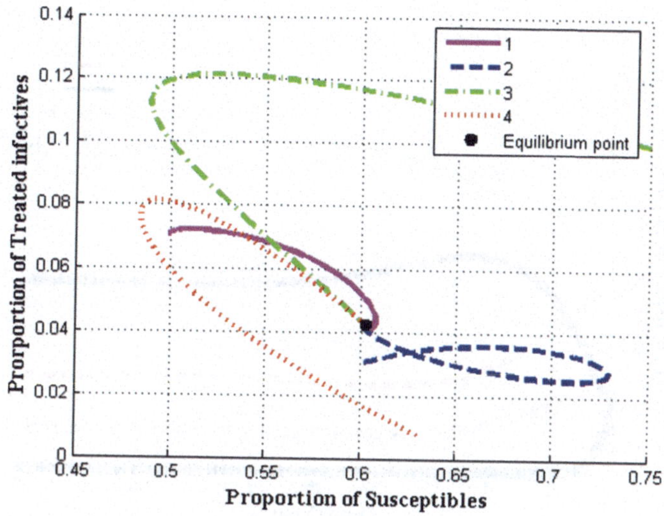

Fig. 3.3c Endemic equilibrium of proportion of treated class

population first and then it decreases, as all infectives subsequently develop full-blown AIDS and they die out by natural or HIV related death. The proportion of treated class increased continuously, since the total population is being constant in this case. Figure. 3.4b showed the variation of proportion of population in all classes with both recruitment of susceptibles and fraction of newborn children, which were infected at birth. It was found that susceptibles first decrease with time after using ARVs (they prolong lifetime), and they increase and then reach their equilibrium

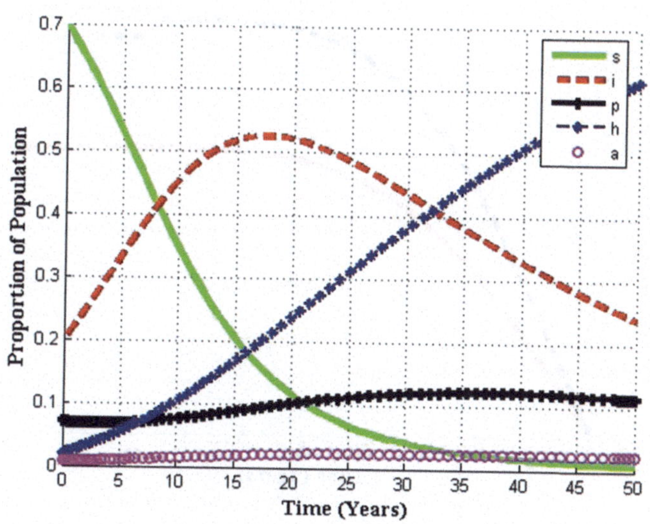

Fig. 3.4a Variation of population in different classes for $\pi = 0$ and $\theta = 0$

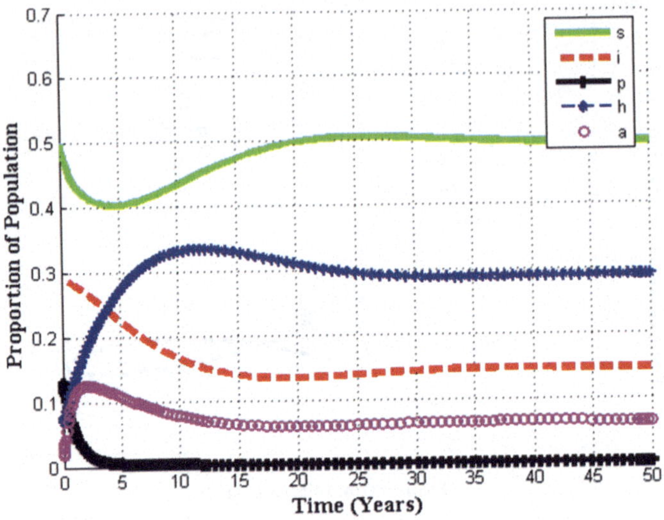

Fig. 3.4b Variation of population in different classes for $\pi = 0.10$ and $\theta = 0.20$

position. Due to vertical transmission from infectives, susceptible population increase continuously; therefore infection becomes more endemic, following that $R_0 > 0$.

The role of vertical transmission in the model, i.e., the rate of recruitment of infected children directly into infective class, is explicitly shown in Figs. 3.5a, 3.5b and 3.5c. It was seen that in Fig. 3.5a as the rate of infected children born θ increases,

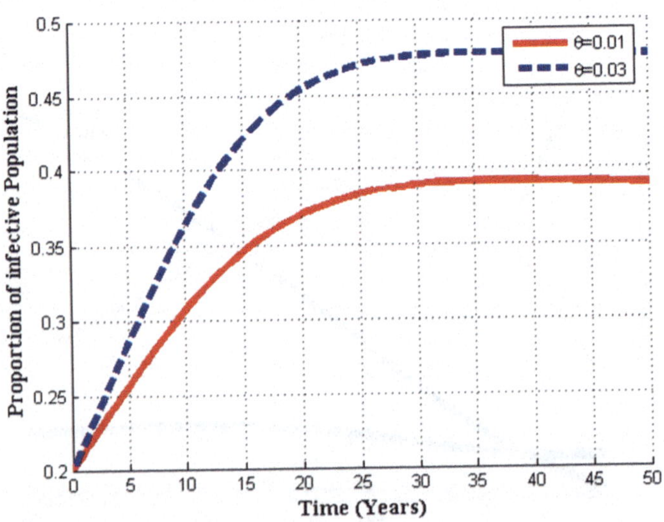

Fig. 3.5a Variation of infected population for different values of θ

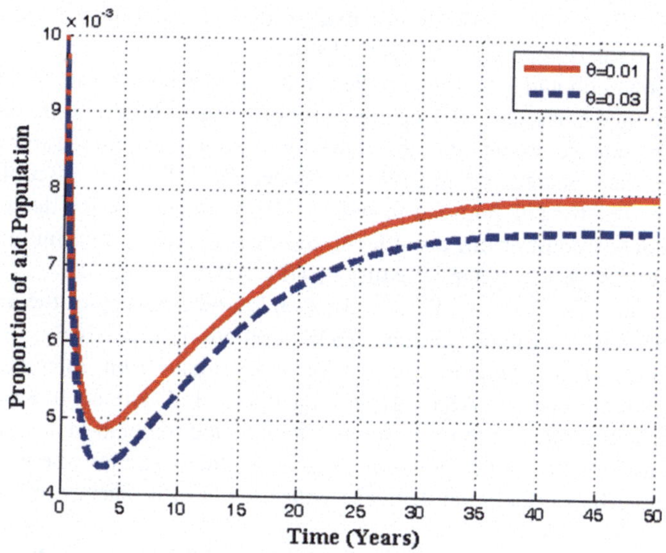

Fig. 3.5b Variation of AIDS population for different values of θ

the proportion infective population also increases. It was noted that the birth of infected children makes the infective population increase. In Fig. 3.5b if there is increase in the value of θ, the proportion of AIDS population decreases with time, and then it increases until it reaches its equilibrium position. Thus, if the birth of infected children is controlled by treatment, the overall infective population will remain under control. This formulated model will help in reducing the AIDS

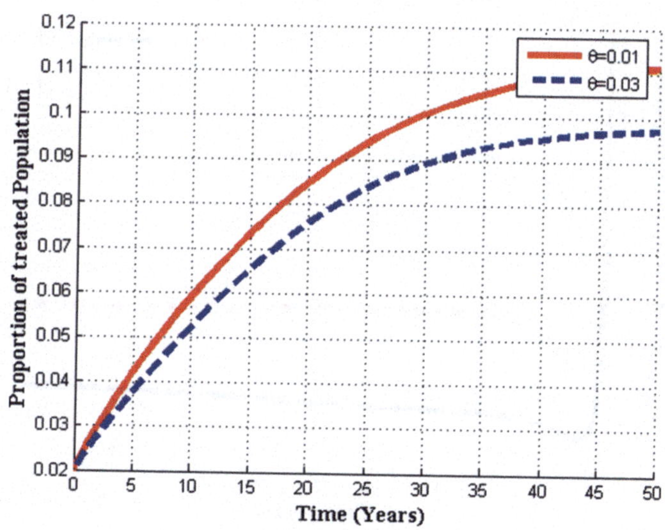

Fig. 3.5c Variation of treated class for different values of θ

population. In Fig. 3.6a it was found that as the rate of infected children born increases, the treated population tends to decline.

Figures 3.6a, 3.6b and 3.6c showed the impact of recruitment rate for susceptible population, treated class, and AIDS patients for different values of π. It was seen that as recruitment rate increases, also the susceptible population increases when compared, rather than decreasing the rate π. Since, the inflow of susceptible cases increases, but the treated population and AIDS population were decreased with time till it reaches equilibrium point/level and then decreases continuously due to HAART treatment in the dynamic nature of HIV/AIDS.

Figures 3.7a, 3.7b, 3.7c, 3.7d, 3.8a, 3.8b, 3.7c and 3.8d depict the variation of infectives, pre-AIDS, treated class, and AIDS population, respectively, with time for different values of movement rate (δ) of individuals from infective class to pre-AIDS, treated class, or AIDS depending upon viral counts. It was seen that with increase in the value of movement rate, the infected population decreases which in turn increases the treated population. Also if we increase movement rate δδ, the pre-AIDS and AIDS population decrease with time until it reaches the equilibrium and stabilizes the model.

Figures 3.8a, 3.8b, 3.8c, 3.8d, 3.9a, 3.9b, 3.9c and 3.9d showed the variation of population in the classes with fraction of movement rate from infectious class σ. It was seen that from the figures when σ_1 increases, the pre-AIDS population also decreases continuously; it might be of treatment which is provided to the patients, but for the AIDS class this is different; it was found that as $\sigma_1$increases, the AIDS population decreases with time then reaches its equilibrium level and increased simultaneously. This was caused by ARVs by prolonging the lifespan, then the patient joins full-blown AIDS, and therefore disease persists. Also it was found from

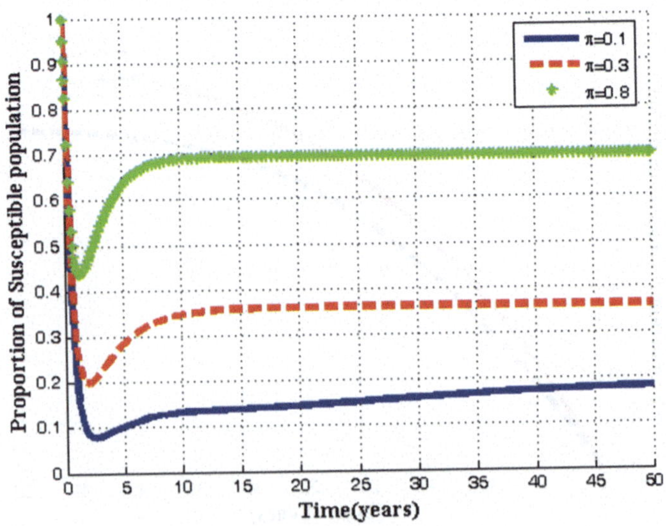

Fig. 3.6a Variation of the susceptible for different values of π

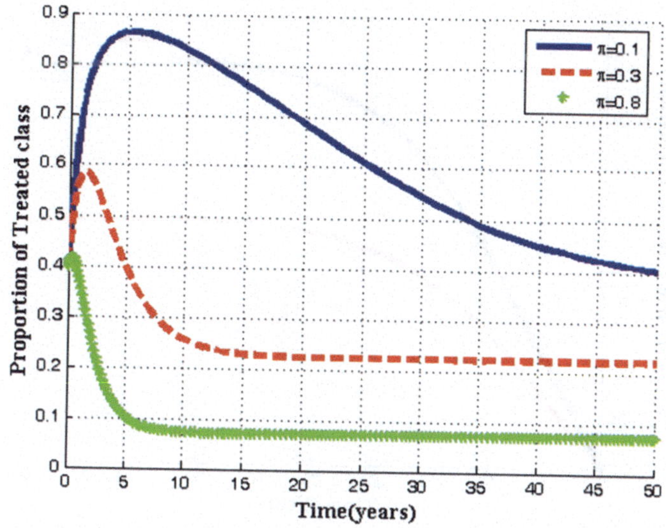

Fig. 3.6b Variation of treated population for different values of π

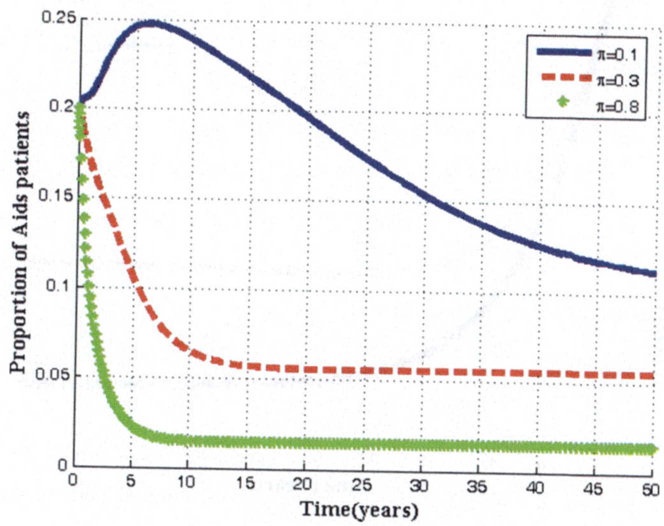

Fig. 3.6c Variation of AIDS population for different values of π

the graph that as σ_2 increases, treated population initially increase, as time gone then it decreases, but in AIDS patients, they decrease continuously up to equilibrium, then they increase because disease still illness exist.

Figures 3.9a, 3.9b, 3.9c, 3.9d, 3.10a, 3.10b, 3.10c and 3.10d predicted the variation of the contact rates of susceptible population with infectives β_1 and susceptible with treated class β_3 in the susceptible and infective population. The

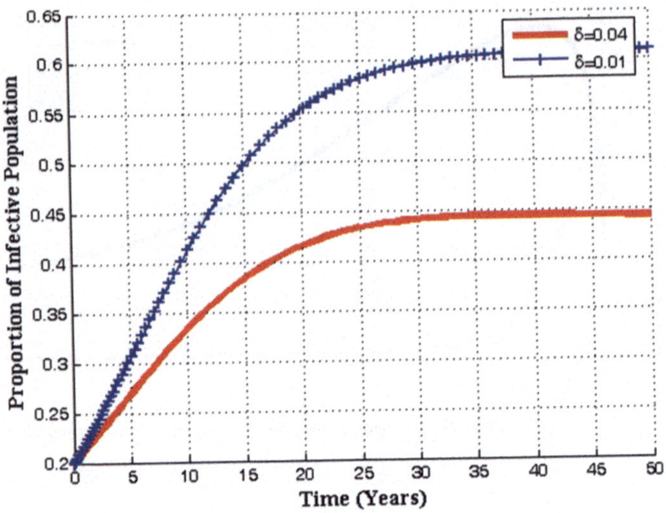

Fig. 3.7a Variation of infective population for different values of δ

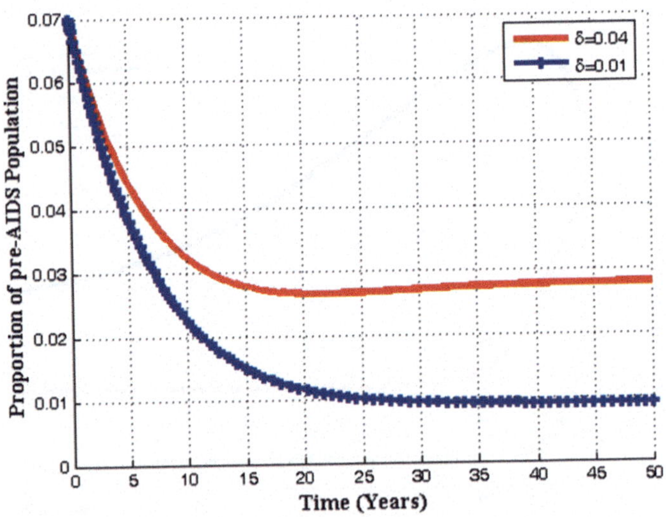

Fig. 3.7b Variation of pre-AIDS population for different values of δ

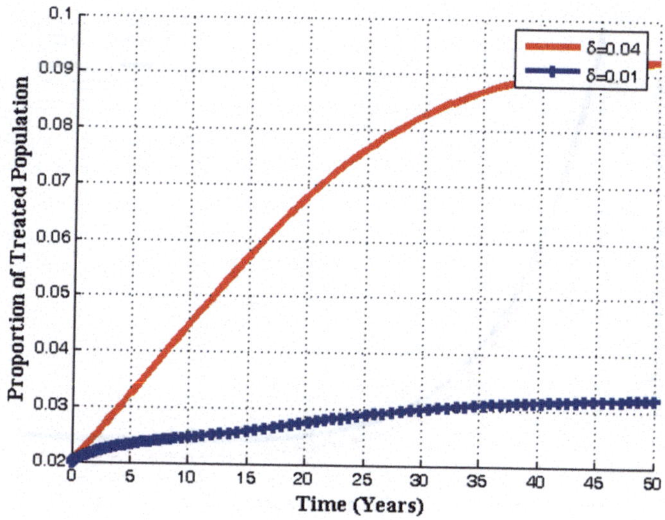

Fig. 3.7c Variation of treated class for different values of δ

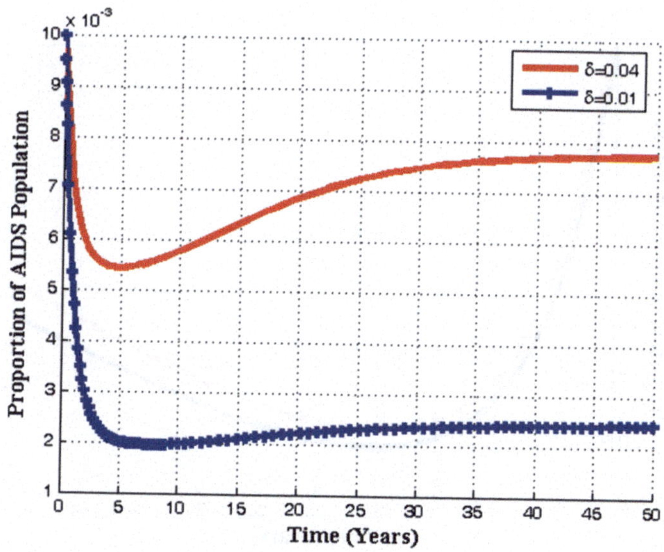

Fig. 3.7d Variation of AIDS population for different values of δ

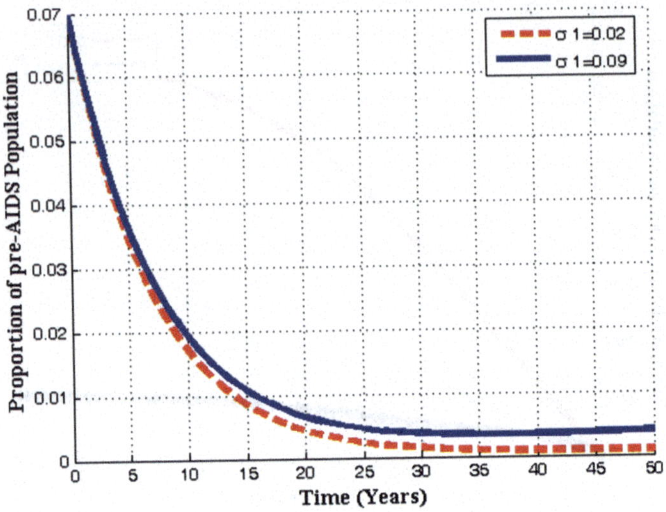

Fig. 3.8a Variation of pre-AIDS population for different values of σ_1

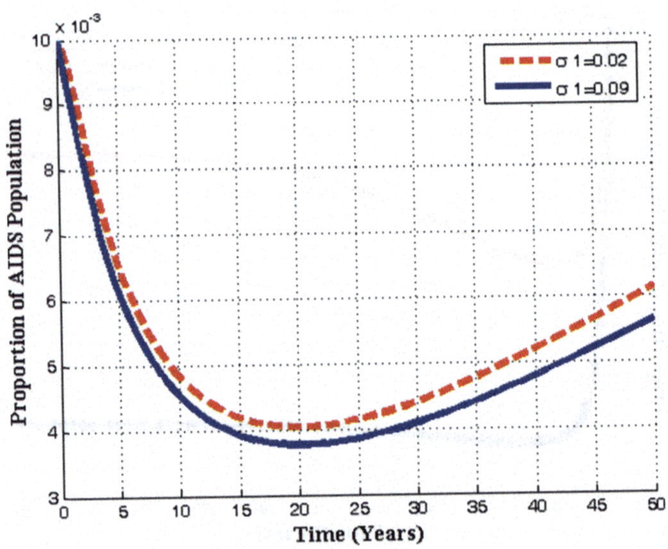

Fig. 3.8b Variation of AIDS population for different values of σ_1

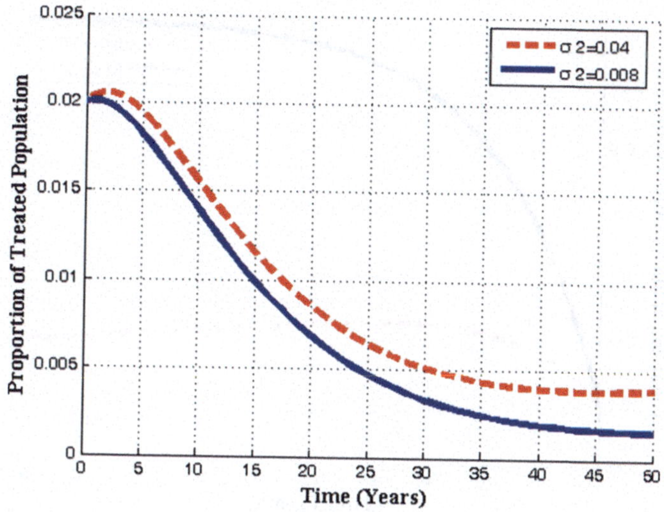

Fig. 3.8c Variation of treated population for different values of σ_2

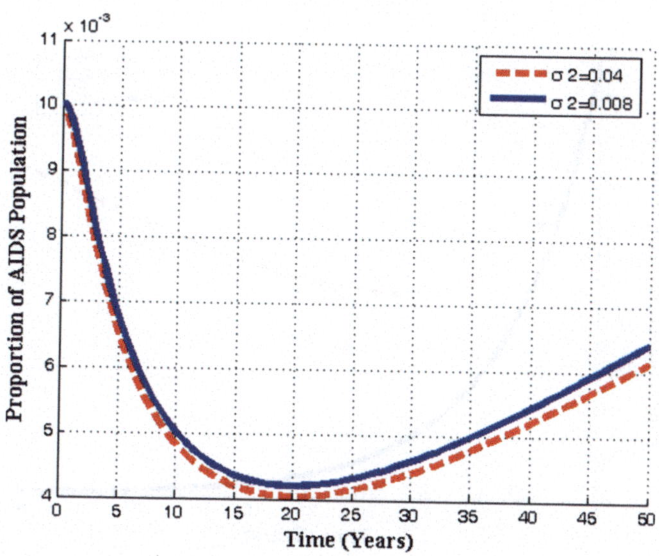

Fig. 3.8d Variation of AIDS population for different values of σ_2

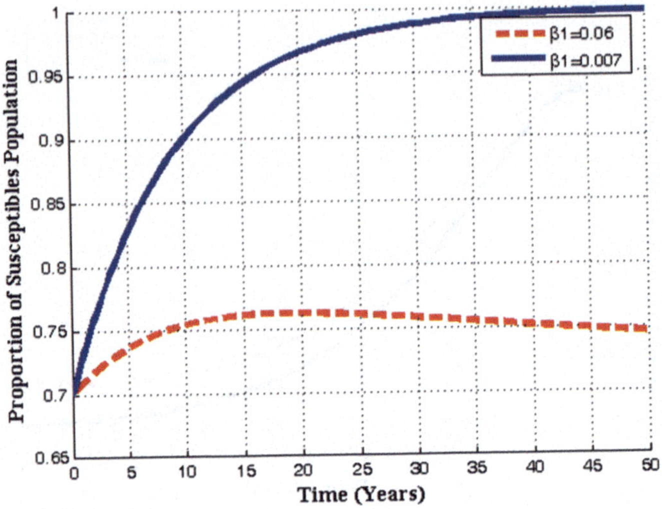

Fig. 3.9a Variation of susceptible population for different values of β_1

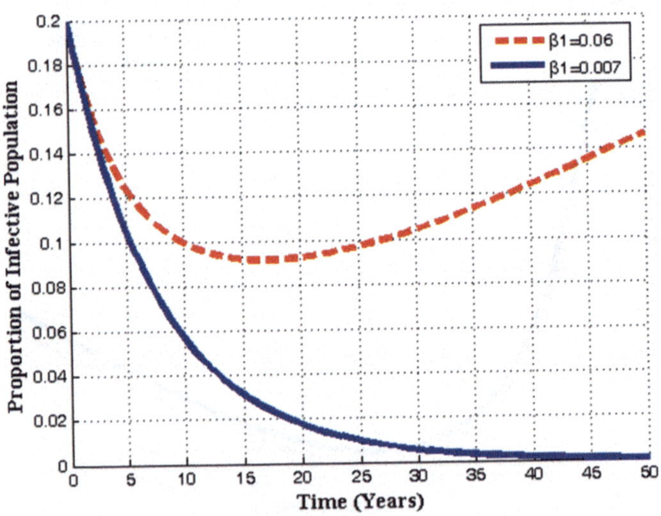

Fig. 3.9b Variation of infective population for different values of β_1

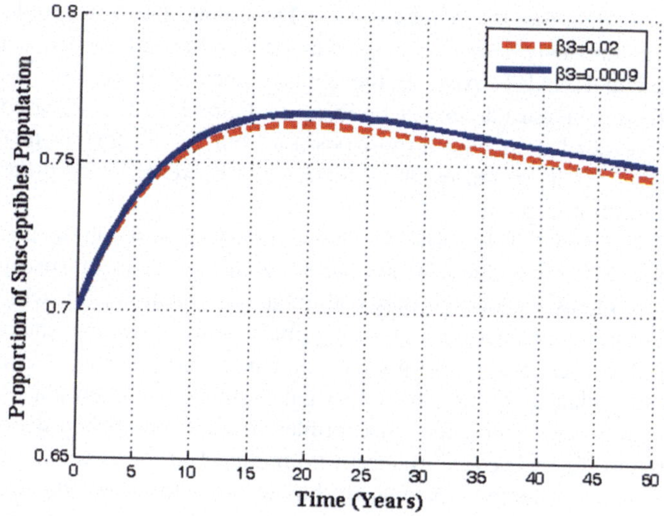

Fig. 3.9c Variation of susceptible population for different values of $\beta 3$

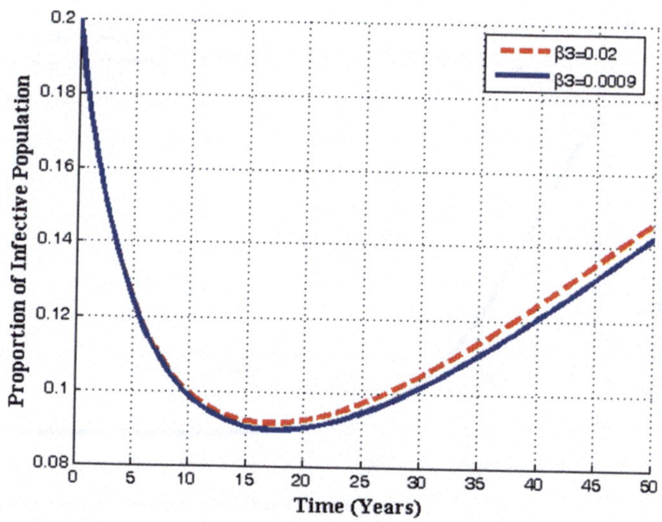

Fig. 3.9d Variation of infective population for different values of β_3

figures indicate that the β_1 increased by CD4 count, the susceptible rate was declined, simultaneously infective class was decreased, and treated classes were well compiled in HAART. Also as the contact rates of susceptible with treated population β_3 were increased, the susceptible population initially increased with time "t" and then reached their equilibrium position, but this differs from that of the infective classes. As β_3 increases, the infective rate decreased with time t and then reached its equilibrium point.

Figures 3.10a and 3.10b showed the variations of susceptible and infective population for different values of number of sexual partners of susceptible with infectives c_1 and between susceptibles with treated population c_3. It was found that as the number of sexual partners of susceptibles with infectives $c_1$increased with time, susceptibles decreased continuously and infectives increased continuously. Also it was seen that if the number of sexual partners of susceptible with treated population c_3 increases with time, susceptibles first increased then decreased with time as shown in Fig. 3.10c due to loss of immunity. But for infectives, it was seen that as c_3 increases, infectives increased; thus in order to reduce the spread of the disease, the number of sexual partners as well as unsafe sexual contact with an infective has to be restricted (Fig. 3.10d).

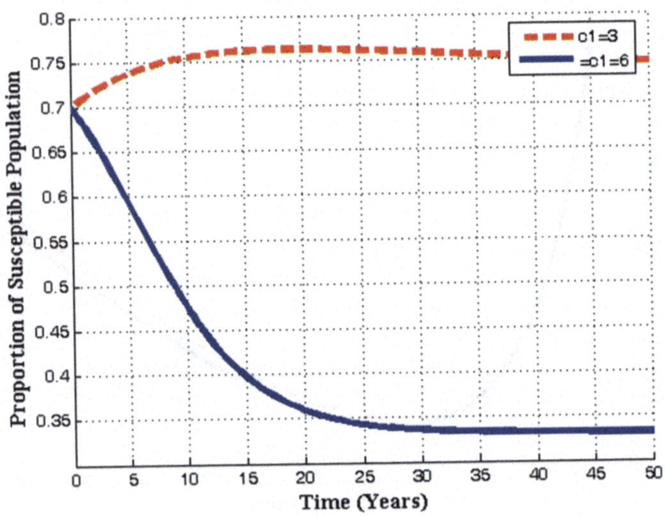

Fig. 3.10a Variation of susceptible population for different values of c_1

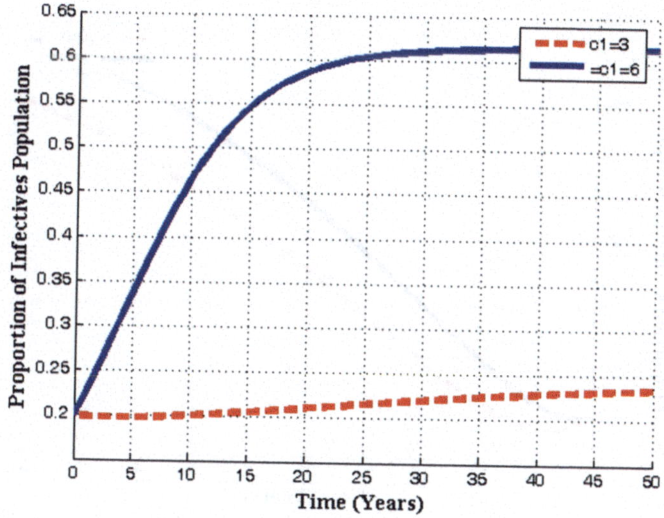

Fig. 3.10b Variation of infective population for different values of c_1

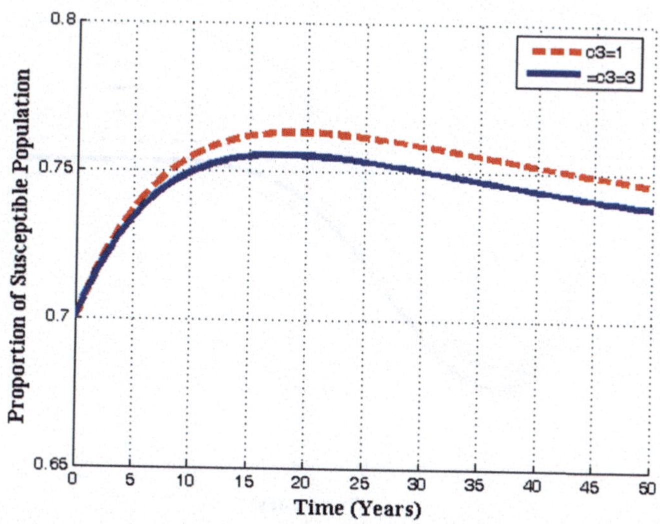

Fig. 3.10c Variation of susceptible population for different values of c_3

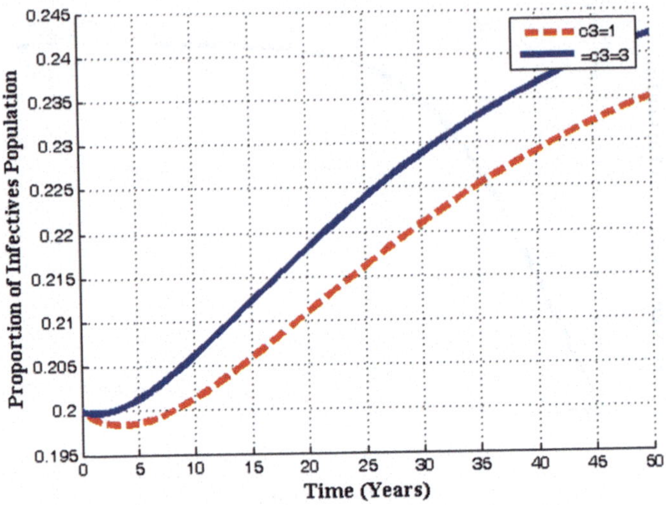

Fig. 3.10d Variation of infective population for different values of c_3

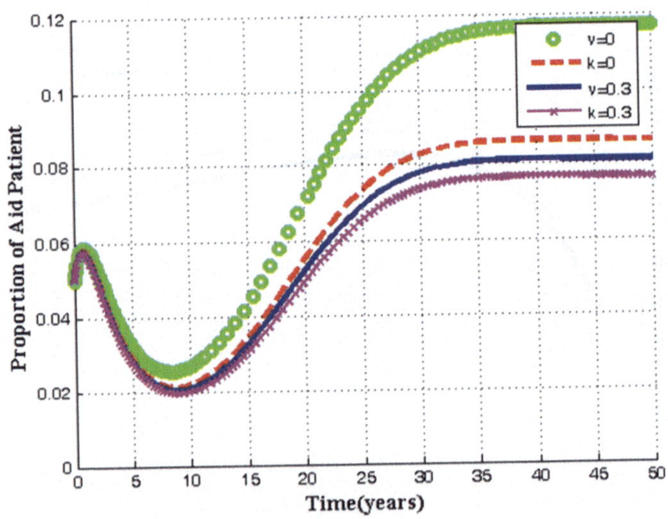

Fig. 3.11a Variation of AIDS patients for different values of k *and* v

Figures 3.11a, 3.11b and 3.12 showed the variation of treatment rates in treated class and AIDS population. It was found that if treatment rate was zero, the disease increased with time, whereas treatment population decreased. Also the graphs showed that as the rates of treatment increased, the AIDS patients decreased due to treatment measures which increased the immune system and prolonged life of the AIDS population; therefore this increased the treated class, respectively.

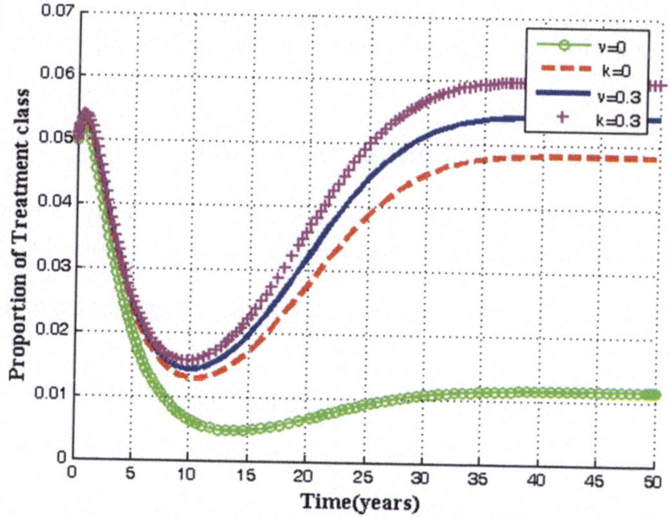

Fig. 3.11b Variation of AIDS patients with varied parameters simulated values of *k and v*

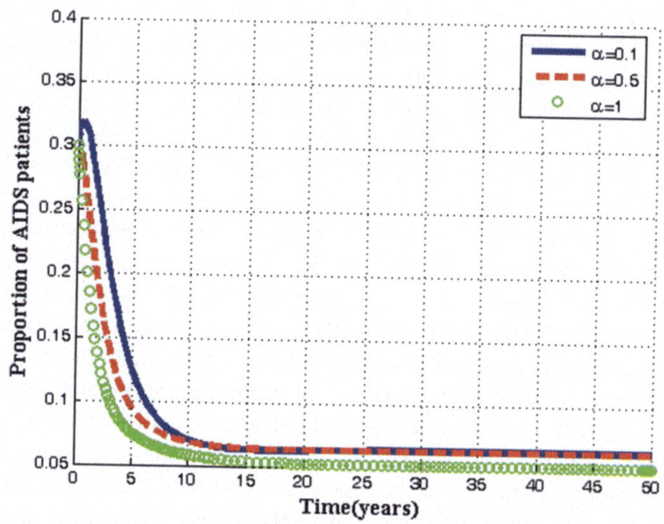

Fig. 3.12 Variation of AIDS populations for different values of α

In Fig. 3.12 the effect of disease-induced death rate α was shown, and it was found that as α increases, the population of AIDS patients decreased. It was found that the AIDS induced death rate α could be controlled by providing antiretroviral drugs (ARVs) to AIDS patients or by advising AIDS patients to follow healthy habits about the AIDS disease. From the figures, it can also be seen that the respective populations were tending to the equilibrium level. This has also been observed for different initial values of the variables. Hence, the endemic equilibrium $E*$ was globally asymptotically stable for the above set of parameter values (Rivadeneira et al. 2012; Royce et al. 1995; Rivadeneira et al. 2014; Ramratnam et al. 1999).

3.13 Numerical Simulations of the Model

To study the dynamical behavior of the model 3.3 numerically, the system was integrated by using Runge-Kutta method using the following set of parameter values:

$$\theta = 0.30\ \varepsilon = 0.20\ v = 0.10\ \beta_1 = 0.40\ \beta_3 = 0.05\ \sigma_1 = 0.20\ \sigma_2 = 0.01\ k = 0.08\ \gamma = 0.90\ c_1 = 3$$

$$c_3 = 1\ m = 0.4\ \pi = 0.40\ \delta = 0.6\ \alpha = 9$$

With initial values

$$S(0) = 0.50\ I(0) = 0.30\ p(0) = 0.12\ h(0) = 0.07\ a(0) = 0.01$$

The endemic equilibrium values are computed as shown graphically in Fig. 3.12. It was shown that i^*, p^*, h^*, and a^* were plotted against the proportion of susceptible populations*. The results of numerical simulation were shown graphically in Figs. 3.11a and 3.12; the distribution of proportion of population with time was shown in different classes with neither new infected children into the population nor recruitments, i.e., $\pi = 0$ and $\theta = 0$ (Simwa et al. 2008; Sattenspiel et al. 1990; Shim et al. 2003). It was seen that in the absence of vertical transmission into the community, the proportion of susceptible population decreased continuously as the population was closed, which resulted in an increase in the proportion of infective population first and then it decreased as all infectives subsequently developed into full-blown AIDS and they die out by natural or disease-induced (Elaiw et al. 2017; Naresh et al. 2006; Stan et al. 2008; Tireito et al. 2018; Vernazza et al. 1997). The proportion of treated class was increased continuously, since the total population is being constant in this case. Figure 3.2 showed the variation of proportion of population in all classes with both recruitment of susceptibles and fraction of newborn children, which were infected at birth. It was found that susceptibles first decreased with time after using ARVs (they prolong lifetime), and they increased and then reached their equilibrium position (Huang et al. 2010; Vassena et al. 2007; Wawer et al. 2005). Since due to vertical transmission from infectives, susceptible population increase continuously; therefore infection becomes more endemic, following that $R_0 > 1$ (White et al. 2004; Williams et al. 2006; Yue et al. 2005; Yang et al. 2015; Zhang et al. 2008).

3.14 Summary

In this chapter, a nonlinear mathematical model was proposed and fitted to know the transmission of HIV/AIDS in a population of varying size with HIV treatment aspects and vertical transmission under the assumption laid down; due to sexual interaction of susceptibles with infectives, the infected babies were born to infected mothers, and this directly increased the infective population. It was assumed that people in pre-AIDS and AIDS classes are exposed and incapable of producing children. By analyzing the model, we have found a threshold parameter $R0$. It was noted that when $R_0 < 1$, $R_0 > 1$ the disease dies out and when $R_0 > 1$ the disease becomes endemic. The model had two non-negative equilibria, namely, the disease-free equilibrium $E_0(1, 0, 0, 0, 0)$ and the endemic equilibrium $E^* = (s,^*i,^*p,^*h,^*a^*)$. It was found that the disease-free equilibrium $E0^*$ was locally asymptotically stable, if $R_0 < 1$ and for $R_0 > 1$ it is unstable, and the infection was maintained at the population level. The endemic equilibrium $E*$, which exists only when $R_0 > 1$, was always locally asymptotically stable. The equilibrium was also shown to be globally asymptotically stable under certain conditions. It was found that an increase in the rate of vertical transmission leads to increased infective population, which in turn increases the pre-AIDS and AIDS population, respectively.

References

Adams BM, Banks HT, Kwon HD et al (2004) Dynamic multidrug therapies for HIV: optimal and STI approaches. Math Biosci Eng 1:223–241

Agarwala BD et al (2002) On two ODE models for HIV/AIDS development in Canada and a logistic SEIR model. J Appl Math 6(Suppl 1):25–70

Anderson RM, Medly GF, May RM, Johnso AM (1986) A preliminary study of the transmission dynamics of the human immunodeficiency virus (HIV), the causative agent of AIDS. IMA J Math Appl Med Biol 3:229–263

Anderson RM, May RM, Boily MC et al (1991) The spread of HIV-1 in Africa: sexual contact patterns and the predicted demographic impact of AIDS. Nature 352:581–589

Anderson RM et al (1998) The role of mathematical models in the study of HIV transmission and the epidemiology of AIDS J. AIDS 18:241–256

Anndelman R et al. (2010) Mother to child HIV transmission in Africa. Policy Fact. AVERT, HIV treatment. http://www.avert.org/treatment.htm. Retrieved on 24th December 2010

Auvert B, Taljaard D, Lagarde E et al (2005) Randomized, controlled intervention trial of male circumcision for reduction of HIV infection risk: the ANRS 1265 trial. PLoS Med 2:298

Bailey RC, Moses S, Parker CB et al (2007) Male circumcision for HIV prevention in young men in Kisumu, Kenya: a randomised controlled trial. Lancet 369:643–656

Berger A, Scherzed L, Stürmer M et al (2005) Comparative evaluation of the COBAS Amplicor HIV-1 monitor™ ultrasensitive test, the new COBAS AmpliPrep/COBAS Amplicor HIV-1 monitor™ and the versant HIV RNA 3.0 assays for quantitation of HIV-1 RNA in plasma samples. J Clin Virol 33:43–51

Boily MC, Bastos FI, Desai K et al (2004) Changes in the transmission dynamics of the HIV epidemic after the wide-scale use of antiretroviral therapy could explain increases in sexually transmitted infection results from mathematical models. Sex Transm Dis 31:100–112

Chen SS, Cheng CY, Takeuchi Y et al (2016) Stability analysis in delayed within-host viral dynamics with both viral and cellular infections. J Math Anal Appl 442(Suppl 2):642–672

Corey L, Wald A, Celum CL et al (2004) The effects of herpes simplex virus-2 on HIV-1 acquisition and transmission: a review of two overlapping epidemics. J Acquir Immune Defic Syndr 35:435–445

Costanza V, Rivadeneira PS, Biafore F et al (2009) A closed-loop approach to antiretroviral therapies for HIV infection. Biomed Signal Process Control 4:139–148

Detels R, Munoz A et al (2005) Patterns of the hazard of death after AIDS through the evolution of antiretroviral therapy. AIDS 19(17):2009–2018

Dietz K, Hadeler K et al (1988) Epidemiological models for sexually transmitted diseases. J Math Biol 26(1)

Elaiw AM et al (2017) Stability of general virus dynamics models with both cellular and viral infections and delays. Math Methods Appl Sci 40(Suppl 16):5863–5880

Galli R, Merrick L, Friesenhahn M et al (2005) Comprehensive comparison of the versant HIV-1 RNA 3.0 (bDNA) and COBAS Amplicor HIV-1 monitor 1.5 assays on 1000 clinical specimens. J Clin Virol 34:245–252

Garnett GP, Anderson RM (1993) Factors controlling the spread of HIV in heterosexual communities in developing countries: patterns of mixing between different age and sexual activity classes. Philos Trans R Soc Lond Ser B Biol Sci 342:137–159

Goodreau SM, Goicochea LP, Sanchez J et al (2005) Sexual role and transmission of HIV type 1 among men who have sex with men, in Peru. J Infect Dis 191(Suppl 1):S147–S158

Gray RH, Kigozi G, Serwadda D et al (2007) Male circumcision for HIV prevention in men in Rakai, Uganda: a randomised trial. Lancet 369:657–666

Gregson S, Nyamukapa C, Garnett GP et al (2002) Sexual mixing patterns and sex-differentials in teenage exposure to HIV infection in rural Zimbabwe. Lancet 359:1896–1903

Haberman S et al (1990) Actuarial review of models for describing and predicting the spread of HIV-infection and AIDS. JIA 117:319–405

Hernandez-Vargas E, Colaneri P, Middleton R et al (2011) Discrete-time control for switched positive systems with application to mitigating viral escape. Int J Robust Nonlinear Control 21:93–111

Hoffmann C et al. (2007) HIV medicine. Flying Publishers, 2007. Available at http://hivmedicine.com/hivmedicine2007.pdf

Huang Y, Wu H, Acosta EP et al (2010) Hierarchical Bayesian inference for HIV dynamic differential equation models incorporating multiple treatment factors. Biom J 52:470–486

Israel-Ballard K, Ziermann R, Leutenegger C et al (2005) Taqman RT-PCR and versant HIV-1 RNA 3.0 (bDNA) assay quantification of HIV-1 RNA viral load in breast milk. J Clin Virol 34:253–256

Korenromp EL, Bakker R, de Vlas SJ et al (2002) HIV dynamics and behaviour change as determinants of the impact of sexually transmitted disease treatment on HIV transmission in the context of the Rakai trial. AIDS 16:2209–2218

Kupriyashkina M et al (2010) The effect of the grants from the global foundation on the policy in HIV/SPID in Ukraine. J Rak i Obshch 142(Suppl 24):7–12

Li MY et al (1996) A geometric approach to global-stability problems. J Math Anal 27(Suppl 4):1070–1083

Longini M, Clark WS, Byers RH et al (1989) Statistical analysis of the stages of HIV infection using a Markov model. Stat in Med 8:831–843

Luo R, Piovoso MJ, Martinezpicado J et al (2012) HIV model parameter estimates from interruption trial data including drug efficacy and reservoir dynamics. PLoS One 7:e40198

Markowitz M, Louie M, Hurley A et al (2003) A novel antiviral intervention results in more accurate assessment of human immunodeficiency virus type 1 replication dynamics and T-cell decay in vivo. J Virol 77:5037–5038

Mhawej MJ, Moog CH, Biafore F et al (2010) Control of the HIV infection and drug dosage. Biomed Signal Process Control 5:45–52

Morris M (1997) Sexual networks and HIV. AIDS 11(Suppl A):S209–S216

Morris M, Handcock MS, Miller WC et al (2006) Prevalence of HIV infection among young adults in the United States: results from the add health study. Am J Public Health 96:1091–1097

Naresh R, Tripathi A, Omar S et al (2006) Modelling the spread of AIDS epidemic with vertical transmission. Appl Math Comput 178:262–272

Newell ML et al (1998) Mechanism and timing of mother to child transmission ofHIV-1 J. AIDS 12:832–837

Nordic Medical Research Council's HIV Therapy Group (1992) Double blind dose-response study of zidovudine in AIDS and advanced HIV infection. BMJ 304:13–17

Nosova EA, Obukhova OV, Romanyukha AA et al (2010) HIV transmission and social disadaptation of the population in Russia *SPID*. Rak i Obshch Zd 14(Suppl 2):13–32

Palella FJ, Delaney KM et al (1998) Declining morbidity and mortality among patients with advanced human immunodeficiency virus infection. N Engl J Med 338(13):853–860

Pankavich S et al (2016) The effects of latent infection on the dynamics of HIV. Differ Equ Dyn Syst 24(Suppl 3):281–303

Perelson AS, Essunger P, Cao Y et al (1997) Decay characteristics of HIV-1-infected compartments during combination therapy. Nature 387:188–191

Phillips L, Potterat J, Rothenberg R et al (1980) Focused interviewing in gonorrhea control. Am J Public Health 70:705–708

Porco TC, Martin JN, Page-Shafer KA et al (2004) Decline in HIV infectivity following the introduction of highly active antiretroviral therapy. AIDS 18:81–88

Prud'homme IT, Kim JE, Pilon RG et al (1998) Amplicor HIV monitor, NASBA HIV-1 RNA QT and quantiplex HIV RNA version 2.0 viral load assays: a Canadian evaluation. J Clin Virol 11:189–202

Putter H, Heisterkamp SH, Lange JMA et al (2002) A Bayesian approach to parameter estimation in HIV dynamical models. Stat Med 21:2199–2214

Ramratnam BS, Bonhoeffer S, Binley J et al (1999) Rapid production and clearance of HIV-1 and hepatitis C virus assessed by large volume plasma apheresis. Lancet 354:1782–1785

Rivadeneira PS, Moog CH et al (2012) Impulsive control of single-input nonlinear systems with application to HIV dynamics. Appl Math Comput 18:8462–8474

Rivadeneira PS, Moog CH, Stan GB et al (2014) Mathematical modeling of HIV dynamics after antiretroviral therapy initiation: a clinical research study. AIDS Res Hum Retrovir 30:831–834

Royce RA, Sena A, Cates W, Cohen MS et al (1995) Sexual transmission of HIV new. Eng J Med 336(15):1072–1078

Sattenspiel L, Koopman J, Simon CP et al (1990) The effects of population structure on the spread of the HIV infection. Am J Phys Anthropol 82:421–429

Shim H, Han SJ, Chung CC et al (2003) Optimal scheduling of drug treatment for HIV infection: continuous dose control and receding horizon control. Int J Control Autom Syst 1:282–288

Simwa R, Pokhariyal GP et al (2008) A dynamical model for stage-specific HIV incidences with application to sub. Saharan Afr IJAMS 18(Suppl 4):184–189

Stan GB, Belmudes F, Fonteneau R et al (2008) Modelling the influence of activation-induced apoptosis of CD4+ and CD8+ T-cells on the immune system response of a HIV infected patient. IET Syst Biol 2:94–102

Tireito FA, Lawi GO, Kaka OA et al (2018) Mathematical analysis of HIV/AIDS prophylaxis treatment model. Appl Math Sci 12(Suppl 18):893–902

Vassena L, Proschan M, Fauci AS et al (2007) Interleukin 7 reduces the level of spontaneous apoptosis in CD4+ and CD8+ T cells from HIV-1 infected individuals. Proc Natl Acad Sci U S A 104:2355–2360

Vernazza PL, Gilliam BL, Dyer J et al (1997) Quantification of HIV in semen: correlation with antiviral treatment and immune status. AIDS 11:987–993

Wawer MJ, Gray RH, Sewankambo NK et al (2005) Rates of HIV-1 transmission per coital act, by stage of HIV-1 infection in Rakai Uganda. J Infect Dis 191:1403–1409

White RG, Orroth KK, Korenromp EL et al (2004) Can population differences explain the contrasting results of the Mwanza, Rakai, and Masaka HIV/sexually transmitted disease intervention trials: a modeling study. J Acquir Immune Defic Syndr 37:1500–1513

Williams BG, Lloyd-Smith JO, Gouws E et al (2006) The potential impact of male circumcision on HIV in sub-Saharan Africa. PLoS Med 3:1032–1040

Yang Y, Zou L, Ruan S et al (2015) Global dynamics of a delayed within-host viral infection model with both virus-to-cell and cell-to-cell transmissions. Math Biosci 270:183–191

Yüe FY, Kovacs CM, Dimayuga RC et al (2005) Preferential apoptosis of HIV-1 specific CD4+ T cells. J Immunol 174:2196–2204
Zhang X et al (2008) Backward bifurcation of an epidemic model with saturated treatment function. J Math Anal Appl 348(Suppl 1):433–443

Large Data Matrices: Random Walk Model and Application of Entropy in HIV Mother to Child Transmission (MTCT)

4

4.1 Introduction

Random walk model (RWM) is one of the important models that help to reduce massive data sets, which can be used for data reduction techniques (Brand et al. 1998; Hanley and McNeil 1982, 1983; Guisan et al. 2002; Fischer et al. 2002; Duba and Hart 1974; Dewar et al. 2003). In (RWM) formulated model, each variable of HIV mother to child transmission will reduce massive data sets without loss of any information (variables, namely, ARV prophylaxis at the time of onset and before birth of neonatal baby, prolonged breastfeeding, placental abruption and high RNA plasma viral load, drug-induced toxicity, HIV-associated illness, lower CD4 counts, WHO advanced clinical stage, opportunistic infections (OIs), etc., were taken randomly) (Agarwal et al. 1998; Ahuja et al. 1993; Andrijich et al. 2001; Artho et al. 2004). The main goal of highly active anti-retroviral therapy (HAART) infers to increase the length of longevity and sustain good quality of life (QOL)—improving their immune function (Hutchinson et al. 1957; Holdridge et al. 1997; Hirzel et al. 2002; Hershkovitz et al. 1998). This was achieved by reducing the large amount of replicating virus VL to as low as possible in all sites where HIV-infected cells are present, thereby preventing infection of new cells and further damage to the immune system. The amount of replicating virus in plasma can be assayed by measuring the concentration of HIV RNA, referred to as the viral load (VL) (Aspinall et al. 1993; Beggs and Plenz 2004; Cheng et al. 1999; Chaovaliwongse 2003; Busby et al. 1986; Brown and Lomolino 1974). In practice, increased trend of viral load (VL) has been observed in pregnant mothers when they are not adhered to the "HAART" treatment. In addition, consideration of a plan for salvage or second-line regimen is required if initial therapy fails. However, HIV is a deadly disease, and it requires a lifelong treatment (Blake et al. 1998; Bellingham et al. 2002; Beggs and Plenz 2004; Aspinall et al. 1993). Usually it is presumed that various parametric and non-parametric high-dimensional life data sets have been generated from the treatment follow-up records. Practically indeed, clinicians and researchers have been facing many problems while carrying out the analysis of high-dimensional data sets to draw the meaningful interpretations of the results to take

D. M. Basavarajaiah, B. Narasimha Murthy, *HIV Transmission*,
https://doi.org/10.1007/978-981-15-0151-7_4

appropriate and necessary clinical decisions about the population (Bellingham et al. 2002; Berry et al. 1997; Blake et al. 1998; Anderson et al. 2002). Many researchers and investigators have been using various techniques of data reduction by traditional methods, i.e., divergent analysis (DA), principal component analysis (PCA), factor analysis, etc. Many authors reported that the analytical intervention is a very essential domain to solve the realistic problems of HIV progression; this research gap will need to be tested and formulate new analytical mathematical models for smoothening of driven HIV data sets (Berry et al. 1997; Blake et al. 1998; Brand et al. 1998). In order to overcome these problems, the present chapter aims to fit random walk model for massive data sets on HIV mother to child transmission (MTCT), and also an attempt was made to explore the application of various entropy deviation methods (Busby et al. 1986; Chaovaliwongse et al. 2003; Cheng et al. 1989; Cormen et al. 2001; Dewar et al. 2003; Fischer et al. 2002).

4.2 Model Formulation

In HIV MTCT, apparently very unique structured and unstructured large data sets were generated from the patients' follow-up records (retrospective and prospective basis). The traditional theoretical data reduction techniques were fluctuating correlation values. The present chapter describes how we can reduce the large dimensional/ massive HIV data sets with complex situations. Know we have consider the correlation matrix 50 × 5 entries with random variables "X" ($X_{ij} =$ ith; CLHIVs were tested HIV at jth interval, the interval period j = tested at 1 week, 6 weeks, 12 weeks, 24 weeks, 36 weeks, 50 weeks, etc.). $1 \leq i \leq 50$, $1 \leq j \leq 5$ was assumed to be norm one vector α∗ (maximization of the variance number $\{\alpha, X_1\}_{i=1}^{56\text{ weeks}}$). The norm one vector was considered as the first principal component (PC), similarly vector a^{**} as the second PC, and so on. As per Wishart and Fisher, each "PC" observation was normally distributed with nxp matrix, and all observations are independent and identical in nature (*i.i.d*) (Tang et al. 2007).

The empirical distribution of the whole collection of singular values throughout of such matrix model is as follows: $P^{-1}\{\#\text{ eigen value} \leq \text{nt}\}$ an absolutely continuous functions. G (t), n, and $P \uparrow \infty$ were asymptotically increased with infinity values of $(\frac{n}{p} \rightarrow \gamma > 0)$. Although "H" will be assumed to be nxn real symmetrical matrix with i.i.d, Gaussian $N\left(1, \frac{1}{n}\right)$ entries with matrix family H_n (non-commutative random variable) were distributed in real expectation value $\mathcal{T}_n(H_n) = \frac{1}{n}\sum_{i=1}^{50\text{ weeks}} E(H_{nii}), \frac{1}{n}E(t_r, H_n)$, where "E" is $\mathcal{T}_n = \left(H_n{}^2\right) = 1$.

4.2.1 Theorem (1)

$(H_{\Lambda 2m}) \rightarrow 1/(m+1)(2m * m)$, Catalan numbers, as $n \uparrow \infty$ which are the $2m^{th}$ moments of the semicircle distribution density $\omega : \omega(x) = ([2\pi]\Lambda(-1)(4 - [x\Lambda 2]^{-1}))$ for $\| x \| \leq 2$ and $= 0$ other.

Proof A symmetrical real matrix nxp (with Gaussian assumptions) assumed only non-negative values of real vector; we have considered "H" is *nxn* random matrix with *i.i.d* N ~ (0, 1) entries of finite moments of all orders of $\lambda_1(H)$, $\lambda_2(H)$, ……λ_N(H). The random variables of each individual "H" observation (HIV tests) will be distributed with Gaussian families with real vectors 'δ'. The real vectors of Gaussian families were measured by $\frac{1}{n}[\delta(\lambda_1(H)) + \delta(\lambda_2)(H)) + \cdots + \delta(\lambda_n(H))]$. For each real vector, "δ" can reproduce the set of norm vectors δ^{**} by the law of semicircle distribution (SSD) and also can alienate long-standing effect of Eigen values with respect to expectation values of associated attributes (CLHIV diagnosis test). In order to reduce HIV massive data sets, we have assumed semicircle distribution law with density "ω" of H nxp matrix; the "H" would generate full-blown expectation values with norm vectors from the equation $\mu_H = \frac{1}{n}\mathbb{E}\left(\sum_{j=1}^{n}\delta_1\left(\lambda_j(H)\right)\right)$. However, in case if the real matrix has not been distributed *i.i.d* of Gaussian assumptions, the values of norm vector of δ^{**} will be derived from the following equation:

$$\int x^m \mu_H(x)\,dx = \frac{1}{n}\mathbb{E}\,tr(H^m) = \tau_n(H^m).$$

4.2.2 Theorem (2)

Let $\{H_n\}$ *be* the independent real symmetrical matrix with finite moments such that $\mathbb{E}\left(H_{n,ij}\right) = 0$ and $\mathbb{E}\left(H_{n,ij}^2\right) = \frac{1}{n}$ for $1 \le i \le j \le n$ if furthermore, $Sup_{1<i<j\le n}\mathbb{E} \mid H_{n,ij} \mid k = 0\left(n^{-\frac{k}{2}}\right)$ *for* each $k \in \mathbb{N}$ as $n \to \infty$

Proof μ_H is the mean Eigen value distribution of "H" that tends to the semicircle law; the way of interpreting result was $\{H_n\}$ is a family of non-co-commutative random variable with certain distribution family $\{\varphi_n\}$ (positive linear functional on the $* -$ *algebra* is generated by H and φ_n will converge to the semicircle law and weak $*$ topology) (Cheng et al. 1999; Cormen et al. 2001; Dewar et al. 2003; Guisan et al. 2002; Pulliam et al. 2000; Ponder et al. 2001; Phillips et al. 2004).

4.3 HIV Random Walk on Disease-Free Groups and Free Probability Model

A disease-free group population "Fn" will provide "nth" values of generation with free probability, viz., g_1, g_1, $\cdots g_n$ and $F_n = \sum_{i=1}^{n} gm^{-1}$ for the set of all individuals' "HIV"-infected children ("n" population). Overwhelmingly, the free probability will be considered as a random walk "Fn." The families of random walks started from the unit of one step, and it was moved from the group elements g with probability $(2n^{-1})$; if $h \in (\mathcal{g}_1, \mathcal{g}_1, \cdots \mathcal{g}_1{}^{-1} \ldots\ldots \mathcal{g}_m{}^{-1})$, then the probability of the return unit was "m" steps; the formulated equation becomes:

$$P(n, m) = P(n, m) = \frac{1}{(2n)^m}\left\langle\left(\sum\nolimits_{i-1}^{n} L\mathcal{g}_n^{-1}\right) m\delta_e, \delta_e\right\rangle,$$

However, the above model will explore the equation $L_2(G)$, $g \rightarrow L_g$ in a unitary representation of $(L_g, \xi)(g^1) = \xi(g^{-1}, g^1)$ for $\xi \in l^2(G)$ and δ_g. In data reduction of large HIV massive data sets, the fitted model would also explore the ideas of long-standing characteristic functions (CF) of the element "*g*". Finally, the representation of theoretical concept of the model was distributed in the form of $p(n, m) = 0$ if m is odd and n = disease free and m = infected odd (Fischer et al. 2002; Root et al. 1998; Reddy et al. 2003; Ratnaparkhi et al. 1998).

$p(n, 2m) = (2n)^{-2m} n^{-m} \left\langle\left(\sum\nolimits_{j=i\,week}^{50\,weeks} Xn, j\right) 2m, \delta e, \delta e\right\rangle$, where 2 m = odd (HIV infected at different intervals).

$X_{n,j} = \frac{1}{\sqrt{2}}\left(L\mathcal{g}_i + Lg_i{}^{-1}\right)$, asymptotic behavior as $n \rightarrow \infty$.

$p(n, m) \approx \frac{1}{(2n)^m}\frac{1}{(m+1)}\binom{2m}{m}$; as compared with theorem (Abello et al. 2002), the above equation was minimized by using central limit theorem (CL) of large entries of HIV data sets triggered by the diagnosis/testing of HIV at different defined time intervals like 1st week, 2nd week, 3rd week, and so on. The HIV diagnosis testing was tested by the following random variable equations:

$(X_{n1(i\,I\,week)}, X_{n2(II\,Week)}, X_{n3(III\,Week\,test\,done)}, \ldots\ldots X_{n(50\,Weeks)})$, was non-computing variables of HIV.

Then the above equation converges with semicircle law.

$\varphi(x) = \langle X\delta_e\delta_e\rangle$, than $X_{n,\,j}$, which could satisfy the following properties:

$$\varphi(P1X_n, i(1))P2X_n, i(2) \ldots\ldots\ldots Pk(X_n, i(k)) = 0$$

$$\varphi(x) = \sum_{i=1}^{n} p_k(X_n, i(k)) = 0$$

For all polynomial random variables, P_1, $P_2 \ldots\ldots P_K$ was driven with $\varphi(P1X_n, i(j)) = 0$ and $i(1) \neq i(2) \ldots\ldots \neq i(k)$ for non-commuting random variables, generated with finite entries (disease-free equilibrium). The successive random variables were distributed normally $N(\mu, \sigma^2)$ and *i.i.d's.* The family of P_1, $P_2 \ldots\ldots P_K$ strongly converges with weak topology of P (n, m).

4.4 Entropy in HIV Model Formulation

In contrast with above fitted model, we have considered the classical cases of random variables. $\xi_1, \xi_2 \ldots \xi_n$ is an independent and standard real Gaussian variable of "G" with open space $\mathbb{M}(\mathbb{R})$ of the probability measures $\mathbb{R}$ (with weak topology). The standard Gaussian's was measured in terms of $\vartheta \notin \overline{G}$; the probability gives rise to

$$\text{prob}\left(\text{the HIV testing measures at different interval } \frac{1}{n}\sum_{j=1}^{n}\delta_J(\xi_J)\in G\right)$$
$$\approx \exp(-n(v,G))$$

Where "G" is the subsets of prohibition measures with δ_J random variable.

Where $C(v,G) = \inf\{I(\mu):\mu\in G\}$ and $I(\mu)$ are denoted as the rate of HIV testing done at different time intervals (relative entropy)

$$I(\mu) = -\int p(x)\log p(x)dx + \frac{1}{2}\int x^2\mu(dx) + \frac{1}{2}\log 2x$$

$$-\int p(x)\log p(x)dx + \frac{1}{2} \quad \text{........ Entropy function.}$$

$$\frac{1}{2}\int x^2\mu(dx) + \frac{1}{2}\log 2x \text{ ---------------- Moments.}$$

and $\mu(dx) = p(x)dx$. The first part of the entropy of the weak topology converges by the Boltzmann-Gibbs entropy method $S(\mu) = -\int p(x)\log p(x)dx$.

The above theorem concludes that the probability of the large deviation from Gaussianity would decrease "nxp" entries, and their coefficients were multiplied with real Gaussianity of weak topology (an infimum of an expression) (Abello 2002). Although the large deviation of HIV testing was done among newborn individuals derived from the real Gaussian entries, the manner of expression was fitted by the following equation (Fisher 1939; Dewar et al. 2003; Zweig and Campbell 1993; Wu et al. 1999; Welk et al. 2002; Wagenaar et al. 2005; Stoppini et al. 1991).

$\text{Prob}\left\{\frac{1}{n}\sum_j \delta\delta(\lambda_j(H_n)\in G\right\} \approx e^{-n^2C(\omega,g)}$, for each entropy will follow *i.i.d* and $\frac{n}{n}$ with real matrix, where "G" is an open set $\mathbb{M}(\mathbb{R})$ which has not been distributed to the semicircle law ω and $C(\omega,G) = \text{Inf}\{I(\mu)/\mu \in G\}$ with

$$I(\mu) = -\frac{1}{2}\iint \log|x-y|\mu(dx)\mu(dy) + \frac{1}{4}\int x^2\mu(dx) + \text{constant}$$

In the analogy of the classical cases, the equation becomes $S^f(\mu) = -\frac{1}{2}\int\int \log|x-y|\mu(dx)\mu(dy)$ as the HIV non tested free entropy. As per the model equation, the important key points were noted that the probability of the empirical Eigen values was distributed in different forms with semicircle law of large numbers exp $(-n^2C(\omega,G)$ in association with different classical cases. The probability of "large deviation" of random set of observations, the equations will become $\exp(-n^2C(v,G)$[14].

4.5 Model Proof

HIV mother to child transmission (MTCT) is a scourge. The valid treatment is an important factor to prevent HIV geometric progression; MTCT rate increases due to high RNA plasma viral load, prolonged duration of labor and delivery, etc. Mother with high plasma viral load between 5000 and 185,000 copies per ml will be more likely to transmit HIV to her young ones; child transmission was more likely to occur during labor and delivery period. However, the frequency of transmission rate was distributed very less; the PLHIVs expressed undetectable viral load (VL). In addition to that, the PLHIV mother who has not received ARV prophylaxis at the time of pregnancy at onset and before birth, prolonged breastfeeding, placental abruption, drug-induced toxicity, illness, lower CD4 count, etc. will be more favorable parameters to transfer HIV MTCT (transmission rate was traumatically increased). In this context, the present fitted model will provide a suitable analytical approach for simulation of HIV MTCT at long standing entries of nxp matrix. We have considered the linear model in the form of $y = H_x + n$, where "x" is K input variables of children who underwent HIV testing at different time intervals and "y" is the "N" large-dimensional output vector (n is the N output results reactive or non-reactive) (Hershkovitz et al. 1998; Hirzel et al. 2002). Since the family of the observations was distributed orthogonally with symmetrical Gaussianity, "H" can also permit the complex values of random input *NXK* matrix with continuous long-standing entries of random variables *rv*. Similarly, the "K" is the number of HIV-transmitted children, and "N" is the same fraction of HIV infection received from mother side at varied time interval in the form of long-standing entries of K = ≠ of not HIV reactive and N = the HIV reactive/infection (Holdridge et al. 1997; Hutchinson et al. 1957).

Obviously, the first "H" denoted propagation coefficient on each reactive and non-reactive pairs of the observations accordingly. For trivial changes of each entropy, H should follow the above equation (concurred on the HIV transmission/ not transmission coefficient) $K = n_T J$, $n = nR_G$ with n_T and n_R (test done and test not done algorithms received from children) and J and g are the number of ANCs for simulation of HIV fraction at larger population size. In spite of the HIV-infected mothers who did not receive a single dose of NVP at the time of labor, the proportion of infection rate increases. In the present fitted model, the entries of H are *'i.i.d'* obtained are realistically true and accurate; the model was distributed with $\mathrm{F}_{\mathrm{A}}^{\mathrm{N}}(\mathrm{x}) = \frac{1}{n}\sum_{j=1}^{N} \mathrm{X}(\lambda_j(\mathrm{A}) \leq \mathrm{x})$ so that, the family of equations were distributed in the form of $\mathrm{F}_{\mathrm{HH*}}^{\mathrm{N}}(\mathrm{x}) - \mathrm{Ne}(\mathrm{X}) = \mathrm{KF}_{\mathrm{HH*}}^{\mathrm{N}}(\mathrm{x}) - \mathrm{Ne}(\mathrm{X})$, where θ is a heavy side function, this was generated non-zero Eigen values of HH∗ and h∗ H; it was expressed in terms of homogeneity.

4.6 Summary

The random walk model and application of entropy will be able to compile and reduce high-dimensional data sets without loss of any information. This method would be more useful for large data sets having distributed with weak law of large numbers that also strongly converge with high density. Another important aspect of this method, the HIV data sets do not fluctuate at the inception of model, whose results are easy to be interpreted by semicircle law of large numbers. Fitted model will undergo further algebraic and mathematical treatment at population level.

References

Abello PM, Pardalos MG, Resende C et al (2002) Handbook of massive data sets. Kluwer Academic Publishers, Norwell

Agarwal R, Gehrke JD, Raghaven P et al (1998) Automatic subspace clustering of high dimensional data for data mining. ACM Sigmod 27(Suppl 2):94–105

Ahuja RK, Magnanti TL, Orlin JB et al (1993) Network flows- theory on algorithm and applications, vol 185. Prentice Hall, Englewood Cliffs, pp 1851–1856

Anderson RP, Gomez-Laverde M, Peterson AT (2002) Geographical distributions of spiny pocket mice in South America: insights from predictive models. Glob Ecol Biogeogr 11:131–141

Andrijich SM, Caccetta L et al (2001) Solving the multisensor data association problem. J Nonlinear Analysis 47:5525–5536

Artho P, Hirase H, Monoconduit L, Zugaro M et al (2004) Characterization of neocortical principal cells and interneurons by network interactions and extracellular features. J Neurophys 92:600–608

Aspinall R et al (1993) An inductive modeling procedure based on Bayes' theorem for analysis of pattern in spatial data. Int J Geogr Inf Syst 6(2):105–121

Beggs JM, Plenz D (2004) Neuronal avalanches are diverse and precise activity patterns that are stable for many hours in cortical slice cultures. J Neurosci 24:5216–5229

Bellingham J, Richards A et al (2002) Receding horizon control of autonomous aerial vehicles. In: Proceedings of the American control conference, Anchorage, AK, pp 8–10

Berry MJ, Lino G et al (1997) Data mining techniques for marketing, sales and customer support. Wiley, New York

Blake CL, Merz CJ et al (1998) UCI repository of machine learning databases

Brand M et al (1998) Pattern discovery via entropy minimization, Uncertainty 99: Inter-national workshop on artificial intelligence and statistics. IJMS 98:21–25

Brown JH, Lomolino MV Biogeography, 2nd edn. Sinauer Associates, Sunderland

Busby JR (1986) A biogeographical analysis of Nothofagus cunninghamii (Hook.) Oerst. in southeastern Australia. Aust J Ecol 11:1–7

Chaovaliwongse W (2003) Optimization and dynamical approaches in nonlinear time series analysis with applications in Bioengineering. Ph.D Thesis. University of Florida

Cheng C, Fu AW, Zhang Y et al (1999) Entropy-based subspace clustering for mining numerical data. In: Proceedings of international conference on knowledge discovery and data mining 18:84–93

Cormen T, Leiserson C, Rivest L (2001) Introduction to algorithms. MIT Press, Cambridge

Dewar R et al (2003) Information theory explanation of the fluctuation theorem, maximum entropy production and self-organized criticality in non-equilibrium stationary states. J Phys A Math Gen 36:631–641

Duba RO, Hart PE (1974) Pattern classification and scene analysis. Wiley-Interscience, New York

Fischer Y, Wittner L, Freund TF, Gahwiler BH (2002) Simultaneous activation of gamma and theta network oscillations in rat hippocampal slice cultures. J Physiol Lond 539:857–868
Fisher RA (1939) The sampling distribution of some statistics obtained from nonlinear equations. Ann Eugenics 9:238–249
Guisan A, Edwards TC, Hasti T (2002) Generalized linear and generalized additive models in studies of species distributions: setting the scene. Ecol Model 157:89–100
Hanley J, McNeil B (1982) The meaning and use of the area under a receiver operating characteristic (ROC) curve. Radiology 143:29–36
Hanley J, McNeil B (1983) A method of comparing the areas under receiver operating characteristic curves derived from the same cases. Radiology 148:839–843
Hershkovitz P et al (1998) Report on some sigmodontine rodents collected in southeastern Brazil with descriptions of a new genus and six new species. Bonner zoologische Beitrage 47:193–256
Hirzel AH, Hausser J, Chessel D, Perrin N (2002) Ecological niche factor analysis: how to compute habitat-suitability maps without absence data? Ecology 87:2027–2036
Holdridge L, Grenke W, Hatheway W, Liang T, Tosi J Jr (1997) Forest Environments. In: Tropical life zones: a pilot study. Pergamon Press, New York
Hutchinson GE et al (1957) Concluding remarks. In: Cold spring harbor symposia on quantitative biology 22:415–427
Phillips SJ, Dud'ık M, Schapire RE (2004) A maximum entropy approach to species distribution modeling. In: Proceedings of the 21st international conference on machine learning. ACM Press, New York 45:655–662
Ponder WF, Carter GA, Flemons P, Chapman RR (2001) Evaluation of museum collection data for use in biodiversity assessment. Conserv Biol 15:648–657
Pulliam HR et al (2000) On the relationship between niche and distribution. Ecol Lett 3:349–361
Ratnaparkhi A et al (1998) Maximum entropy models for natural language ambiguity resolution. Ph.D. Thesis. University of Pennsylvania, Philadelphia
Reddy S, Davalos LM et al (2003) Geographical sampling bias and its implications for conservation priorities in Africa. J Biogeogr 30:1719–1727
Root T et al (1998) Environmental factors associated with avian distributional boundaries. J Biogeogr 15:489–505
Stoppini L, Buchs PA, Muller D (1991) A simple method for organotypic cultures of nervous tissue. J Neurosci Methods 37:173–182
Tang A, Jackson D, Hobbs J, Chen W, Smith J, Patel H, Beggs JM (2007) Asecond-order maximum entropy model predicts correlated network states, but not their evolution over time (Computational and systems neuroscience, Salt Lake City) Abstract II-62
Wagenaar DA, Madhavan R, Pine J, Potter SM (2005) Controlling bursting with closed-loop multi-electrode stimulation. J Neurosci 25:680–688
Welk E, Schubert K, Hoffmann M et al (2002) Present and potential distribution of invasive mustard (Alliara petiolata) in North America. Divers Distrib 8:219–233
Wiley EO, McNyset KM, Peterson AT, Robins CR, Stewart AM (2003) Niche modeling and geographic range predictions in the marine environment using a machine-learning algorithm. Oceanography 16(3):120–127
Williams PM et al (1995) Bayesian regularization and pruning using a Laplace prior. Neural Comput 7(1):117–143
Wu JY, Guan L, Tsau Y (1999) Propagating activation during oscillations and evoked responses in neocortical slices. J Neurosci 19:5005–5015
Zaniewski AE, Lehmann A, Overton JM (2002) Predicting species spatial distributions using presence-only data: a case study of native New Zealand ferns. Ecol Model 157:261–280
Zweig MH, Campbell G (1993) Receiver-operating characteristic (ROC) plots: a fundamental evaluation tool in clinical medicine. Clin Chem 39(4):561–577

Statistical Models of Postnatal Transmission of HIV Type-I Infection from Mother to Child on Global Perspectives

5

5.1 Introduction

About 5.0 millions of Indians suffer from HIV; the retention rate was <10–15%. Though experimental results have shown the transitions between postnatal transmission and survivability of PLHIVs, little is known about the dynamism of progression of HIV and transmission probability. Therefore, the present chapter demonstrated various statistical models for estimation of HIV postnatal transmission at population level. The incidence rate of postnatal transmission and HIV survival rate of ANCs data was extracted from database of "ART" Karnataka CMIS (obtained from the State AIDS control organization). The models were built for the likelihood estimation and size of the population under the age of 15 years; the data was obtained from ART on monthly intervals, starting from 2005 to 2018. The non-AIDS mortality rate and annual number of births to mothers, who are on HIV-positive and HIV-negative data sets, were originally extracted from the ASSA AIDS database source, and also the demographic data sets were obtained from the patient pre-ART registration card, and ASSA model is a widely used model for estimation of geometric progression of HIV epidemic at population level (Department of AIDS control, 2008). This model will allow for the estimation of incidence of HIV in different modes. Children under the age of 15 years, the transmission from infected mothers on or before birth (intrapartum or intrauterine transmission) and transmission from infected mothers after birth, as a result of breastfeeding (Koepsell and Weiss 2003). In the absence of PMTCT, women who are HIV seropositive at the time of their first antenatal screening were assumed to have an average probability of transmitting the virus at delivery equal to 0.20 (Kuhn et al. 2005) with the probability varying according to the mothers' CD4 count (Homsy et al. 2009). In the absence of PMTCT, women who are HIV seropositive at the time of delivery are assumed to be HIV transmission probability. If the woman acquires HIV while breastfeeding, a higher transmission probability was assumed to apply during the acute phase that follows HIV acquisition reported (Reynolds et al. 2006). PLHIVs who are initiated highly active ART

D. M. Basavarajaiah, B. Narasimha Murthy, *HIV Transmission*,
https://doi.org/10.1007/978-981-15-0151-7_5

(HAART) during pregnancy are assumed to have ($p = 0.03$), the probability of transmitting the virus to their infant at birth. It was assumed that 50% of women, who have received positive test results, elect to formula feed, 45.6% initially practice exclusive breastfeeding (which is assumed to reduce the risk of transmission per month of breastfeeding), and the remaining practiced mixed feeding from birth, for a median duration of 8–10 months (Lawn et al. 2006). In women who know themselves to be positive and elect to practice exclusive breastfeeding (EBF), the median duration of EBF is assumed to be 4 months, after which women either practice abrupt weaning or switch to mixed feeding (Lingappa et al. 2010). If women receive "HAART" while breastfeeding, the monthly postnatal transmission risk is assumed to be reduced by 86%. If the mother does not receive HAART while breastfeeding, but the infant receives extended nevirapine prophylaxis, the rate of transmission is assumed to be reduced by 60% (Lisse et al. 1997).

5.2 Model Formulation

The model produces estimates of the annual mortality probability of children aged "a" (in years) in year "t." The pediatric HIV model includes the growth of the population at monthly intervals, and it is therefore necessary to convert the annual mortality probability into a monthly mortality rate (Lingappa et al. 2009). For children aged 1 year and older, the monthly mortality rate was assumed to be one twelfth of the annual mortality rate, i.e., at "q."

$$-\frac{1}{12}\ln\left(1-\text{qat}\right) \tag{5.1}$$

However, children under the age of 1 year, the annual mortality probability was maximum, and much of the mortality risk was focused in the 1st month of life. Therefore we have to follow the approach of (Lisse et al. 1997; Moodley et al. 1997; Mugo et al. 2011). Weibull distribution model was fitted to calculate the monthly failure or mortality rate from the infant mortality rate in the "ASSA" model (Minkoff et al. 2003). Suppose we had "c r" and "b" which are the rate and shape of the parameters for Weibull distribution. In this chapter, we have described the survival was up to 12 months of age, i.e., the proportion of infants surviving to age "a" (in years) is as follows:

$$\exp\left(-\text{rab}\right) \tag{5.2}$$

Suppose that $q0t$ and $q01t$ represent the infant and neonatal mortality rates, respectively, in year t, i.e., the probabilities of death by 12 months and 1 month, respectively. Then

$$q0t = 1 - \exp(-r) \tag{5.3}$$

$$qo1t = 1 - \exp[(-r(1/12)b] \tag{5.4}$$

From which it follows that

$$r = -\ln(1 - qot) \tag{5.5}$$

$$b = \ln\left[\frac{\ln(1 - q01t)}{\ln(1 - qot)}\right]\left[\ln\frac{1}{12}\right]^{-1} \tag{5.6}$$

Substituting the values of $q0\ t$ and $q0\ t$ estimated from (Mayanja et al. 2004) (0.0454 and 0.0198, respectively, for births in the preceding 5 years) gives $r = 0.0265$ and $b = 0.43$. For convenience, we can use this value of "b" for all years, although the parameter might be expected to vary slightly over time. This makes it possible to estimate the monthly survival probabilities (ignoring AIDS mortality) in each year, given only the "$q0t$" values estimated by the ASSA model and the assumed value of $b = 0.43$.

5.3 Intrauterine and Intrapartum Transmission

This section begins with a review of estimates of mother-to-child transmission at birth; many authors have reported intrauterine and intrapartum transmission (Morrison et al. 2007; Minkoff et al. 2003; Moodley et al. 1997) in the absence of any intervention and the effects of short-course antiretroviral prophylaxis (ARV), as well as antiretroviral treatment (ART) initiated for the mothers own health with CD4 count >250 μ/dl (Matthews and Mukherjee 2009; Mmeje et al. 2012). Evidence on the probability of vertical transmission from mothers, who acquire HIV in late pregnancy, is also reviewed by (Natu 2007). Single-dose NVP was given to the mother after birth for the interval 1–6 h.

5.4 Transmission Probability at or Before Birth, in the Absence of ARV Prophylaxis

Although, there have been several studies in India that have estimated the proportion of pregnant women, who transmit HIV to their children before or soon after birth, it is difficult to estimate the proportion of children who are infected intrauterine/intrapartum. This is because the PCR test typically does not yield a positive result until 12 weeks after HIV transmission has occurred (Department of AIDS control, 2008). It is therefore necessary to wait for at least a month before one can reliably identify almost all of the infants who have been infected before or at birth (Natu 2007). However, over this time period, some infants will have acquired HIV through breastfeeding and might also be PCR-positive at the time of testing (Morrison et al.

2007). This makes it difficult to identify the infants, who were truly infected at or before birth. It is possible to estimate the proportion of children who become infected at or before birth, based on what is known about the rate of transmission through breast milk and the rate at which newly infected infants develop detectable virus. In the present chapter, we consider $R(a)$ the proportion of infants born to HIV-positive mothers, who test positive at age "a" (in months) on a "PCR" test and further suppose that "π" is the proportion of infants, who acquire HIV at or before birth, in the absence of any antiretroviral drug (ARV), and also the model was consider "f' is the proportion of HIV-positive mothers, who formula feed exclusively $\beta(a)$ and the probability of breastfed child acquires HIV postnatal and has PCR-detectable virus by age "a" is equal to

$$R(a) = \pi + (1 - \pi)(1 - f)\beta(a) \tag{5.7}$$

It was assumed that the infants that were infected at or before birth have PCR-detectable virus by age a (this would generally be the case for $a \geq 1.5$). From this it follows that

$$\pi = \frac{R(a) - (1 - f)\beta(a)}{1 - (1 - f)\beta(a)} \tag{5.8}$$

Assumed, breastfed infants acquire HIV at rate "h," and newly infected infants develop PCR-detectable virus at rate γ. Then the model becomes

$$\beta(a) = \int_0^a h \exp(-\mathrm{ht})(1 - \exp(-\gamma(a - t)) \, \mathrm{dt} \tag{5.9}$$

$$1 - \frac{\gamma \exp(-\mathrm{ha}) - h \ \exp(-\gamma a)}{r - h} \tag{5.10}$$

The parameters "h" and "γ" have been estimated to be $0.014 \times 1/12$ and 2.0 per month, respectively (see Eq. 5.31). In all of the studies that were considered, "a" is 1.5 months and hence is 0.012, which relate only to women who were not receiving any antiretroviral prophylaxis. Similar studies by Mugo et al. (2011), Moodley et al. (1997), Lingappa et al. (2009), and Matthews and Mukherjee (2009) reported that the average estimate of the proportion of infants, who acquire HIV intrauterine or intrapartum, is 19.7% only fractionally lower than the proportion of infants who have detectable virus at the age of 4–6 weeks.

5.5 Model Results

Since rates of vertical transmission of HIV are dependent on the maternal CD_4 count and uptake of "HAART" relative to short-course ARV drugs will depend on the pregnant woman's CD_4 count, it is necessary to estimate rates of vertical transmission that would be expected in each CD_4 stage and to re-express the effect of the short-course ARV regimens in terms of percentage reductions in transmission. This is based on review of CD_4 distributions in pregnant, HIV-ANCs, and relative rates of vertical transmission in different CD_4 intervals. In the present chapter, it was demonstrated that the average rate of transmission at or before birth, in the absence of "PMTCT," was 46.0%, if the mother has a CD_4 count less than 100–200 μ/dL;19.80%, if the mother has a CD_4 count of 201 to <250 μ/dL; 8.60%, if the mother has a CD_4 count of 251–350 μ/dL; 2.5%, if the mother has a CD_4 count greater than >500 μ/dL; and 1.4%, if the mother has a CD_4 count >500 μ/dL. The proportions of ANCs in the CD_4 <200, 200–349, 350–500, and >500 categories were estimated to be 14.0%, 24.9%, 24.5%, and 36.6%, respectively (Reynolds et al. 2006). Single-dose nevirapine has been assumed to reduce the transmission probability by 40% and when combined with AZT from 28 weeks (previous guidelines NACO) assumed to reduce the probability by 80%. The efficacy of "AZT" drug was alone and assumed to be 35%. And also it was assumed that the percentage reduction due to short-course ARV prophylaxis is the same regardless of the maternal CD_4 count, as there is little consistency in the relationship between efficacy and CD_4 count between different studies which were reported by Pattanapanyasat and Thakar (2005), Padmapriyadarshini et al. (2009), (Shah, eds) etc (Tables 5.1 and 5.2) (Figs. 5.1 and 5.2).

Table 5.1 Proportions of infants infected at 4–6 weeks after birth to mothers on HAART

Timing of HAART initiation	HAART initiation criteria	No. of ANC's cases	% HIV+
At 28 weeks	None	532	1.1%
Before conception	CD4 <250, WHO stage III/IV	118	0.0%
During pregnancy	CD4 <200, WHO stage IV, CD4 <350 + stage III	107	1.0%
During pregnancy	None	809	0.8%
During pregnancy	CD4 <250, WHO stage IV	495	2.8%

Table 5.2 Probability of transmitting of HIV from mother to child in Bangalore city

Antenatal care	Probability of transmission determined from fitted model
HIV seropositive at 1st antenatal visit, no prophylaxis	0.621
Receiving single-dose nevirapine	0.140
Receiving AZT from 28 weeks	0.338
Receiving single-dose nevirapine and AZT from 28 weeks	0.245
Receiving highly active HAART – started during pregnancy	0.446
HIV seronegative at 1st ANC visit	0.743
Not receiving ARV prophylaxis	0.845

Included in the uncertainty analysis (Mean of 0.35, standard deviation 0.08)

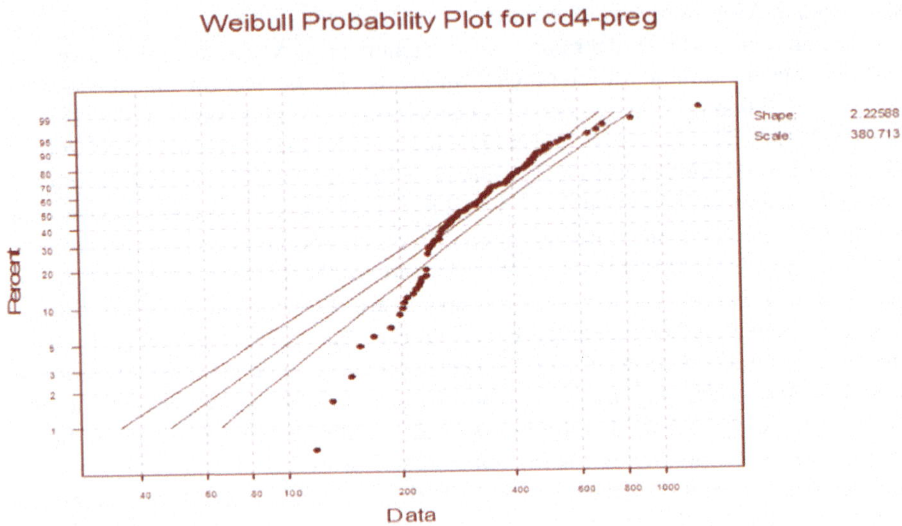

Fig. 5.1 Probability plot for baseline CD4 count at the time of HAART initiation

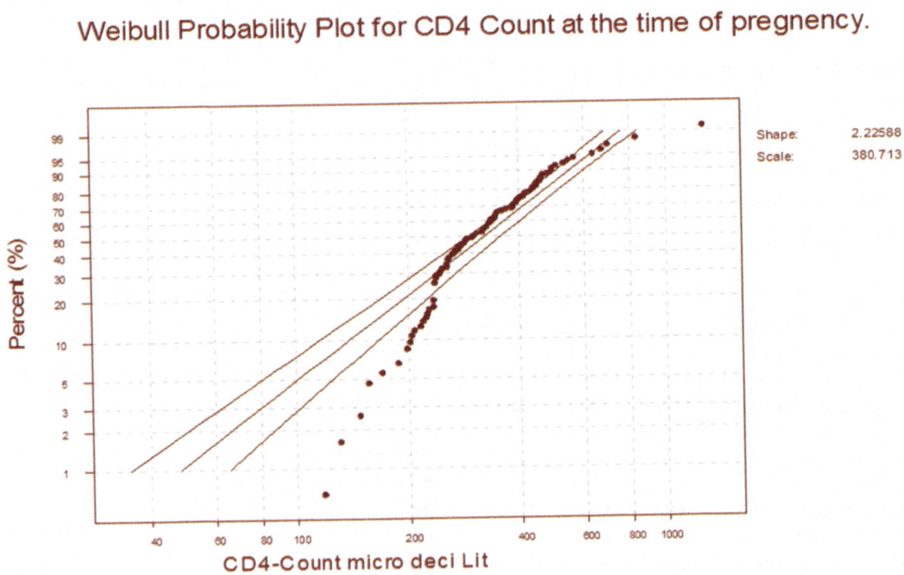

Fig. 5.2 Probability plot for CD4 count at the time of pregnancy

5.6 Model Discussion

Demographic profile: a total of 78% were illiterate; 63.35% were below poverty line; and 10.65% were in high-income group. The mean age of the ANCs was 24.65 ± 4.8 years (IQR 21.25–26.14). About 25% of pregnant women's families migrated from other parts of the state for seasonal employment, and 80% of the patients were heterosexual. Primigravida was 55.26% and gravida II 13.26% and the remaining were gravida III. A total of 82.36% of patients' husband had seroconversion. Mean baseline CD_4 count was 116.35 ± 56.25 μ/dL (CI 95%;102.23–123.65%) before inception of HAART. Increasing trend of CD_4 count was found after 1 year completion of HAART therapy, and at the onset of pregnancy, CD_4 count mean was 289 ± 45.22 μ/dL (CI95% 265.20–301.28%). Shah (2007) reported that CD_4 cell counts <100 μ/dL at the time of inception of HAART can get better chance of transmission of HIV from mother to child. This analysis suggests that the level of HIV prevalence in children and the unmet need for ART in children are substantially greater (Universal access to AIDS treatment, 2010). A similar study was reported by (Van der Paal et al. (2007). In part, this is because most other models have assessed the rate of mother-to-child transmission using the HIV prevalence in pregnant women at their first antenatal screening and have ignored the very significant ($p < 0.001$) vertical transmission that can occur in women, who seroconvert after their first antenatal visit, either before delivery or while breastfeeding (World health organization, 2002).

The high HIV prevalence rate was estimated by present fitted model; it is partly due to the lower rate of AIDS mortality, particularly in children who acquire HIV at or before birth. Although it is possible that our model estimates of AIDS mortality rates are understated, the estimates are projected based on empirical data and assuming significantly ($p < 0.001$) higher AIDS mortality rates would result in model estimates of pediatric HIV prevalence lower than those observed in the high-risk groups (HRGs) household surveys. Watanabe et al. (1996) studied the HIV prevalence levels measured between 2005 and 2008 household surveys; it would be exaggerated by false-positive reactions, since confirmatory testing of all reactive specimens was conducted in both surveys. It is also unlikely that the high levels of pediatric HIV prevalence observed in the HRGs' surveys would be due to nosocomial transmission ($p < 0.001$). This analysis suggests that the "PMTCT" program in India has already had a significant impact on HIV incidence and that the recent adoption of new "PMTCT" protocols 2012 is expected to lead roughly 60% reduction in pediatric HIV incidence by 2015. Further reductions in HIV incidence could be achieved through better implementation of existing protocols. However, a significant problem is the high proportion of vertical transmission occurring from mothers, who are recently seroconverted and are undiagnosed. New interventions will need to be developed to address these problems. Our fitted model is best fit for the estimation of diseases progression of "MTCT," mortality of ANCs, and epidemic status of "HIV" progression.

5.7 HIV Vertical Transmission Statistical Model-Model Description

Mother-to-child transmission indicates that transfer of virus is from HIV-positive mother to newborn baby (Van der Paal et al. 2007; Shah 2006; Padmapriyadarshini et al. 2009; Pattanapanyasat and Thakar 2005; Matthews and Mukherjee 2009; Agarwal et al. 2008; Mugo et al. 2011; Gray et al. 2005). This can occur during pregnancy, labor and delivery, or breastfeeding. Usually 5–20% of children will be infected through breastfeeding. It is known that 15–30% of newborn babies delivered by HIV-positive women will be infected (Mugo et al. 2011). In 2015, globally around 700,000 children less than 15 years of age were infected with HIV, mainly through mother-to-child transmission (Mayanja et al. 2004). The high prevalence of HIV infections in many developing countries has give rise to increasing concern about the risk of transmitting the virus through breastfeeding. In a recent review, breastfeeding is recognized as an important cause of mother-to-child transmission (MTCT) and accounts for 7–14% of the overall transmission rate. However, so far there have been no changes to policies, which advocate that "breast is best" in the health profession, even where HIV infection rates are known to be high (Mugo et al. 2011). Due to many perceived physiological and psycho-social advantages of breastfeeding compared to feeding with infant formula milks, as well as awareness of the risks of diarrhea and associated mortality (which are even more pronounced in emergency situations), where formula feeds are used. Yet there is unease among some health professionals and policymakers about this subject, as in areas where HIV infection is highly prevalent, there is a significant risk that breast milk will be the medium through which the deadly virus is passed. India's one-third of infants born to HIV-positive mothers contract HIV through mother-to-child transmission and become infected during their mothers' pregnancy, childbirth, or breastfeeding. In 2015, 80,000 children under the age of 15 contracted HIV, over 90% of them through mother-to-child transmission of HIV (MTCT). Between 15% and 25% of children born to HIV-infected mothers get infected with HIV during pregnancy or delivery, while about 15% of the children get infected through breastfeeding (Natu 2007).

5.8 Formulation of the Model

The prospective and retrospective secondary data sets were obtained from ART centers in Karnataka during 2009–2013. Structured questionnaires were used to obtain the primary information on physical, psychological, level of independence and environmental factors, which influence on mothers, who are exposed to breastfeeding in infants. The laboratory parameters like baseline CD_4 count at the time of inception of HAART and successive serial CD_4 counts at 6 months, 1 year, 24 months, etc. were documented. WHO clinical stage anthropometric parameter, status of gravida, clinical history, adverse drug reactions and treatment failure, ARV prophylaxis at the onset of pregnancy, and infant delivery were systematically documented at greater accuracy and less SE. The propounded parameters were analyzed by using SPSS-16.50 version software. The chi-square 2×2 contingency, specificity, and sensitivity test was employed to know the actual predicted prevalence rate of "MTCT" through breastfeeding. Retrospective and prospective data sets were obtained from "ART" center of Karnataka; demographic, clinical profile, ADV, and SDV drug reaction data were extracted from white cards and patients' green books; follow-up CD_4 count at 6 months and 12 months was recorded in a separate master chart.

5.9 Poisson Distribution Model

A random variable "X" (HIV-infected mother) can follow Poisson distribution, if it assumes only non-negative values; the probability density function (PDF) was formulated as follows:

$$P(X = x) = \sum_{i=1}^{N=100 \text{ HIV infected mother}} \frac{e^{-\lambda i} \lambda i^{xi}}{xi!} \tag{5.11}$$

where:

xi= number of babies infected from their mother over a period of time
λi = mean and variance of the parameters
e= exponential term ($e = 2.71$)

The relative risk of infection rate will be largely distributed over a period of time; the Eq. (5.10) tends to normal approximation (Table 5.3):

$$x_i \tilde{N}(n, p) \tag{5.12}$$

The above fitted model, the margin $n + 1$, $n + 2$ is fixed numbers, and counts n_{11}, n_{12} are random variables having the following distribution:

Table 5.3 Relative risk of infected mother-associated parameters was tested by using 2 × 2 contingency models

Sl. No.	Variables	(D) Baby HIV infected	($\overline{D}$) Baby HIV not infected	Total
1.	With breastfeeding(E)	n_{11}	n_{12}	$n_{11} + n_{12}$
2.	Without breastfeeding ($\overline{E}$)	n_{21}	n_{22}	$n_{21} + n_{22}$
	Total	$(n + 1)$	$(n + 2)$	(N)

$$n_{11}\left\{\text{Bin }(n+1, p\left[\frac{E}{D}\right], n_{12}\tilde{\text{Bin}}(n+1, \left[\frac{E}{\overline{D}}\right]\right\} \quad (5.13)$$

The relative risk of HIV MTCT was calculated by following formula:

$$\psi = \sum_{I=1}^{n}\left\{\widehat{P}\left(\frac{D}{E}\right)|\widehat{P}\left(\frac{D}{\overline{E}}\right)\right\} \quad (5.14)$$

where $\widehat{P}\left(\frac{D}{E}\right) = \frac{n_{11}}{n_{11}+n_{12}}$, and $\widehat{P}\left(\frac{D}{\overline{E}}\right) = \frac{n_{21}}{n_{21}+n_{22}}$

Hypothesis testing. the predicted HIV MTCT risk factors were tested by using null hypothesis

$H_o = \pi_1, \pi_2 = \ldots\pi_k$. This is equivalent to $H_o = \text{Sin}^{-1}\sqrt{\pi_k}$

If $\text{p}_\text{i} = \frac{x_i}{n_i}$ is the sample proportion of infected mother in responding to complications at i^{th} intervalTest statistics, $\text{Sin}^{-1}\sqrt{\text{p}_\text{i}}\tilde{N}\left(\text{Sin}^{-1}\sqrt{\text{p}_\text{i}}, \frac{1}{4n_i}\right)$

$$\tau_n = \sum_{i=1}^{N=\text{HIV infected mother}} 4n_i\left(\text{Sin}^{-1}\sqrt{\text{p}_\text{i}} - \overline{A_P}\right)2 \quad (5.15)$$

where $\overline{A_P} = \frac{\sum_{i=1}^{N=\text{HIV infected mother}} 4n_i(\text{Sin}^{-1}\sqrt{\text{p}_\text{i}}}{\sum_{i=1}^{n} n_i}$ is distributed with $(k - 1)$ df

Positive predicted value of HIV MTCT with respect to risk factors was calculated by the

$$\text{PPV}(\%) = \frac{n_{11}}{(n_{11}+n_{12})} \times 100 \text{ Specificity } (\%) = \frac{n_{22}}{(n_1+n_{22})} \times 100$$

$$\text{NPV }(\%) = \frac{n_{22}}{(n_{21}+n_{22})} \times 100$$

The null hypothesis was tested $\tau_n > \chi^2$, $(k - 1)$df rejects the null hypothesis (Table 5.4)

Four focus group, eight direct, and two in-depth interviews were conducted with written consent; collected numerical data were transformed into Epi info software and analyzed by suitable test statistics. As per the analysis, the mean age of the patients was 24.58 ± 1.50 years, CI-95%, 22.99–26.52 ($p < 0.05$). Age groups were classified based on the mean ± 0.5 SD and mean ±1SD. (Table 5.3) it was showed that the age between 18 and 25 years (85.0%; $p < 0.05$), 26–32 years (15.0%; $p > 0.05$), Marital status; Married, 87% (CI 95% −83.25–88.92, $p < 0.05$), Unmarried, 3.00% (CI 95% 0.80–4.26 $p > 0.05$), Discordant couple, 8.0% (CI 95%-5.06–9.22, $p > 0.05$), Unknown, 2.0% (CI 95% 0.96–3.08, $p > 0.05$). The same study reported by Thamatoor et al. examined the individual and district level variables that could characterize HIV positivity among ANCs across 24 districts in

Table 5.4 Demographic features of HIV-infected pregnant mothers

Sl. No	Variables	No	CI-95%	P-value
1	Age (years)			
	18–25	85	80.01–87.22	$P < 0.05$
	26–32	15	14.02–16.88	$P > 0.05$
2	Marital status			
	Married	87	83.25–88.92	$P < 0.05$
	Unmarried	3.00	0.80–4.26	$P > 0.05$
	Discordant couple	8.0	5.06–9.22	$P > 0.05$
	Unknown	2.0	0.96–3.08	$P > 0.05$
3	Educational status			
	Literate	45	44.22–46.99	$P < 0.05$
	Illiterate	56	53.62–58.20	$P < 0.05$
	Unknown			
4	Economic status			
	Low income	55	53.26–56.21	$P < 0.05$
	Medium income	35	32.66–36.78	$P < 0.05$
	High income	10	9.01–11.23	$P > 0.05$
5	Risk factors			
	Heterosexuality	74	73.26–75.61	$P < 0.05$
	IDU's	03	0.86–4.21	$P > 0.05$
	Unknown	23	22.66–24.26	$P > 0.05$
6	Status of spouse HIV status			
	+Ve	65	63.26–68.76	$P < 0.05$
	−Ve	18	17.28–19.03	$P < 0.05$
	Not attended	06	4.02–7.88	$P > 0.05$
	Unknown	11	10.01–12.56	$P > 0.05$
7	Gravida			
	Primigravida	66	64.23–67.56	$P < 0.05$
	Gravida II	23	21.02–24.56	$P < 0.05$
	Gravida III	07	6.23–8.11	$P > 0.05$
	Gravida IV	04	3.41–4.56	$P > 0.05$
8	Types of delivery			
	Caesarian	28	27.63–29.22	$P < 0.05$
	LSCS	03	2.01–4.28	$P > 0.05$
	MTP	01	0.12–1.56	$P > 0.05$
	Normal	68	65.22–69.87	$P < 0.05$
9	Place of delivery			
	Govt. tertiary care center	85	84.55–87.26	$P < 0.05$
	Pvt. hospitals	10	8.01–11.63	$P > 0.05$
	Resident	05	3.01–6.58	$P > 0.05$

Significant ($p < 0.05$)

4 southern Indian states using a multilevel statistical modelling approach. A present study characterized younger women and illiterate women, those employed in agricultural occupation or housekeeper and helper, which were found to be significantly ($p < 0.01$) HIV positive. HIV prevalence among FSWs and the percentage of women marrying below 18 years were significantly ($p < 0.01$) associated with a higher HIV positivity among ANCs. Study has shown that educational status contributed to literate was 45.0% (CI 95%; 44.22–46.99, $p < 0.05$) and Illiterate was 55% (CI 95%; 53.62–58.20, $P < 0.05$). With regard to economic status, contribution to low income was 55.0% (CI 95%; 53.26–56.21 $p < 0.05$), medium income was 35% (CI 95% 32.66–36.78 $p < 0.05$), and high income was 10% (CI 95% 9.01–11.23 $P > 0.05$). Thus, primarily heterosexual transmission from the ANCs to the core group of bridge population like truck drivers, hotel keepers, and unmarried regular clients with heterosexually 74% (CI 95%;73.26–75.61 $p < 0.05$), IUD's 3.0% (CI 95%; 0.86–4.21 $p > 0.05$) and Unknown origin 23.0% (CI 95% 22.66–24.26 $p > 0.05$); Status of spouse HIV reactive was 65.0% (CI; 95% 63.26–68.76 $p < 0.05$), Non reactive was 18 0.0% (CI 95%; 17.28–19.03,$p > 0.05$), not attended was 6.0% (CI 95% 4.02–7.88 $p > 0.05$) and unknown was 11% (CI 95% 10.01–12.56 $p > 0.05$); Status of gravida was primigravida, 66% (CI 95% 64.23–67.56 $p < 0.05$), gravida II, 23.0% (CI 95% 21.02–24.56 $p < 0.05$), gravida III; 7.00% (CI 95% 6.23–8.11, $p > 0.05$) and gravida IV, 4.0% (CI 95%; 3.41–4.56, $p > 0.05$); Mode of delivery was Caesarian, 28.0% (CI 95%;27.63–29.22 $p < 0.05$), LSCS; 3.0% (2.01–4.28, $p > 0.05$), MTP; 1.0% (0.12–1.56, $p > 0.05$) and normal delivery, 68.0% (CI 95% 65.22–69.87 $p < 0.05$). Study documented the place of delivery based on geographical location, and it was government tertiary care center 85.0% (CI 95%; 84.55–87.26, $p < 0.05$), private hospitals 10.0% (CI 95%; 8.01–11.63, $p > 0.05$), and own resident 5.0%(CI 95%; 3.01–6.58, $p > 0.05$). Early sexual activity, of which age at marriage is a proxy in the Indian context, is the known risk factor for HIV both in India and globally. This is partly due to vulnerability of young women due to sensitive nature of their genital tract. In a study by Bhattacharya, 97% of women surveyed in India during 1992–1993 did not use any contraception before their first child was born (Table 5.5).

Positive predictive value (PPV) $= \frac{a}{a+b} \times 100 = 15.68\%$, Negative predictive value (NPV) $= \frac{d}{c+d} = 91.83$, Specificity (%) $= \frac{d}{b+d} \times 100 = 51.13\%$, Sensitivity (%) $= \frac{a}{a+c} \times 100 = 66.66\%$. From (Table 5.3) it depicts that, the prevalence of HIV MTCT through breastfeeding was 15.68%, without breastfeeding was 8.16%, with sensitivity (66.66%), specificity (51.13%), and NPV (91.83%).

Table 5.5 Rate of infection with or without breastfeeding

Sl No.	Variables	Baby HIV infected	Baby HIV not infected	Total
1.	With breastfeeding	08 (a)	43 (b)	51 (a+b)
2.	Without breastfeeding	04 (c)	45 (d)	49 (c+d)
	Total	12 (a+c)	88 (b+d)	100 N

Chi-square value-5.69 $p < 0.05$

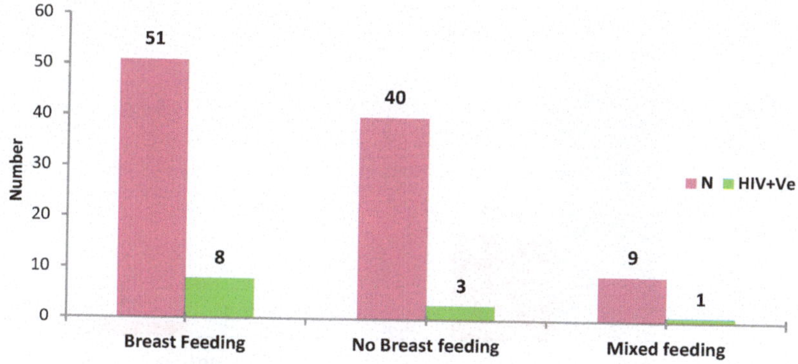

Fig. 5.3 HIV status of baby with different types of feeding

A total of a hundred HIV-infected mothers were prospectively recruited for the study; out of 51 breastfeeding mothers, 8 babies were HIV infected. Out of 40 mothers who were not feeding the baby, the rate was found to be 3%. In the case of mixed feeding, out of nine mothers, only one baby was infected and presented in Fig. 5.3. Children who are breastfed for a longer duration grow better than those breastfed for a shorter period (Guthrie et al. (2010). Hamadache et al. reported that, fewer episodes of neonatal and childhood morbidity such as fever, acute diarrhea, and upper respiratory infections than non-breastfed babies (Gray et al. 2005). Children aged 9–18 months, who were never breastfed or stopped breastfeeding, experienced approximately four times higher mortality than those who were able to continue breastfeeding (Cooper et al. 2009). There is continued concern that infants born to HIV-infected mothers may acquire HIV through breastfeeding, depending on duration and other underlying risk factors. A present study showed that the frequency of breast milk transmission of HIV-I was 8.0% and that 40.0% of infant infection could be avoided by the use of breast milk substitutes (Asnake and Amsalu 2005). Similar findings were reported by John et al. According to an Indian study on infant feeding and HIV-I transmission, it was observed that an exclusive breastfeed was found to have significantly lower risk of HIV-I transmission when compared with mixed feeding. A present study showed that only one child was infected in mixed feeding option. Any form of trauma to the gastrointestinal tract or its immature state may therefore make the infants more vulnerable to infection (French and Brocklehurst 1998). Replacement feeding carries increased risk of morbidity and mortality associated with malnutrition and infectious diseases other than HIV. This is especially high in the first 6 months of life and decreases thereafter. The risk and feasibility of replacement feeding are affected by the local environment and the individual mother's situation. When HIV-infected mothers choose not to breastfeed from birth or stop breastfeeding later, they should be provided with specific guidance and support for at least the first 2 years of the child's life to ensure adequate replacement feeding. NACO program would strive to improve conditions that will make replacement feeding safer for HIV-infected

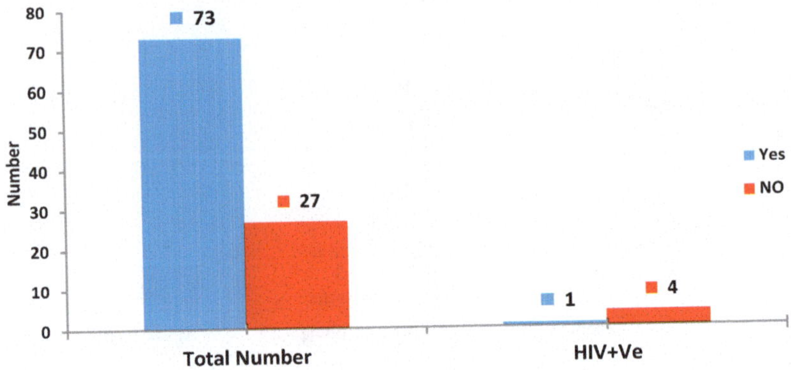

Fig. 5.4 HIV status of baby for ARV prophylaxis received at onset of birth

mothers and families. Shortening this transition period however may have negative nutritional consequences for the infants and psychological consequences for the infant and mother and expose risk of breast pathology, which may increase the risk of HIV transmission if cessation of breastfeeding is not abrupt. The best duration for this transition is not known and may vary according to the age of the infants and/or environment. Therefore, the present study suggests that HIV-infected mothers who breastfeed should be provided with specific guidance and support when they cease breastfeeding to avoid harmful nutritional and psychological consequences and to maintain breast health.

Figure 5.4 determined that the transmission rate was measured in terms of definable characteristics, viz., with or without ARV prophylaxis given to mother and baby at the time before and onset of delivery (within 6 h). A present study showed that only one baby gets infected after receiving ARV prophylaxis and also revealed that four babies were infected, who were not receiving ARV prophylaxis. Bekker et al. (2011), Celum et al. (2010) reported that in the efficacy of ARV drugs in reducing MTCT of HIV-I, the present study found more promising results; the intrapartum and neonatal single-dose nevirapine reduced MTCT during the first trimester and onset of baby birth. Nevirapine is a non-nucleotide reverse transcriptase inhibitor. Its long life in pregnant women and babies makes it simple and easy to administer as a single oral dose (Gray et al. 2005) (Table 5.6).

HIV-infected mothers' clinical-associated parameters were presented in Table 5.5; the mean age of the patients 24.58 $\pm$ 1.50 years (CI 95% 22.99–26.52 $p < 0.050$) study showed that the younger age group mothers highly expressed transfer of HIV infection to their babies. WHO clinical staging was hallmarked, and it was explained in terms of stage (I) 9(9.0%) (CI-95% 8.56–10.33 $p > 0.05$), stage (II) 25(25.0%) (CI-95% 23.56–26.45, $p < 0.05$), stage (III) 54(54.0%) (CI-95% 52.19–55.63, $p < 0.05$), and stage (IV) 12(12.0%) (CI-95% 36.21–39.15, $p < 0.05$). A total 38% of the patients which were on HAART with CI 95% was 36.21–39.15, $p < 0.05$. The immunological markers were measured based on mothers' CD4 count μ/dL. The baseline CD_4 counts (at the time of inception of HAART), CD4 count at 6 months, and 12 months follow-up data were recorded, and

Table 5.6 Associated clinical parameters of HIV-infected mothers' univariate model

Sl. No.	Variables	Mean±SD	CI-95%	P-value
1.	Age(years)	24.58 ± 1.50	22.99–26.52	$P < 0.05$
2.	WHO clinical stage			
	Stage I	09(9.0%)	8.56–10.33	$P > 0.05$
	Stage II	25(25.0%)	23.56–26.45	$P < 0.05$
	Stage III	54(54.0%)	52.19–55.63	$P < 0.05$
	Stage IV	12(12.0%)	11.58–13.54	$P < 0.05$
3.	On HAART	38.00%	36.21–39.15	$P < 0.05$
	While on HAART	62.00%	60.15–63.88	$P < 0.05$
4.	CD4 count at baseline	158.90 ± 98.13	156.22–161.15	$P > 0.05$
	CD4 count at 6 months	296.31 ± 65.42	293.44–297.82	$P > 0.05$
	CD4 count at 12 months	365.99 ± 34.22	362.01–368.12	$P < 0.05$
5.	Comorbidity			
	Yes	24.00%	22.01–26.09	$P > 0.05$
	No	76.00%	74.20–77.88	$P < 0.05$
6.	Adverse ARV drug reaction	18.02%	17.00–19.14	$P > 0.05$
	Serious adverse ARV drug reaction	7.63%	6.01–8.11	$P > 0.05$
7.	CD4 count at time onset of pregnancy	389 ± 20.02	376.02–390.10	$P < 0.05$
8.	CD4 count at time baby delivery	255.10 ± 56.12	254.22–257.86	$P > 0.05$

SD standard deviation, *CI* confidence interval

it was expressed in terms of mean. The average CD4 count at baseline was 158.90 ± 98.13 μ/dl (CI 95%; 156.22–61.15, $p > 0.05$), CD4 count at 6 months was 296.31 ± 65.42 μ/dL (CI 95%; 293.44–297.82, $p > 0.05$), and CD_4 count at 12 months was 365.99 ± 34.22 μ/dL (CI 95%; 362.01–368.12, $p < 0.05$). About 24% patients had comorbid conditions out of which 7.63% were inflamed by serious adverse reactions, viz., NVP rashes, AZT-induced anemia, and lactic acidosis. The immunological biomarkers like baseline CD_4 count were positively correlated with the onset of pregnancy and time of baby delivery; the CD4 count was negatively correlated with onset of delivery ($r = -0.56$). The elevated CD_4 count at the time of pregnancy was 389 ± 20.02 μ/dL (Table 5.7) (Fig. 5.5).

The KPM model was bound to express the duration of breastfeeding and HIV infection. In Fig. 5.6 it was determined that the interval duration of breastfeeding was practiced for 10–12 months. In the case of HIV-infected mothers, who have practiced for 16.25 ± 0.936 months (CI 95% 12.01–18.66), the Omnibus test of Model -2Loglikelihood 86.98 with coefficient of determination was $R^2 = 77.0\%$. In Table 5.6 the transmission rate was statistically significant ($p < 0.05$).The average body weight of a neonatal baby was 2.79 ± 0.206 kg (CI 95%; 2.02–3.16), Omnibus tests of 56.28 with $R^2 = 55.0\%$. The babies' mean APGAR score was 8.06 ± 0.36, and -2Loglikelihood was 56.28 with coefficient determination which was 55.0%.

Table 5.7 Associated parameters of HIV-infected neonatal baby

Sl	Variables	Estimates of survival mean±SE	Mean duration CI 95%		IQR	Omnibus tests of model	R-square (%)
			Lower bound	Upper bound		-2Loglikelihood	
1	Age of the baby (weeks)	45.11 ± 1.18	42.92	47.30	45–55	701.89	0.68*
2	Body weight of neonatal baby (Kgs)	2.79 ± 0.206	2.02	3.16	2.0–3.2	56.28	0.55
3	Duration of breastfeeding (months)	10.24 ± 0.572	9.12	11.36	8–12	44.66	0.72*
4	Duration of breastfeeding of HIV-infected baby (months)	16.25 ± 0.936	12.01	18.66	11–20	86.98	0.77*

Significant $p < 0.01$

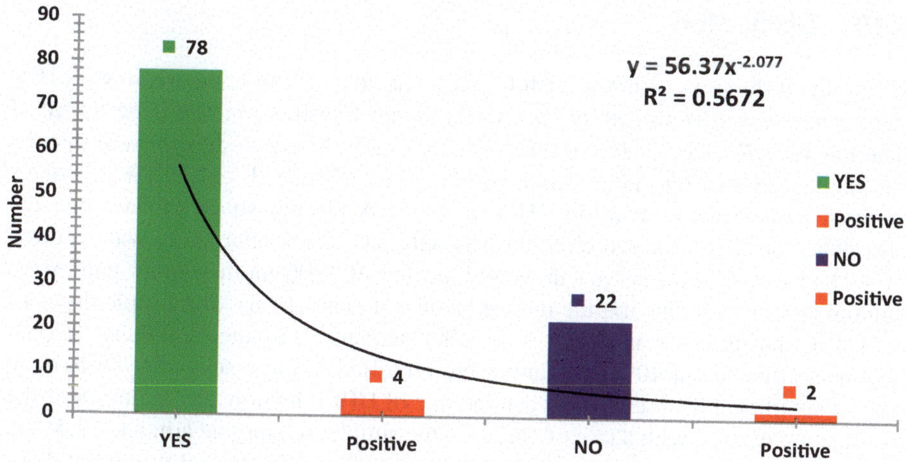

Fig. 5.5 DBS results at 6 weeks of baby age

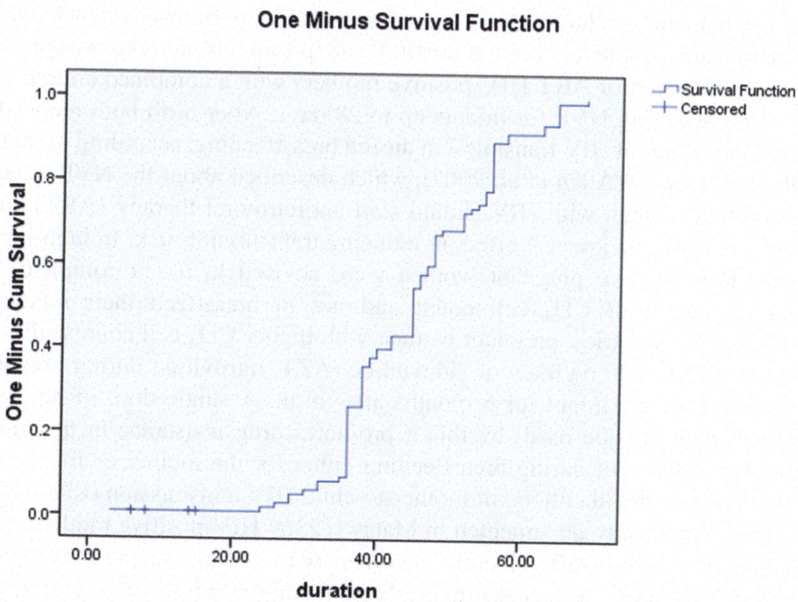

Fig. 5.6 Survival function of HIV-infected baby (KPM model)

5.10 Discussion

When infant duration of breastfeeding (BF) was analyzed in comparison with HIV status, there was a significantly ($p < 0.01$) higher transmission rate [Coefficient of determination $R^2 = 0.72$, $P = 0.0012$, log-rank test]. Many studies showed that the nevirapine regimen was able to reduce MTCT by 47%, with only 8.1% of infants exposed to nevirapine acquiring HIV at birth. A present study showed that the prevalence of NVP-exposed children was only 5.0%; a similar study was reported by a Hamadache et al. As per the study, a total of 1306 mother/infant pairs were randomized to either nevirapine during labor and postdelivery or multiple doses of AZT/3TC during labor and for 1 week after delivery to mother and baby. In both treatment arms, about 40% of infants were breastfed. Eight weeks after birth, there was no significant difference between the rate of HIV infection and death across the two treatment arms, with a rate of 14.3% in the simpler nevirapine arm and 12.5% in the more involved and expensive dual therapy arm. Antiretroviral prophylaxis for neonates and for women during pregnancy and delivery has been the cornerstone for prevention of MTCT. Antiretroviral prophylaxis reduces perinatal transmission by several mechanisms, including lowering of maternal prepartum viral load and pre- and postexposure prophylaxis of the infant. Postexposure prophylaxis was provided through administered of ART HIV-positive mothers with a combined antiretroviral regimen or suggesting NVP for infants up to 28 days. After birth both reduced the risk of mother-to-child HIV transmission during breastfeeding, according to findings from the BAN study (Allen et al. 2007), which described about the NVP issues. It was found that women with HIV should start antiretroviral therapy (ART) during pregnancy to have the greatest effect in reducing transmission risk. In high-income countries, HIV-positive pregnant women were advised to use a complete ART regimen regardless of CD_4 cell count and not to breastfeed their infants. In resource-limited countries, pregnant women with higher CD_4 cell counts still often receive the ACTG 076 regimen of zidovudine (AZT, retrovirus) during pregnancy and labor and for the infant for 6 months after birth. A single dose of nevirapine (Viramune) may also be used; by this it promotes drug resistance in the mother. Antiretroviral treatment during breastfeeding either for the mother or for the baby can help to reduce the likelihood of mother-to-child HIV transmission (Koepsell and Weiss 2003). In a study documented in Malawi, 2369 HIV-positive mothers with a CD_4 count of at least 250 cells/mm^3, women with anemia or pre-existing liver impairment, and those who had previously used antiretroviral drugs during pregnancy were excluded. All women received oral single-dose nevirapine during labor, followed by zidovudine/lamivudine (Combivir) for both mothers from the onset of labor and babies from birth, continuing for 7 days. Mothers were counselled to breastfeed exclusively for 6 months and then wean the baby rapidly between 24 and 28 weeks, since studies have shown that mixed feeding of breast milk and alternative foods increases HIV transmission risk. In one more population-based study reported in Botswana, the study revealed that HIV-positive pregnant women in Botswana, who had a CD4 cell count above 200 cells/mm, starting at 26–34 weeks of pregnancy and continuing through infant weaning at 6 months, were randomly assigned to receive either zidovudine/lamivudine/abacavir (Trizivir combination pill) or else lopinavir/ritonavir plus zidovudine/lamivudine; in addition, 170 women with a CD4 cell count <200 cells/mm^3 started zidovudine/lamivudine plus nevirapine. All infants received single-dose nevirapine after delivery and zidovudine for 4 weeks, and risk of transmission was very less. Mother-to-child HIV transmission occurred late in the pregnancy and that in the absence of any intervention, between 20% and 45% of the infants become infected from their HIV-positive mothers. Major international guidelines on HIV and infant feeding were released in 2001 by an interagency task team on mother-to-child HIV transmission comprising WHO, UNICEF, UNFPA, and UNAIDS. These guidelines promote different infant feeding options for women with differing socioeconomic status. In the guidelines, so-called formula feeding is recommended for women for whom replacement feeding was considered "acceptable, feasible, affordable, sustainable, and safe." HIV-positive women were encouraged to exclusively breastfeed for the first 6 months of their child's life (Morrison et al. 2007).

5.11 Summary

Mother-to-child HIV cumulative transmission rate was 23.84%. In the HIV context, the routine breastfeeding was associated with antiretroviral therapy; it could help to decrease the rate of MTCT. Appropriate measures should be provided for prevention of mother-to-child transmission (PMTCT) among HIV-infected mothers. Highly active antiretroviral therapy (HAART) can be used for preventing mother-to-child transmission.

5.12 Genetic Model Approach to Plasma RNA Viral Load (VL) and CD4 Count for MTCT Transmission

Highly active antiretroviral therapy (HAART) has been harnessed as one of the key interventions for mitigating HIV epidemic at global level. The primary goal of HAART is to decrease HIV-related morbidity and mortality. While on HAART, it was expected that the patient experiences fewer number of HIV-related illnesses, their CD4 count should rise and remain above the baseline, and the viral load (VL) should become undetectable (<47 copies/ml). The main aim of the study is to correlate the virological suppression (HIV viral load $\leq$47 copies/mL) and immunological functions, when the CD4 count >500 μ/dL at 24 and 48th week follow-up intervals from inception of HAART with NNRTI+PI-based regimen. Further, we have studied correlation between baseline variables associated with virological suppression (VL). We have fitted various genetic models and demonstrated by using massive HIV data sets and also evaluate the efficacy of the fitted models on the basis of theoretical and practical approach.

5.13 Model Formulation

A cohort data was extracted in the month of March 2009 from different government hospitals, functionally working in Bangalore city; a total of 168 children have been initiated on HAART. All cases fulfilled the inclusion criteria; the age group was between 5 and <16 years at time of HAART inception. At least 12 months of follow-up data or one known viral load (VL) measurement, and CD_4 count were available after initiation of HAART, prior exposure to HAART, except exposure through prevention of mother-to-child transmission (PMTCT).

5.14 Formulation of the Model

$$Y_{ijk} = \mu + \alpha_i + \varepsilon_{ijkl}$$

Y_{ijkl} = Observed value for *i*th mother *j*th period *k*th baby
μ = General mean
α_i = Effect of *i*th mother – HIV infected
β_{ij} = Effect of *i*th HIV infected mother and *j*th period
ε_{ijkl} = Error associated with *i*th mother *j*th period *k*th baby CD4 – adjusted factor

5.15 Assumption of the Model

The observations are independent and identical (iid), each CD_4 and viral load (VL) testing follow-up period was mutually exclusive in nature, and the tested experimental error for each follow-up period is normally distributed with μ, common variance $\sigma^2 \varepsilon_{ijkl} \sim N(\mu, \sigma^2)$. All possible CD_4 and viral load (VL) pairs of means were compared with the same precision even though differences between may be large (Table 5.8).

Table 5.8 Analysis of variance table for estimation of heritability

Sl. No.	Source of variation	df	SS	MSS	EMS	Variance ratio "F" @1% level
1.	Between groups (mothers)	M-1	S_B^2	MSB=$\frac{S_B^2}{M-1}$	$\sigma_W^2 + K_1\sigma_M^2$	$F=\frac{MSB}{MSW}$
2.	With in groups (CD4 count)	K-M	S_W^2	MSW=$\frac{S_W^2}{K-M}$	σ_W^2	
	Total	N-1	TSS			

5.16 Analytical Methods

Correction factor= $\frac{\left(\sum Y_{Yij}\right)^2}{N}$ or
TSS= $\sum Y_{ij}^2$ – CF
Group SS= $\frac{Y_{1.}^2+Y_{2.}^2+Y_{t.}^2}{r}$ – CF
Error SS= TSS-Group–SSB

5.17 Genetic Correlation ($-1 \leq r^2 \leq 1$)

The genetic correlation was derived to know the resemblances between mother CD4 count and RNA plasma viral load for HIV transmission rate. He pointed out that the lower CD4 count and high plasma viral load were strongly associated with in utero transmission, and similar studies were conducted by Mayanja et al. (2004), Minkoff et al. (2003), Lingappa et al. (2009), and Lawn et al. (2006). In this proximity of the research, present hypothesis has fitted different genetic model approaches to know the transmission rate of HIV MTCT. Let X_1 be the variable considered as mother CD4 count or RNA plasma viral load at inception of HAART, and $X_2, X_3, \ldots X_n$ is considered as follow-up CD4 count or RNA plasma viral load at different intervals like 6 months, 12 months, 24 months, etc. The resemblance of the CD4 count and RNA viral load is modelled as below (Table 5.9).

The genetic correlation was obtained by using the following theoretical approach:

Table 5.9 ANOVA and covariances of CD_4 count and RNA viral load

Source of variation	df	Variance		Covariance
		X1	X2. . . .Xn	X1, v/s X2. . . .Xn
Between CD4 count and RNA viral load	S-1	σ_{gx1}^2	σ_{gxn}^2	$\sigma_{gx1\ xn}$
Between CD4 count and RNA viral load	N-S	σ_{ex1}^2	σ_{exn}^2	$\sigma_{ex1\ xn}$

$$r_g = \frac{\sigma_{\mathrm{gX1\ Xn}}}{\sqrt{\sigma^2{}_{\mathrm{gx1}}\sigma^2{}_{\mathrm{gxn}}}} \tag{5a}$$

$$r_p = \frac{\sigma_{\mathrm{gX1\ Xn}} + \sigma_{\mathrm{eX1\ Xn}}}{\sqrt{\sigma^2{}_{\mathrm{gx1}} + \sigma^2{}_{\mathrm{gxn}} + \sigma^2{}_{\mathrm{ex1}} + \sigma^2{}_{\mathrm{exn}}}} \tag{5b}$$

$$r_e = \frac{\sigma_{\mathrm{eX1\ Xn}}}{\sqrt{\sigma^2{}_{\mathrm{ex1}}\sigma^2{}_{\mathrm{exn}}}} \tag{5c}$$

As per the above the fitted model 5a, 5b, and 5c, the final equation of the model becomes

$r_p = r_g + r_e$
Phenotypic Correlation = Genotypic correlation + Environmental Correlation
Variance of $\sigma_p{}^2 = \sigma_W{}^2 + \sigma_M{}^2$

5.18 Estimation of Heritability ($0 \leq h^2 \leq 1$)

Heritability (h^2): The rate of MTCT is determined by using heritability, it is denoted by h^2, and heritability lies between $0 \leq h^2 \leq 1$

$$h^2 = \frac{\sigma_M{}^2}{\sigma_W{}^2 + \sigma_M{}^2}, k = \frac{1}{M-1}\left(N - \frac{\sum n_i{}^2}{N}\right)$$

where k is the number of HIV-infected children produced from the mothers (Tables 5.10, 5.11, 5.12 and 5.13) (Figs. 5.7 and 5.8)

$$t = \frac{\sigma_M{}^2}{\sigma_W{}^2 + \sigma_M{}^2} = h^2 = 4(t), \mathrm{SE}(h^2) = \frac{\sqrt[4]{2(1-t)^2\{1 + (k-1)t\}\ 2}}{k(k-1)(m-1)}$$

5.19 Numerical Results of Genetic Models

Table 5.10 Genetic correlation matrix of CD4 count follow-up of an infected mother who transfers HIV infection to her child

Follow-up	Inception HAART	6 months	12 months	24 months	36 months	48 months	At time of delivery
Inception HAART	$1h^2 = 0.12$[a]	0.04	0.39	0.74	0.75	−0.08	0.56
6 months	0.20+−0.16	$1h^2$=0.36[a]	−0.25	0.74	0.44	0.73	0.31
12 months	0.21+−0.18	−0.36+0.11	$1h^2$=0.55	0.49	0.23	0.37	−0.34
24 months	0.52+0.22	0.11+−0.63	−0.18+0.67	$1h^2$=0.62	−0.05	0.75	0.48
36 months	0.62+−0.13	0.28+0.16	−0.19+0.42	−0.16+0.11	$1h^2$=0.59	0.57	0.49
48 months	0.14+−0.22	0.11+0.62	−0.26+0.63	0.28+0.47	0.33+−0.24	$1h^2$=0.68	−0.41
At time of delivery	0.18+−0.38	−0.32+0.63	0.10+−0.44	0.63+[a]−0.15	0.63+−0.14	0.22+−0.63	$1h^2$=0.16[a]

[a]Diagonal elements that denoted heritability (h^2) lie between $0 \le h^2 \le 1$, above diagonal elements denoted phenotypic correlation r_p, and below diagonal elements denoted genotypic and environmental correlation $r_{g+}r_e$

Table 5.11 Genetic correlation matrix of RNA plasma viral load of an infected mother who transfers HIV infection to her child

Follow-up	Inception HAART	6 months	12 months	24 months	At time of delivery
Inception HAART	$1h^2 = 18*$	0.61	0.37	0.78	−0.55
6 months	0.23 + 0.38	$1h^2$=0.12*	0.35	0.48	−0.23
12 months	0.11 + 0.26	−0.21 +0.56	$1h^2$=0.23	−0.26	−0.38
24 months	0.26 + 0.52	−0.24 + −0.72	0.26 +0.52	$1h^2$=0.44	0.14
At time of delivery	−0.13 + −0.42	−0.42 +0.19	0.18 + −0.56	−0.32 + *0.46	$1h^2$=0.13*

Diagonal elements that denoted heritability (h^2) lie between$0 \leq h^2 \leq 1$, above diagonal elements denoted phenotypic correlation r_p, and below diagonal elements denoted genotypic and environmental correlation $r_{g+}r_e$
*Significant at 1% level

Table 5.12 Analysis of variance of CD4 count (micro/dL) follow-up from inception of HAART till baby delivery of an HIV-infected mother who does not transfer infection to her child

Source of variation	df	Sum of square (SS)	Mean sum of square (MSS)	F-variance ratio
CD4 count follow-up period	6	5,647,864	941,311	37.19** ($P = 0.000$)
Error	252	6,377,512	25,308	
Total	258	12,025,376		

Table 5.13 Analysis of variance of CD4 count (micro/dl) follow-up from inception of HAART till baby delivery of an HIV-infected mother who transfers infection to her child

Source of variation	df	Sum of sqaure (SS)	Mean sum of square (MSS)	F-variance ratio
CD4 count follow-up period	6	3,291,554	548,592	24.89* ($p = 0.002$)
Error	147	3,253,381	22,132	
Total	153	6,544,934		

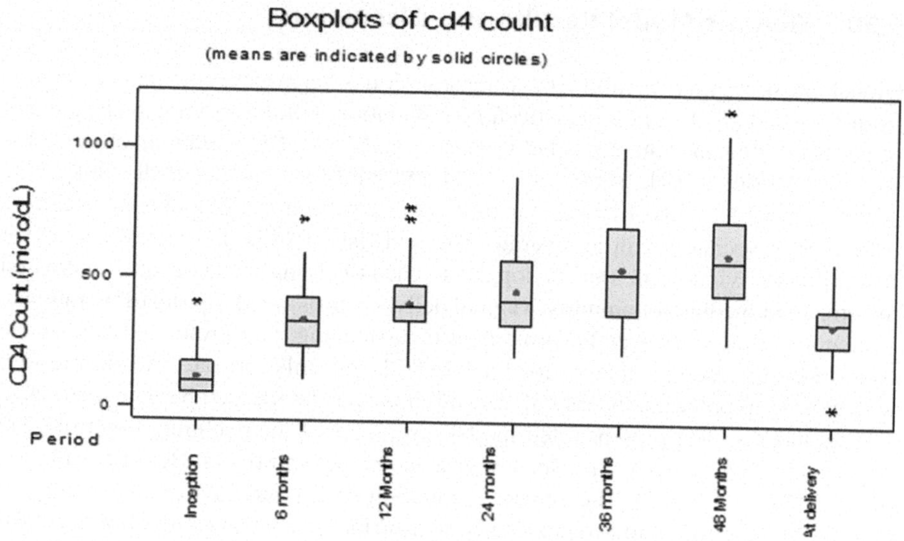

Fig. 5.7 CD4 means box plot on HIV-infected mother who does not transfer HIV infection to her child

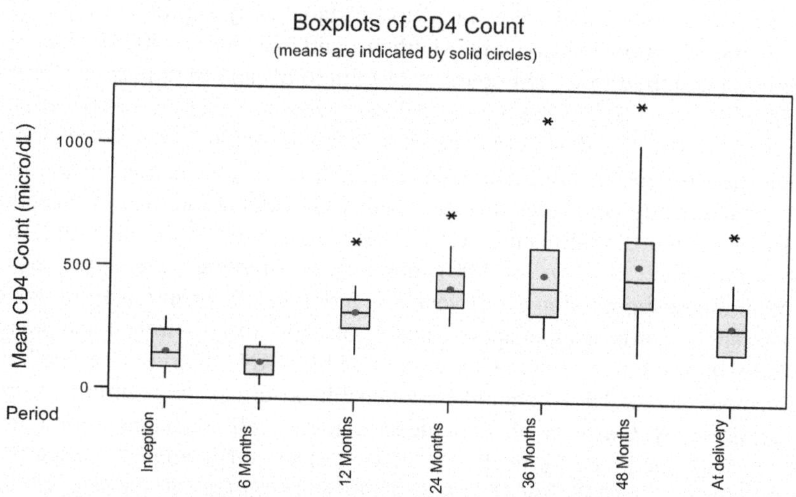

Fig. 5.8 CD4 means box plot on HIV-infected mother who transfers HIV infection to her child

5.20 Genetic Model Results and Discussion

Global rate of mother-to-child HIV-1 transmission is heterogeneous; estimates range from 14% to 48%. In a non-breastfeeding population with fewer viral loads, the risk of perinatal transmission rate is between 15% and 25%. The variations of transmission may be due to risk factors or to CD4 and viral load characteristics in specific populations and also to differences in timing of transmission. Although many factors have been associated with an overall increased risk of MTCT, increased maternal RNA plasma viral load (>3.26 $\log_e 10^4$), CD4+T–lymphocyte count, decreased maternal cell mediated immunity, vaginal delivery, prolonged rupture of membrane, prematurity, low birth weight, prolonged breastfeeding, and prolonged labor were considered as creeping factors for HIV MTCT transmission rate. According to a widely used hypothesis, the rate of transmission was determined by new intervened genetic models. The present fitted model revealed that the declining trend of CD4 count and RNA plasma viral load was at more proximity for HIV transmission ($h^2 = 0.13*$, $p < 0.001$). The genetic correlation (0.23) and environmental correlation (0.38) were found to be statistically significant ($p < 0.001$) with HIV transmission. At the time of inception of HAART, the viral load was relatively more and laid down the immunity of the mother. In Tables 5.8 and 5.9, it is depicted that the follow-up CD4 count and RNA plasma viral load and the heritability estimates expressed lower values and were found to be statistically significant ($p < 0.001$), when compared to transmission rate. Matthews and Mukherjee (2009), Natu (2007) reported that maternal low CD4 count (<250 micro/dl) and high plasma RNA viral load ($3.80 \log_e 10 \times 10^6$) at the time of delivery were risk factors for HIV transmission, and also decreased maternal cell mediated immunity was associated with perinatal transmission and hypothesized to be risk factors for in utero transmission.

The present study concludes that the lower CD4 cells at the time of inception of HAART were more significantly ($p < 0.05$) associated with increased risk of transmission ($h^2 = 0.18$, $p = 0.00$) and further supported the hypothesis that maternal immunosuppression at delivery was a risk factor for intrapartum transmission. This study confirmed that approximately 30–40% of HIV-infected infants were infected by their mother's lower CD_4 count and high RNA plasma viral load; this is because maternal viral load should be amenable to direct intervention. A similar study reported by Grace et al. concluded that the cell mediated immunity was correlated with increased vertical transmission. The cell mediated immunity may directly influence transmission or may be a surrogate marker for maternal viral load. As per this fitted logistic regression model, prolonged breastfeeding, lower CD_4 count and high plasma viral load, prematurity, low birth weight, maternal immunity, and deficiency of vitamin C were significantly ($p < 0.001$) associated with HIV transmission. Another European collaborative study suggested that HIV RNA dynamics over pregnancy differs by time, type of HAART therapy, drug adherence, and WHO clinical stage.

5.21 Robustness of Genetic Model

The model robustness was tested by using maximum likelihoods (MLEs). A fitted model in the present study was found to use more MLEs (-2loglikelihood was 120.16), it signifies the new intervened model, and the fitted model was considered as best fit ($R^2 = 90.63\%$). The fitted model was shown to be more positive for estimation of heritability (h^2) and genetic correlation. The assumption of the model can easily estimate the interaction effects with respect to different biological and laboratory parameters. The homogeneity of both variables, CD4 count and RNA plasma viral load, was tested with analysis of variance (ANOVA) and was statistically significant ($p < 0.001$), and observations were normally distributed.

5.22 Summary

In summary, this study demonstrated that lower maternal viral load and CD_4 count were statistically significant with increase of transmission rate. This fitted model will help to explain the success of NACP program, and the genetic model serves as a tool for clinicians, researchers, and policymakers for implementation of a new innovative program for prevention of MTCT.

5.23 Modelling on RNA Plasma Viral Load and CD4 Count (Micro/dL)

5.23.1 Linear Model

CD4 count and RNA plasma viral load were varied parameters. The series of data matrix was not always stationary; instead, the parameters will make changes on ANCs' population based on body condition, OIs, and drug adherence. This pattern was observed by using linear model fitting:

$$Y_{t=0 \text{ to } 56 \text{ months}} = \alpha + \beta^t,$$

where:

$t =$ interval of time (inception of HAART to 56 months)
$\alpha =$ intercept
$\beta =$ slope of the curve

5.23.2 Exponential Model

$$Y_{t=0 \text{ to } 56 \text{ month}} = c\, e^{\mathrm{kt}} \quad k > 0$$

where $C=$ initial value increases without bound to asymptotic to Y

5.23.3 Logarithmic Model

The logarithmic model was developed to know the monotonicity of CD_4 count and RNA plasma viral load.

$$Y_{t=0 \text{ to } 56 \text{ monts}} = a + b \ \ln(x)$$

where $t =$ interval of time (inception of HAART to 56 months), $\alpha =$ intercept, and $\beta=$ slope of the curve.

5.23.4 Power Model

The power model was used to know the strength of the relation between follow-up CD4 count and RNA plasma viral load. The model was distributed in a wide range of magnitude; these include size of the population and scale invariance (Table 5.14).

$$Y_{t=0 \text{ to } 56 \text{ months}} = \alpha X^{\beta}, \text{Take log on both sides}$$

$$\text{Log } Y_t = \text{Log } \alpha + \beta \ \log \ X, \text{Finally, the power model becomes}$$

$$Y_{t=0 \ to \ 56 \text{ monts}} = e^{\alpha + \beta X}$$

5.24 Simulated Numerical Results

Table 5.14 Simulation of different distribution models based on ANC's CD4 count (micro/dL) with different follow-up periods

Sl. No.	Model	Simulated equation for an HIV-infected mother who does not transfer HIV infection to her child ($t = 0$–56 months follow-up)	R^2 (%)	Simulated equation for HIV-infected mother who transfers HIV infection to her child ($t = 0$–56 months follow-up)	R^2 (%)
1.	Linear	$Y_t = 89.49x$	10.0	$Y_t = 51.28x$	27.10
2.	Exponential	$Y_t = e^{1.211^x}$	21.40	$Y_t = e^{1.041^x}$	29.80
3.	Logarithmic	$Y_t = 180.80 \ln(x) + 180.3$	60.70	$Y_t = 103.5 \ln(x) + 100.3$	89.99*
4.	Polynomial	$Y_t = -5.13x^3 + 19.45x^2 + 117.2x$	89.00*	$Y_t = -1.26x^3 + 3.56x^2 + 90.12x$	99.91*
5.	Power	$Y_t = 165.1x^{0.645}$	66.71	$Y_t = 105.7x^{0.573}$	90.09*

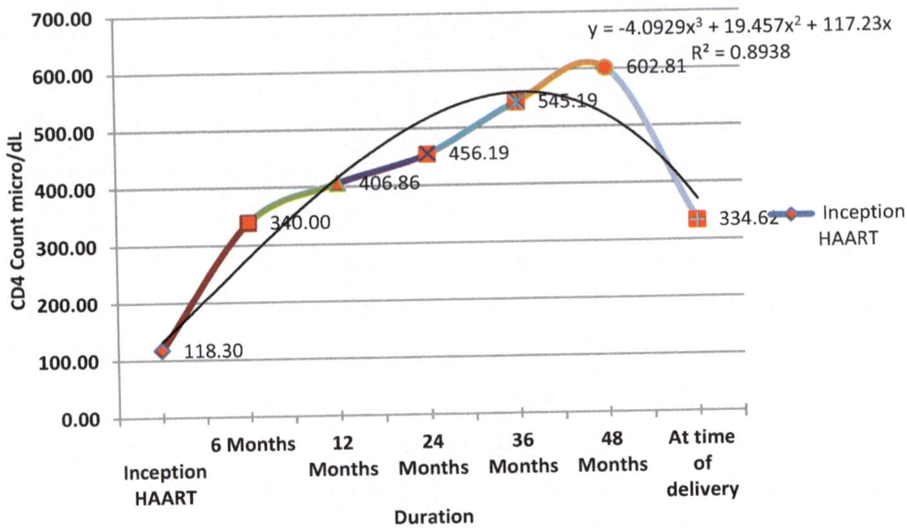

Fig. 5.9 Mean CD4 count for different follow-up periods of ANC polynomial model

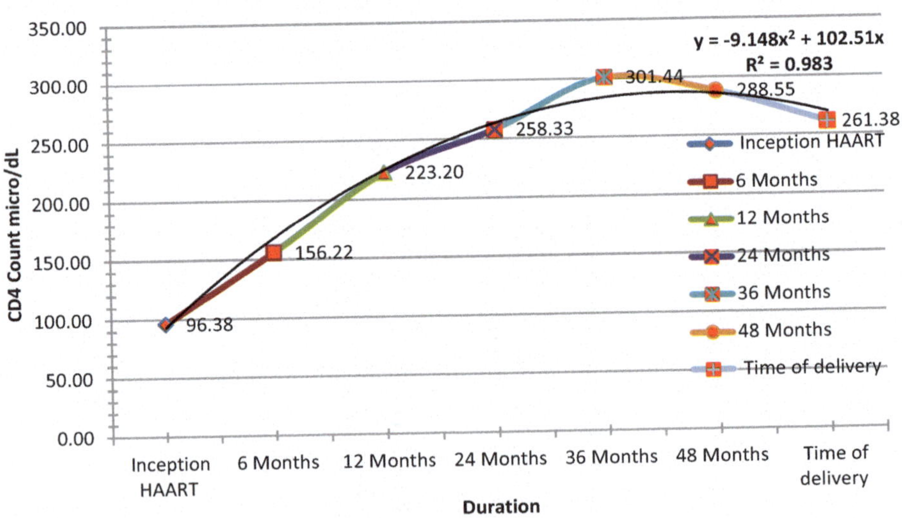

Fig. 5.10 HIV-infected child – mothers' CD4 count polynomial model

5.25 Results and Discussion of the Model

The CD_4 count and RNA plasma viral load were critical measures of immune suppression system and were used as important biomarkers for describing the progress of AIDS-defining illness and mother-to-child transmission rate. Usually, ANCs have reported better CD4 count with good immune system and adherence level >95% and HAART initiation with very good CD4 count. Otherwise, it follows a declining trend. The two parameters (CD4 count and viral load) were directly proportional to the immune system. The distribution of the rate at which CD_4 cell counts and RNA plasma viral load declines as predicted by our fitted model is presented in (Table 5.13). The fitted model had demonstrated a good agreement between the predicted and observed distribution of both parameters and biomarkers. As per the findings, third degree polynomial ($Y_t = -5.13x^3 + 19.45x^2 + 117.2x$) model was considered as the best model for the distribution of the CD4 count for increased level of MTCT ($R^2 = 89.0\%$). The same model was fitted for RNA viral load biomarker; the logarithmic ($Y_t = 103.5 \ln(x) + 100.3$), polynomial ($Y_t = -1.26x^3 + 3.56x^2 + 90.12x$), and power distribution models ($Y_t = 105.7x^{0.573}$) were found to be good predictors ($R^2 = 89.99\%$, $R^2 = 99.91\%$, $R^2 = 90.09\%$, respectively) for the estimation of progression rate of MTCT (Figs. 5.9 and 5.10).

5.26 Summary

The fitted model showed most of the variability in rates at which CD4 count and RNA viral load declines can be explained by the coefficient of determination values. The present fitted model is found to express the greater accuracy, more consistency, and reduced time for prediction of disease progression rate by using various HIV biomarkers.

References

Agarwal D, Chakravarty J, Sundar S, Gupta V, Bhatia BD (2008) Correlation between clinical features and degree of immunosuppressant in HIV infected children. Indian Pediatr 45:140–143

Allen S, Stephenson R, Weiss H, Karita E, Priddy F, Fuller L et al (2007) Pregnancy, hormonal contraceptive use, and HIV-related death in Rwanda. J Womens Health (Larchmt) 16:1017–1027

Asnake S, Amsalu S (2005) Clinical manifestations of HIV/AIDS in children in Northwest Ethiopia. Ethiop J Health Dev 19:24–28

Bekker L-G, Black V, Myer L, Rees H, Cooper D, Mall S et al (2011) Guideline on safer conception in fertile HIV-infected individuals and couples. South Afr J HIV Med 12:31–44

Celum C, Wald A, Lingappa JR, Magaret AS, Wang RS, Mugo N et al (2010) Acyclovir and transmission of HIV-1 from persons infected with HIV-1 and HSV-2. N Engl J Med 362:427–443

Cooper D, Harries J, Myer L, Orner P, Bracken H, Zweigenthal V (2007) "Life is still going on": reproductive intentions among HIV-positive women and men in South Africa. Soc Sci Med 65:274–283

Cooper D, Moodley J, Zweigenthal V, Bekker LG, Shah I, Myer L (2009) Fertility intentions and reproductive health care needs of people living with HIV in Cape Town, South Africa: implications for integrating reproductive health and HIV care services. AIDS Behav 13(Suppl 1):38–46

Department of AIDS Control, Ministry of Family Welfare, Government of India (2008) Annual report2008–2009. http://nacoonline.org/upload/Publication/Annual_ Report_NACO_2008–09.pdf. Accessed on 27 Feb 2010

French R, Brocklehurst P (1998) The effect of pregnancy on survival in women infected with HIV: a systematic review of the literature and meta-analysis. Br J Obstet Gynaecol 105:827–883

Gray RH, Li X, Kigozi G, Serwadda D, Brahmbhatt H, Wabwire-Mangen F et al (2005) Increased risk of incident HIV during pregnancy in Rakai, Uganda: a prospective study. Lancet 366:1182–1188

Guthrie BL, Choi RY, Bosire R, Kiarie JN, Mackelprang RD, Gatuguta A et al (2010) Predicting pregnancy in HIV-1-discordant couples. AIDS Behav 14:1066–1071

Hamadache D (n.d.) HIV testing guidelines for children of confirmed or suspected HIV positive parents. http://www.chiva.org.uk/health/guidelines/hiv-testing. Accessed on 27 Feb 2010

Homsy J, Bunnell R, Moore D, King R, Malamba S, Nakityo R et al (2009) Reproductive intentions and outcomes among women on antiretroviral therapy in rural Uganda: a prospective cohort study. PLoS One 4:4149

Koepsell TD, Weiss NS Epidemiologic methods: studying the occurrence of illness. Oxford University Press, Oxford, p 2003

Lawn SD, Myer L, Bekker LG, Wood R et al (2006) CD4 cell count recovery among HIV-infected patients with very advanced immunodeficiency commencing antiretroviral treatment in sub-Saharan Africa. BMC Infect Dis 6:59

Lingappa JR, Kahle E, Mugo N, Mujugira A, Magaret A, Baeten J et al (2009) Characteristics of HIV-1 discordant couples enrolled in a trial of HSV-2 suppression to reduce HIV-1 transmission: the partners study. PLoS One 4:5272

Lingappa JR, Baeten JM, Wald A, Hughes JP, Thomas KK, Mujugira A et al (2010) Daily acyclovir for HIV-1 disease progression in people dually infected with HIV-1 and herpes simplex virus type 2: a randomised placebo-controlled trial. Lancet 375:824–833

Lisse IM, Aaby P, Whittle H, Jensen H, Engelmann M, Christensen LE (1997) T-lymphocyte subset in West African children: impact of age, sex, and season. J Pediatr 130:77–85

Matthews LT, Mukherjee JS (2009) Strategies for harm reduction among HIV-affected couples who want to conceive. AIDS Behav 13(Suppl 1):5–11

Mayanja BN, Shafer LA, Van der Paal L, Kyakuwa N, Ndembi N, Hughes P et al (2004) Effect of pregnancy on immunological and virological outcomes of women on ART: a prospective cohort study in rural Uganda. Tropical Med Int Health 2(Suppl 12):168–170

Minkoff H, Hershow R, Watts DH, Frederick M, Cheng I, Tuomala R et al (2003) The relationship of pregnancy to human immunodeficiency virus disease progression. Am J Obstet Gynecol 189:552–559

Mmeje O, Cohen CR, Cohan D (2012) Evaluating safer conception options for HIV- serodiscordant couples (HIV-infected female/HIV-uninfected male): a closer look at vaginal insemination. Infect Dis Obstet Gynecol 2012:587651

Moodley D, Bobat RA, Coovadia HM, Doorasamy T, Munsamy S, Gouws E (1997) Lymphocyte subset changes between 3 and 15 months of age in infants born to HIV-seropositive women in South Africa. Tropical Med Int Health 2:415–421

Morrison CS, Wang J, Van Der Pol B, Padian N, Salata RA, Richardson BA (2007) Pregnancy and the risk of HIV-1 acquisition among women in Uganda and Zimbabwe. AIDS 21:1027–1034

Mugo NR, Heffron R, Donnell D, Wald A, Were EO, Rees H et al (2011) Increased risk of HIV-1 transmission in pregnancy: a prospective study among African HIV-1-serodiscordant couples. AIDS 25:1887–1895

Natu SA (2007) Daga SR et al antiretroviral therapy in children: Indian experience. Indian Pediatr 44:339–343

Padmapriyadarshini C, Poornagangadevi N, Chadrasekaran K, Subramanian S, Thiruvalluvan C, Bhavani PK et al (2009) Prevalence of underweight, stunting, and wasting among children infected with human immunodeficiency virus in south India. Int J Pediatr 2009:837627

Pattanapanyasat K, Thakar MR (2005) CD4+ T cell count as a tool to monitor HIV progression and anti retroviral therapy. Indian J Med Res 121:539–549

Reynolds HW, Janowitz B, Homan R, Johnson L (2006) The value of contraception to prevent perinatal HIV transmission. Sex Transm Dis 33:350–356

Shah I (2006) Correlation of CD_4 count, CD_4% and HIV viral load with clinical manifestations of HIV in infected Indian children. Ann Trop Paediatr 26:115–119

Shah I (2007) Antiretroviral therapy. In: Shah I, Shah NK, Manglani M (eds) IAP speciality series on pediatric HIV, 1st edn. Indian Academy of Pediatrics, Mumbai, pp 63–69

Shah N et al (2007) Clinical diagnosis of pediatric HIV, IAP Speciality Series on Pediatric HIV, 1st edn. Indian Academy of Pediatrics, Mumbai, pp 21–29

Shah D, Gupta P, Ghai OP Nutrition and health. In: Gupta P, Ghai OP (eds)

Universal Access to AIDS Treatment: Targets and Challenges (n.d.). http://www.avert.org/universal-access.htm. Accessed on 27 Feb 2010

Van der Paal L, Shafer LA, Mayanja BN, Whitworth JA, Grosskurth H (2007) Effect of pregnancy on HIV disease progression and survival among women in rural Uganda. Tropical Med Int Health 12:920–928

Watanabe M, Iwatani Y, Hidaka Y, Mitsuda N, Amino N (1996) Changes in soluble CD4 and CD8 proteins in healthy pregnant and postpartum women. Am J Reprod Immunol 36:220–227

World Health Organization (2002) Scaling up antiretroviral therapy in resource limited settings: guidelines for a public health approach. WHO, Geneva

Survivability and Growth Model Approach to CD_4 Counts of PLHIVs

6

6.1 Introduction

Low CD4+T lymphocyte counts (CD4 counts) in ANCs women's are likely to be associated with a variety of complication, including many viral infections, bacterial infections, parasitic infections, sepsis, tuberculosis, coccidiomycosis, burns, trauma, intravenous injections of foreign proteins, malnutrition, over-exercising, pregnancy, corticosteroid use, normal daily variation, psychological stress, and social isolation. It is also possible that anti-HIV medications can lower CD_4 counts, when used for long periods, and the short-term rise in CD_4 counts that is associated with its use may be due to a variety of factors that are unrelated to any anti-HIV activity. This chapter discussed a brief review of several studies documenting low CD_4 counts in people who are experiencing such conditions explained through statistical model that can serve as a tool for understanding the temporal changes of CD_4 count in HIV-infected pregnant women. This study is meant to be an introduction to AIDS-related mathematical biology for scientists with nonmathematical background. The data on HIV/AIDS patients over 18 years of age group, who had started HAART during April 2004 to March 2007, retrospective cohort data sets, were collected from different government hospitals of Karnataka. Growth models, binary logistic regression, and Weibull distribution model were employed to fit the progression rate of CD_4 count in HIV-/AIDS-infected pregnant women. The mean age of women on ANC was 28.25 ± 7.96 years. About 75.46% of them were infected through their spouses, and mean treatment follow-up time from the onset of pregnancy was 9.70 months. Many patients complied with HAART treatment adherence. The cumulative survival rate after initiation of HAART was 0.95 ($p \leq 0.05$, $R^2 = 79.82\%$). HAART with CD_4 count >350 μ/dL was likely to achieve better survival rate. The CD_4 count is also an important immunological marker for HIV patients and the rate of CD_4 count decline is often much more rapid in inception of HAART <250 μ/dL with clinical stage IV. A more common methodology employed in the field of epidemiology is survival analysis. Survival analysis sometimes referred to as "duration analysis" analyzes the time to failure, where failure signifies a single discrete event. Survival analysis commonly uses panel and cohort surveys with

D. M. Basavarajaiah, B. Narasimha Murthy, *HIV Transmission*,
https://doi.org/10.1007/978-981-15-0151-7_6

repeated interviews on a sample of interest (Ferradini et al. 2006). Unlike logit and probit models, the dependent variable is the “waiting time until the occurrence of a well-defined event” (Nicastri et al. 2005). A unique element of a survival analysis model is that it is able to retain observations for which the event has not occurred and then take the effects of these observations into account, statistically (Phillips et al. 2008). In the context of ARV treatment in NACP Programme (NACO), survival analysis is a helpful tool for determining the duration of time an individual is likely to survive with certain health symptoms and other demographic, physical, health, and clinical domain characteristics. Epidemiological studies have applied survival analysis to examine the time of survival until death. Rosen et al. (2007) used survival analysis to examine gay men with AIDS and how well realistic acceptance or knowledge of the disease predicts the duration of survival. The authors assess the efficacy of HAART treatment, those who had a “low CD_4 count at the time of inception<250 μ/dL” realistic acceptance and those who had a “high- CD_4 count at the time of inception>250 μ/dL” realistic acceptance and find that those who realistically accepted that they were ill experienced a significant decrease in survival time. Similarly, Reynolds et al. (2009a) used survival analysis to determine the effect of clinical and demographic factors on survival, among 901 AIDS cases in Austria. They concluded that there are considerable differences in survival time between different HIV-risk groups (intravenous drug users, heterosexual contact, and homosexual contact). In a more recent study in Brazil, Reynolds et al. (2009b) used survival analysis to look at the effects of gender differences on survival in HIV/AIDS cohorts. Conditional on the fact that men and women have equal and free access to HAART and other drugs that alleviate the mortal effects of HIV/AIDS, they find survival rates to be dramatically different between males and females (holding all other variables constant). In one specification, being female was shown to be a good predictor of shorter survival. Stringer et al. (2006) also employed survival analysis in Asia and the Pacific Region to predict short-term disease progression among HIV-infected patients, half of whom were receiving antiretroviral treatment and the other half who remained as a control group. They reported that compared to patients receiving antiretroviral treatment, patients not on treatment had a higher rate of disease progression. However, all of these studies differ in their employment of survival analysis. They draw notable conclusions about the length of time a person with certain characteristics survives with a particular disease. This in turn leads to specific policy implications. Most of these studies look at the detrimental impact of HIV/AIDS.

6.2 Model Description

The present study used the survival analysis or “time to event analyses, where the focus was on analyzing the time leading up to an event. For this analysis, the event was defined as death, lost to follow-up, and missed treatment. There were two specific elements of survival analysis data, censoring and non-normality. The purpose of using survival analysis for this study was to follow subjects over the 13 years and to observe at which point in time they experience death (Chen et al. 2008).

6.3 Survival Analysis

This generally refers to statistical analysis for time to event data. The outcome variable of interest is time to event, usually called failure time or survival time or lifetime. For example:

(a) Time from the start of treatment to a failure event
(b) Time from birth to death = lifetime
(c) Time from HIV infection to AIDS
(d) Time from birth to onset of a disease = onset age

The distribution of survival times is usually described or characterized by three functions:

Survival Function

$$S(t) = P(\text{an individual survival longer than } t) = P(T > t)$$

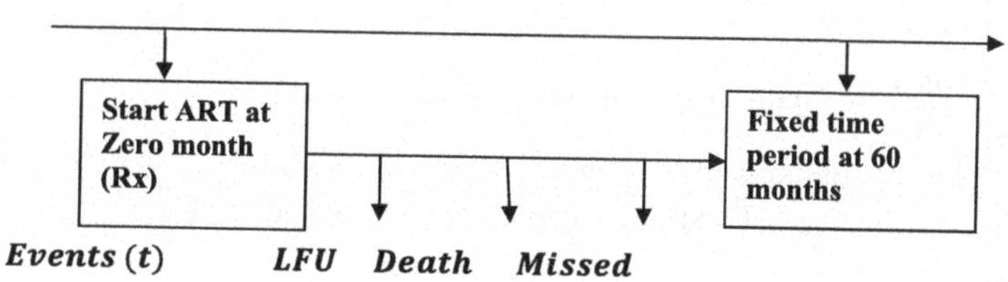

$$S(t) = 1 - P(\text{an individual die before fixed time}).$$
$$S(t) = 1 - F(t).$$

6.4 Concept of the Model

The distribution of survival times is usually described or characterized by three functions.

Survival Function

$$
\begin{aligned}
S(5) &= P(\text{an HIV-infected patient's survival longer than 60 months}) \\
&= P(T > 60 \text{ months})
\end{aligned}
$$

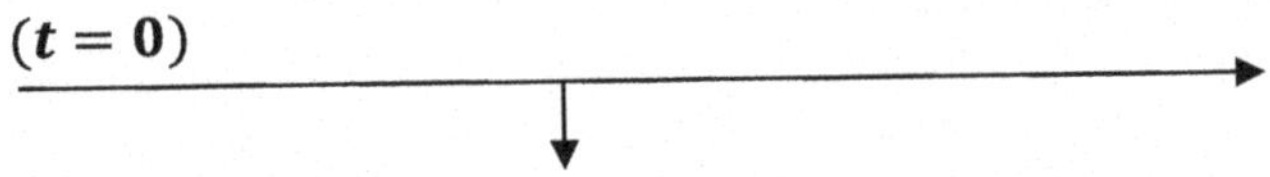

$P(t = 60 \text{ months})$.

$$
\begin{aligned}
S(60) &= 1 - P(\text{an HIV-infected patient dies before 60 months}) \\
&= 1 - F(60 \text{ months})
\end{aligned}
$$

(b) Estimation of $S(t)$:

$$
\widehat{S}(t) = \frac{\text{No. of patients who survive longer than "}t\text{"}}{\text{Total no. of patients in cohort}} \quad (\text{if the observations are not censored})
$$

Probability Density Function

$$
\mathbf{f(t)} = \lim \Delta \mathbf{t} \to 0 \frac{\mathbf{P}(\text{an individual dying in the interval } \mathbf{t,t} + \Delta \mathbf{t},}{\Delta \mathbf{t}}
$$

$$
\mathbf{f(t)} = \frac{-\mathbf{ds(t)}}{\mathbf{dt}} = (\text{The slope of the survival function})
$$

$$
\widehat{\mathbf{f}}(\mathbf{t}) = \frac{\text{No. of patients dying in the interval begining at the time of "}\mathbf{t}\text{"}}{\text{Total no. of patients} \times \text{interval width.}}
$$

(d) Hazard Function(Hz)

$$
\mathbf{h(t)} = \lim \Delta \mathbf{t} \to 0' \frac{1}{\Delta \mathbf{t}} \mathbf{P}(\text{an individual dies in the time interval}(\mathbf{t}, \mathbf{t} + \Delta \mathbf{t})
$$

$$
\begin{aligned}
\mathbf{h(t)} &= \lim \Delta \mathbf{t} \to 0 \frac{1}{\Delta \mathbf{t}} \mathbf{P}((\mathbf{t} < \mathbf{T} < \mathbf{t} + \Delta \mathbf{t})/\mathbf{T} > \mathbf{t}. \\
&= \frac{\mathbf{f(t)}}{1 - \mathbf{f(t)}} = \frac{\mathbf{f(t)}}{\mathbf{S(t)}}
\end{aligned}
$$

Estimation of $h(t)$:

$$\hat{\mathbf{h}}(\mathbf{t}) = \frac{\text{No. of deaths in}(\mathbf{t}, \Delta\mathbf{t})}{\text{No. of alive patients at } \mathbf{t} * \Delta\mathbf{t}} = \frac{\text{No. of deaths in}(\mathbf{t}, \Delta\mathbf{t})/\text{Total pts}}{\Delta\mathbf{t} * (\text{No. of patients at } \mathbf{t})/\text{Total pts}}$$

6.5 Compound Growth Rate Model (CGR)

A number of studies pertaining to HIV progression growth rate have been carried out. The important functional forms employed to study the growth rates were linear, exponential, and logarithmic forms. However, many of the studies have used the geometric forms (compound growth rate) which were given by a well-known method used for the variation of CD_4 count before HAART start (ART) and after 1 year completion of the HAART treatment. However, the compound growth rate is given by $Y = AB^t$, where Y is the variable under the study, B represents the regression coefficient and it is (1 + CGR), CGR is the compound growth rate, and t is time period for assessment of CD_4 count at different time intervals. This model was used to estimate the rate or trend of RNA plasma viral load in the body system, and the incremental changes of CD_4 count over a period of time were calculated by using the equation:

$$\text{CGR} = \frac{b}{\overline{y}} \times 100, \text{ in case of an increase of CD4 count CGR}$$
$$= (\text{Antilog } B - 1) \times 100$$

y: Represents the time period for the assessment of CD4 count at 6 months, 12 months, 24 months, etc.
a, A: Constant values
b, B: Coefficient of regression
CGR: Growth rate,
$\overline{y}$ = Mean of CD4 Count.

6.6 Model Results

In order to capture variations in survival time, the present study used a sample made up of individuals recruited for cohort in 2012 and who were in-depth interviewed (IID) in 2013. There was a total of 202 married women aged between 20 and 29, likely to conceive their pregnancy (Table 6.1).

Table 6.1 Univariate descriptive statistics of CD4 count (age-dependent univariate model)

Sl. no.	Variable	ANCs mean ± SD	*P*-value
1.	Age (year)	23.26 ± 7.18 (202–40.64%)	0.029*
2.	Baseline CD4	116.36 ± 56.46(202)	0.492Ns
3.	CD4 at the end of 6 months	302.01 ± 152.28(196)	0.036*
4.	CD4 at the end of 1-year cohort	372.28 ± 96.73(195)	0.006**
5.	CD4 at the end of 2-year cohort	379.36 ± 65.39(193)	0.021*
6.	CD4 at the end of 3-year cohort	410.00 ± 49.50(191)	0.085*
7.	CD4 at the end of 4-year cohort	445.00 ± 41.29(187)	0.011*
8.	CD4 at the end of 5-year cohort	451.00 ± 36.98(185)	0.003*
(ii)	WHO clinical stage		
(a)	Stage I	Nil	
(b)	Stage II	8(1.60%)	0. 531 ns
(c)	Stage III	85 (17.10%)	0.422 ns
(d)	Stage IV	109 (21.93%)	0.488 ns
(e)	Working assessment up to 5 years	157(31.58%)	0.067*
(f)	Ambulatory assessment up to 5 years	20(4.02%)	0.176 ns
(g)	Bedridden assessment up to 5 years	09(1.81%)	0.402 ns
(h)	Death	16(3.24%)	0.033*
(iii)	HIV-TB co-infection		
(a)	Yes	18(7.24%)	0.203 ns
(b)	No	184(37.02%)	0.891 ns
(iv)	Mean duration of Rx start to end of the fifth cohort		
(a)	Mean days	1738 ± 48.93(186)	0.002**

Significant $p < 0.01$

The average age of the patient was 23.26 ± 7.18 years; mean baseline CD_4 count before start of HAART was lower than the national guidelines; it was recorded as 116.36 ± 56.46 μ/dL; after 1 year of completion of HAART, mean CD_4 count had increased: CD_4 at 6 months (302.01 ± 152.28 μ/dL), CD4 at 1 year (372.28 ± 96.73 μ/dL), CD4 at 2 years (379.36 ± 65.39 μ/dL), CD4 at 3 years (410.00 ± 49.5 μ/dL 0), CD_4 at 4 years (445.00 ± 41.29 μ/dL), and CD4 at 5 years (451.00 ± 36.98 μ/dL). WHO clinical staging was assessed based on national guidelines, WHO stage II, 8(1.60%); stage III, 85 (17.10%); and stage IV, 109 (21.93%), and found to be statistically nonsignificant. Clinical and physical assessment was made by Cronbach scale, the PLHIV, who were in working condition, was 157 (31.58%, $p < 0.05$), ambulatory 20 (4.02%, $P > 0.05$), bedridden 09 (1.81%, $p > 0.05$), death 16 (3.24%, $p < 0.05$), and HIV-TB co-infection 7.24%. Mean duration of HAART initiation at the end of the study was 1738 ± 48.93 days with $p < 0.002$, which was statistically significant (Tables 6.2 and 6.3).

Table 6.2 Survivability of a different CD4 category with HAART duration

Survival time (weeks)	Survival proportion	Standard error	Survival proportion	Standard error
9	–	–	0.947	0.0512
12	0.987	0.0124	0.895	0.0704
13	0.975	0.0175	–	–
14	0.962	0.0212	–	–
18	–	–	–	–
19	0.950	0.0245	–	–
20	0.924	0.0298	–	–
22	0.911	0.0322	–	–
23	0.871	0.0381	0.842	0.0837
24	0.818	0.0440	0.737	0.101
25	0.792	0.0464	–	–
26	0.751	0.0496	–	–
30	0.738	0.0504	–	–
34	0.711	0.0522	0.614	0.116
35	0.697	0.0529	–	–
36	0.599	0.0569	0.553	0.119
38	–	–	–	–
40	–	–	–	–
44	0.541	0.0584	–	–
45	0.351	0.0569	0.484	0.123
46	0.305	0.0553	–	–
47	0.290	0.0546	–	–
48	–	–	–	–
52	0.275	0.0538	–	–
53	0.259	0.0529	–	–
54	0.198	0.0485	0.387	0.131
55	0.183	0.0471	0.258	0.137
56	0.0915	0.0354	0.129	0.114
58	0.0732	0.0327	–	–
60	0.0488	0.0295	–	–
63	0.000	0.000	–	–

Comparison of survival curves (log-rank test)

6.7 Model Discussion

In order to analyze the relative risk of an individual surviving, the data described above were converted into survival data by establishing the two time variables (start, which is age in 2004, and end, which is age at death or age in 2010) and the failure variable (1, if dead). After setting the data to survival analysis mode, there were 488 total failures, with the average entry age of 23 years (time 0:2004) and the

Table 6.3 Survival rate on HAART patients determined by using growth model

Sl. no.	Components	Coefficient	SE	R^2 (%)	Survival growth or rate	P-value
1.	Intercept (year)	4.217	0.080	45.64%	0.652 ns	$P \geq 0.05$
	Rx start (HAART) <250 CD4 cell count (μ/dL)	0.072	0.007			
2.	Intercept (year)	9.382	0.065	89.75%	0.980[a]	$P \leq 0.05$
	Rx start (HAART) >250 CD4 cell count (μ/dL)	0.077	0.004			

[a]Significant at 0.05 level

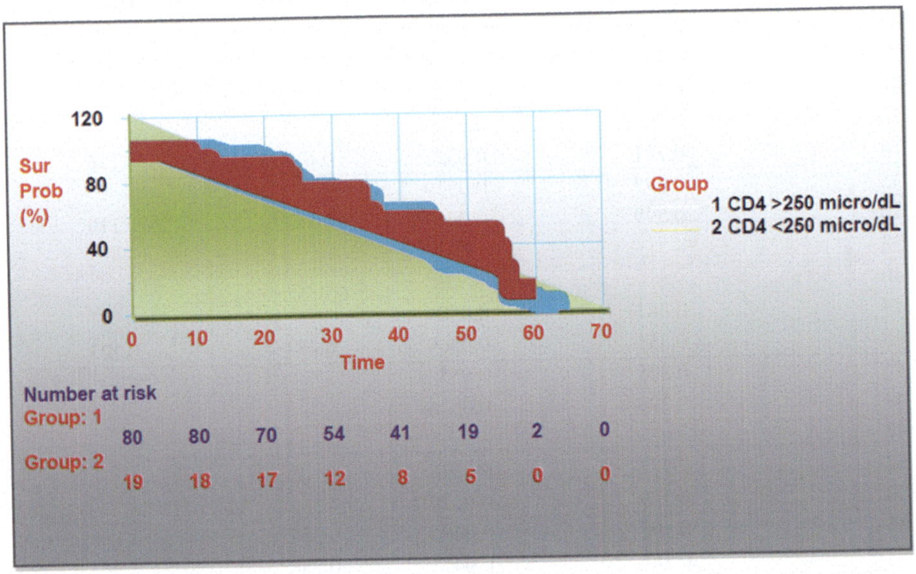

Fig. 6.1 Kaplan–Meier survival curve and its 95% confidence interval for patients initiating therapy from a different CD4 category

average exit age of 30 years (time 1:2010). From 2004, the average survival time for an individual was about 5 years. Overall, 16 individuals were reported to be dead by 2004. Before running a Cox proportional-hazards model, the Kaplan–Meier curve was estimated for two groups, i.e., low CD4 count <250 μ/dL and higher CD4 count >250 μ/dL (Fig. 6.1). The curve showed no significant difference in survival probability between two groups. Results from the statistical test confirmed that there was no statistical significance for CD4 count in survival probabilities (log-rank test $p = 0.20$). Similarly, the Kaplan–Meier survival curve was predicted for previously married individuals (divorced, widowed, or separated) relative to individuals who have either never married or married; the curve showed that there was a significant difference between the two groups of individuals (log-rank test $p = 0.000$).

The Kaplan–Meier model was useful for understanding the differences in survival time for individual exogenous variables. To capture the effects of multiple variables on survival time, the study also used a Cox proportional-hazards model. Cox proportional-hazards ratio for the risk of death of an individual with certain OI symptoms is presented in three different specifications. In the first specification, the effect of the four chronic symptoms on survival time was evaluated. Persistent weight-loss symptom was reported as statistically significant ($p < 0.01$), where the risk of disease progression to death was 16% greater than those who do not report having chronic weight-loss (Stringer et al. 2006). Although not statistically significant, individuals reporting the other three chronic symptoms were predicted to have a greater risk of death, relative to those individuals who do not report a chronic illness. Controlling for other biological and demographic exogenous variables, the second and third specifications showed that there are other factors that contribute to a shorter survival time (Rosen et al. 2007). In the third specifications, individuals experiencing persistent weight loss have a 23% greater risk of death, compared to individuals who do not experienced this chronic illness.

The variable duration of chronic illnesses and OIs was also statistically significant ($p < 0.01$). As hypothesized, individuals who reported having a chronic illness of less than a year were likely to live longer. In the analysis, individuals who experienced a chronic illness between 53 and 104 weeks (1–2 years) presented 64% greater risk of death than individuals who experienced some chronic symptoms between 0 and 26 weeks (6 months). Women who reported between 157 and 209 weeks of illness (3–4 years) had 94% greater risk of death compared to the baseline group and showed no statistical significance or effect on the estimated risk of survival for individuals reporting chronic illness compared to those who do not report any illness (Sungkanuparph et al. 2007; Samb et al. 2007). The quality of the diagnosis cannot be measured in this variable. As a result, doctor's diagnosis for a chronic illness had little effect on the estimated risk of death. Age was only statistically significant for one group of individuals (HAART start >250 CD_4 μ/dL); 21- to 26-year-olds had lower-risk group and survived more. Individuals aged 26–35 years old were found to have a 61% greater risk of progression to death compared to the baseline age group (HAART start <250 CD_4 μ/dL). There was a trend of increased risk of progression to death as age increases (63% greater risk for individuals 18–25 years old and 87.0% greater risk for individuals 26–34 years old). Estimated hazard ratios for other age categories were not statistically significant and therefore are not presented in the table. While the use of the cohort data containing demographic and biological information allows for the analysis of survival time, survivability models have many limitations. First, the variables used to capture the chronic health symptoms are very limited in scope. There is no medical examination or in-depth analysis of each symptom (Tuboi et al. 2007). Further, these data rely heavily on the individual's ability to consistently self-report the chronic and OI symptoms, they have been experiencing and for how long. If the data are reported inconsistently, the results in this analysis are likely to be biased. Second, the CD_4 count was evaluated for chronic symptoms; in this study, chronic weight loss alone was statistically significant ($p < 0.01$) and the strongest predictor of risk of death (World health organization 2010). There are a number of exogenous factors that could be biasing the hazard ratio on the chronic weight loss variable. Some of these factors include poor nutrition, acute or chronic illness, or a disease inherent to the family. Most of the patients well complied with treatment adherence (>95%). The cumulative survival rate after inception of HAART was 0.98 ($p \leq 0.05$, $R^2 = 79.82\%$). HAART with CD_4 count>350 μ/dL was likely to have achieved better survival rate (Weidle et al. 2006). The CD_4 count was also an important immunological marker for HIV-infected patients; the rate of CD_4 count decline was often much more rapid, if inception of HAART was at CD_4 <250 μ/dL with clinical WHO stage IV (Wools-Kaloustian et al. 2006).

6.8 Summary

Growth model can easily calculate the rate of survivability; it is the best model for forecasting the survival rate. The findings of these models are strengthened by the relatively homogeneous as well as heterogeneous study population. While fitting up of survival and growth model, the method of growth analysis provide a good estimate of survival rate ($R^2 = 81.25\%$) with proportion of survival growth of 0.95.

References

Chen SC et al (2008) Increased mortality of male adults with AIDS related to poor compliance to antiretroviral therapy in Malawi. Tropical Med Int Health 13:513–519

Ferradini L, Jeannin A, Pinoges L et al (2006) Scaling up of highly active antiretroviral therapy in a rural district of Malawi: an effectiveness assessment. Lancet 367:1335–1342

Hoffmann CJ, Charalambous S et al (2009) Viremia, resuppression, and time to resistance in human immunodeficiency virus (HIV) subtype C during first-line antiretroviral therapy in South Africa. Clin Infect Dis 49:1928–1935

Kahn JG et al (2011) CD4 cell count and viral load monitoring of antiretroviral therapy in Uganda: cost effectiveness study. BMJ 343:d6884

Kamya MR et al (2007) Predictors of long-term viral failure among Ugandan children and adults treated with antiretroviral therapy. J Acquir Immune Defic Syndr 46:187–193

Keiser O et al (2008) Antiretroviral therapy in resource-limited settings 1996 to 2006: patient characteristics, treatment regimens and monitoring in sub-Saharan Africa, Asia and Latin America. Trop Med Int Health 13:870–879

Lohse N, Kronborg G, Gerstoft J, Larsen CS, Pedersen G, Pedersen C et al (2006) Virological control during the first 6–18 months after initiating highly active antiretroviral therapy as a predictor for outcome in HIV-infected patients: a Danish, population-based, 6-year follow-up study. Clin Infect Dis 42:136–144

Nicastri E, Chiesi A, Angeletti C, Sarmati L, Palmisano L, Geraci A et al (2005) Clinical outcome after 4 years follow-up of HIV-seropositive subjects with incomplete virologic or immunologic response to HAART. J Med Virol 76:153–160

Phillips AN, Pillay D, Miners AH, Bennett DE, Gilks CF, Lundgren JD (2008) Outcomes from monitoring of patients on antiretroviral therapy in resource-limited settings with viral load, CD4 cell count, or clinical observation alone: a computer simulation model. Lancet 371:1443–1451

Reynolds SJ, Nakigozi G, Newell K, Ndyanabo A, Galiwongo R, Boaz I et al (2009a) Failure of immunologic criteria to appropriately identify antiretroviral treatment failure in Uganda. AIDS 23:697–700

Reynolds SJ, Kityo C, Mbamanya F, Ndyanabo A, Galiwongo R, Boaz I et al (2009b) Evolution of drug resistance after virological failure of a first-line highly active antiretroviral therapy regimen in Uganda. Antivir Ther 14:293–297

Rosen S, Fox MP, Gill CJ (2007) Patient retention in antiretroviral therapy programs in sub-Saharan Africa: a systematic review. PLoS Med 4:e298

Samb B, Celletti F, Holloway J, Van Damme W, De Cock KM, Dybul M (2007) Rapid expansion of the health workforce in response to the HIV epidemic. N Engl J Med 357:2510–2514

Stringer JS, Zulu I, Levy J, Stringer EM, Mwango A, Chi B et al (2006) Rapid scale-up of antiretroviral therapy at primary care sites in Zambia: feasibility and early outcomes. JAMA 296:782–793

Sungkanuparph S, Manosuthi W, Kiertiburanakul S, Piyavong B, Chumpathat N, Chantratita W (2007) Options for a second-line antiretroviral regimen for HIV type 1-infected patients whose initial regimen of a fixed-dose combination of stavudine, lamivudine, and nevirapine fails. Clin Infect Dis 44:447–452

Tuboi SH, Brinkhof MW, Egger M, Stone RA, Braitstein P, Nash D et al (2007) Discordant responses to potent antiretroviral treatment in previously naive HIV-1-infected adults initiating treatment in resource-constrained countries: the antiretroviral therapy in low-income countries (ART-LINC) collaboration. J Acquir Immune Defic Syndr 45:52–59

Weidle PJ, Wamai N, Solberg P, Liechty C, Sendagala S, Were W et al (2006) Adherence to antiretroviral therapy in a home-based AIDS care programme in rural Uganda. Lancet 368:1587–1594

Wools-Kaloustian K, Kimaiyo S, Diero L, Siika A, Sidle J, Yiannoutsos CT et al (2006) Viability and effectiveness of large-scale HIV treatment initiatives in sub-Saharan Africa: experience from western Kenya. AIDS 20:41–48

World Health Organization (2010) Antiretroviral therapy for HIV infection in adults and adolescents in resource-limited settings: recommendations towards a public health approach. WHO, Geneva

Predictive Model Approach to HIV TB Co-infection in Vertical Transmission

7

7.1 Introduction

Tuberculosis (TB) is the most common AIDS-defining opportunistic infection worldwide (UNAIDS 2001). HIVTB co-infection is becoming a global emergency especially in India (NACO, 2016). Its diagnosis is notoriously challenging in countries, with poor resources and with limited diagnostic facilities.(Paranjape et al. 1997) defined AIDS as characterized by a number of opportunistic infections (OIs), which are responsible for high morbidity and mortality (Pawlowski et al. 2012; Kumarasamy et al. 2004; Krischner et al. 1999; Lange et al. 2004). In fact, even before the discovery of the causative virus, cases of AIDS were defined as those having certain opportunistic infections (OIs) (Mahe et al. 2005). The spectrum and distribution of opportunistic infections in AIDS patients is ever-expanding. This spectrum varies from continent to continent as also between children and adults (UNAIDS 2001; Nita et al. 2014). There are differences in the pattern of opportunistic infections (OIs) in AIDS patients depending upon the risk group. From the limited studies conducted, it is quite apparent that tuberculosis is the single most important opportunistic infection associated with AIDS in our country (NACO, 2016). It is estimated that an HIV-infected individual is six times at higher risk of acquiring tuberculosis than an HIV-negative individual. In AIDS patients, the incidence of extrapulmonary tuberculosis (EPTB) increases and that of smear positive pulmonary tuberculosis decreases (PTB) making the diagnosis of the disease much more difficult, unless good diagnostic tools are available (Pawlowski et al. 2012). In the present chapter, the prevalence, pattern, and risk factors for HIV TB co-infection among infected children were discussed.

D. M. Basavarajaiah, B. Narasimha Murthy, *HIV Transmission*,
https://doi.org/10.1007/978-981-15-0151-7_7

7.2 Methods and Data Source

Cross-sectional 5-year retrospective cohort data sets were obtained from the ART center between April 2004 and December 2009. Demographic profile, age, sex, family history, occupation, economic status, educational status, and HIV seropositivity of the parents were included. Clinical profile, type of regimen, duration of the regimen, WHO clinical stage, types of OIs, onset of OIs to start of HAART, complication and illness, anthropometric parameters and growth parameters, and immunological markers like CD4 (μ/dL) count at baseline, CD4 (μ/dL) count at onset of TB, and progressive serial CD4 (μ/dL) count were collected with written permission. Collected data was analyzed by using SAS and SPSS16.50 version. Logistic regression and univariate models were used to draw the significant inference.

7.3 Formulation of Model (Logistic Regression Model)

In the present study, setting an outcome as presence/absence of OIs (presence coded 1 and absence coded 0). The focus was on situations in which the outcome variable was dichotomous, although extension of the techniques of LRA (logistic regression analysis) was to outcome with three or more categories (improved CD_4 count), CD_4 remains same or consistently maintained or worsen. (Prasad et al. 2003a; Prasad R et al.2003b; Purohit et al.1996; Quigley et al. 2001; Rajasekharan et al. 2000; Roeger et al. 2009; Samuel et al. 1996; Shah et al. 2013a). In this section, the simple regression model was reviewed and then presented to the model for LRA. The fundamental model underlying logistic regression analysis (LRA) poses that a continuous outcome variable is in theory, a linear combination of a set of predictors (age, sex, CD4 count, etc.). Thus, for an outcome variable, Y and a set of p predictor variables $X_1,\ldots,X_p$, the LRA model is fitted in the following form:

$$Y_{ij} = \alpha_i + \beta_j X_1 + \beta_j X_2 + \ldots \beta_n X_n + \epsilon_{ij} \tag{7.1}$$

where:

Y_{ij}= Observed value of ith infected baby with effect of OIs at j^{th} period
α_i= Effect of OIs on i^{th} infected baby
$\beta_n X_n$= Coefficient values on nth variable or parameter
ϵ_{ij}= Error associated with i^{th} infected baby with effect of OIs at j^{th} period

$$Y_{ij} = \alpha_i + \sum\nolimits_{i=1}^{n} \beta_n X_n + \epsilon_{ij} \tag{7.2}$$

$$E(Y/X_1 X_2 X_P) = Y^1 = \alpha + \sum_{j=1}^{r} \beta_j X_j$$

$$\text{Loge}\left[\frac{\pi}{1-\pi}\right] = \alpha + \beta_1 X_1 + \cdots \beta_P X_P.$$

$$\text{Loge}\left[\frac{\pi}{1-\pi}\right] = \alpha + \sum_{j=1}^{r} \beta_j X_j$$

"Y" variable coded 0 and 1, 0, 1 represented OIs with or without present,

$$\text{ODD ratio of OIs} = \text{Loge}\left[\frac{\pi}{1-\pi}\right]$$

7.4 Model Results

Table 7.1 Descriptive statistics of HIV-infected children on HAART demographic and laboratory profile

Sl	Categorical variable	Male	Female
i	Age(years)	6.2 ± 3.4	5.63 ± 4.80
(a)	<5 years	38(63.33%)	22(36.66%)
ii	Family history		
(a)	Parents' education status		
(b)	Illiterate	32(84.21%)	15(68.10%)
(c)	Literate	06(15.78%)	07(31.81%)
iii	Economic status		
(a)	Low income group	22(36.66%)	12(20.00%)
(b)	Medium income group	09(15.00%0	06(10.00%)
(c)	High income group	07(11.66%)	04(6.66%)
iv	Occupation		
(a)	Employed	15(25.0%)	07(11.66%)
(b)	Unemployed	19(31.66%)	12(20.00%)
(c)	Unknown	04(6.66%)	03(5.00%)
v.	Residence		
(a)	Urban	07(11.66%)	05(8.33%)
(b)	Rural	29(48.33%)	15(25.00%)
(c)	Not known	04(6.66%)	02(3.33%)
vi.	WHO clinical staging		
(a)	Stage-I	05(8.33%)	01(1.66%)
(b)	Stage-II	08(13.33%)	04(6.66%)
(c)	Stage-III	07(11.66%)	07(11.66%)
(d)	Stage-IV	18(30.00%)	10(16.66%)
vii	Regimen		
	S+L+N	13(21.66%)	09(15.0%)
	S+L+E	09(15.0%)	03(5.0%)
	Z+L+N	12(20.0%0	06(10.0%)
	Z+L+E	04(6.66%)	04(6.66%)
viii	Immunological marker		
	CD4 (%)	8.36	7.65 ($P \leq 0.05$)

Table 7.2 TB sites and WHO clinical stage

Sites of TB	No (%)	WHO clinical stage	CD4 cell count	CD4 (%)	P-value
Pulmonary TB	08 (13.33%)	3	242	8.2	$P < 0.05$
Disseminated	02 (3.33%)	4	08	4.8	$P < 0.05$
TBM	03 (5.00%)	4	146	6.3	$P < 0.05$
Lymph node	01 (1.66%)	3	310	11.9	$P < 0.05$
Bone	02 (3.33%)	4	102	5.1	$P < 0.05$
Total	16 (26.66%)	4	161	7.2	$P < 0.05$

Table 7.3 Age-wise distribution and site of TB in co-infected children

Age (years)	PTB	Disseminated	TBM	Lymph node	Bone
0–1 years	02 (12.50%)	0.0	02 (12.50%)	0.0	0.0
>1–2 years	02 (12.50%)	01 (6.25%)	01 (6.25%)	01 (6.25%)	01 (6.25%)
>2–5 years	01 (6.25%)	01 (6.25%)	0.0	0.0	01 (6.25%)
>5–10 years	02 (12.50%)	0.0	0.0	0.0	0.0
>10–15 years	01 (6.25%)	0.0	0.0	0.0	0.0
>15–17 years	00	00	0.0	0.0	0.0
Total	08 (50.0%)	02 (12.50%)	03 (18.75%)	01 (6.25%)	02 (12.50%)

Table 7.4 Sensitivity, specificity, and +ve predictive value for various methods used for diagnosis of TB co-infected children

Sl. No	Variables used for TB diagnosis	(%)	Sensitivity (%)	Specificity (%)	PPV (%)
a	History of chronic cough >1 month	10	44.40	92.50	21.10
b	Positive history of contact (TB)	39	55.6	80.10	11.10
c	+Ve chest X-ray (TB)	3.00	11.1	82.6	2.10
d	History of ingestion of unpasteurized cow milk	5.00	12.2	98.50	40.0
e	Mantoux test >5 mm in diameter	00	00	00	00
f	Gastric lavage for AFB	04	00	00	00
g	Sputum for AFB	05	00	00	00
h	Weight loss(>10 kgs)	29	100	80.0	18.40

Table 7.5 Association between presence and absence of opportunistic infection, categorical variables, and HIV CD4 count marker

Variables	β	SE	Wald	Sig	Exp (β)	CI-95% for Exp(β)
a. Baseline CD4 count	−0.02	0.01	3.91	0.048	0.998	1.00
b. CD4 count after 1 year HAART	0.00	0.02	0.072	0.788	6.00	1.003
c. Age	0.071	0.104	0.464	0.469	1.073	1.315
d. Sex	−0.414	0.668	0.385	0.535	0.661	2.446
e. Opportunistic infection	0.794	1.37	0.335	0.563	2.221	

−2log likelihood function −60.57, Cox-Snell R square = 0.140, Nagelkerke $R^2 = 0.203$, $p \leq 0.05$

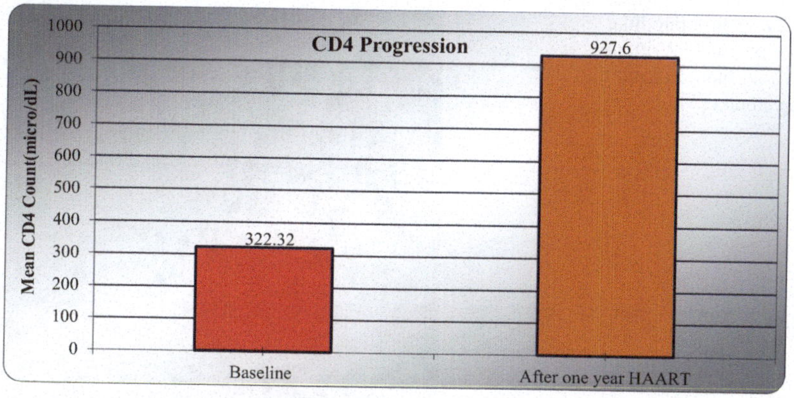

Fig. 7.1 Trend of CD4 count in pediatric TB-HIV co-infected

7.5 Model Proof

Logistic regression method was used to correlate the functions of explanatory variables to the probability of ("Diseases presence1=yes, 0=no"). We had adjusted for the confounding effect of CD4 count and age. The effect of relationship is presented below (Fig. 7.1)

$$\log_e\left(\frac{p_i}{1-p_i}\right) = \alpha_i + \sum_{i=1}^{60\ \text{children}} \beta_j X_j$$

The function $\log_e[p_i/(1 - p_i)]$ is called the "logit." Odds ratio of CD4 count with respect to OIs was six times greater than odd, for those with non TB presented in Table 7.5 younger age groups were highly associated with exposure of TB, nearly 1.07 times greater risk of TB co-infection. From Table 7.1) in a total of 60 HIV-infected children reviewed during the 5 years period, 15 (25.26%) were diagnosed as having coexisting TB. Their mean age, weight, CD4 cell count, and CD4 percentage at the time of diagnosis were 6.3 ± 2.4 years, 14.3 ± 3.4 kg, 262 ± 28.0 cells/ml, and 9.9%, respectively. Pulmonary TB accounted for 14.60% of all TB cases, while disseminated form was seen in 3%, TB meningitis (5.0%) and TB bone (2.5%). TB defaulter at 2 months, 6 months, and 8 months was 0.86%, 1.10%, and 2.56%, respectively. The mean CD4 cell count and percentage of 261.6 ± 28.0 cells/ml and 9.9%, respectively, signify severe immune suppression. From Table 7.1 resulted values were found that there was no statistical significant difference in the characteristics of male and female co-infected children. Table 7.3 depicted that the children in younger age group were found to be more susceptible to TB and they were detected sputum positive (7.60%). Table 7.2 children in the age group of 1–2 years and 2–5 years were statistically significant ($p \leq 0.05$) with TBM

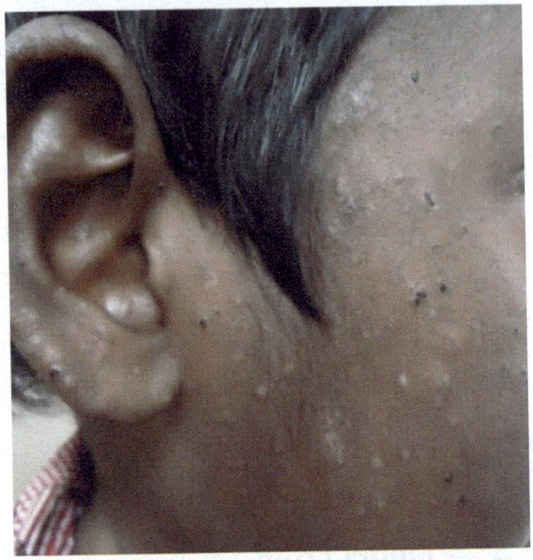

Fig. 7.2a Papulopnodular dermatoses. Note: Written permission obtained from the patient caretaker

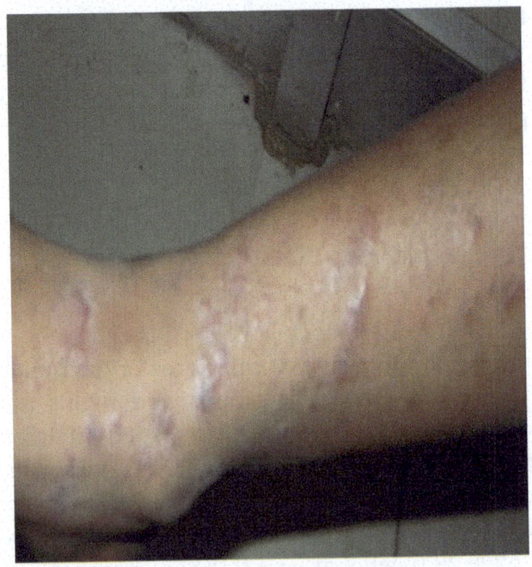

Fig. 7.2b Lichenoid eruption. Note: Written permission obtained from the patient caretaker

and disseminated TB (3.33%). The environment in which the children live and CD4 cell count are two important indicator variables, which were considered to be HIV TB co-infection and also HAART was started at a very low CD4 cell count (<10.62%) and high RNA plasma viral load, the TB manifestation were highly associated with aforesaid parameters presented in (Fig. 7.2a, 7.2b, 7.2c, 7.2d, 7.2e, 7.2f, 7.2g, 7.2h and 7.2i) section.

Table 7.4 concludes that identification of AFB in sputum specimens and radiological diagnosis were used as standards for diagnosis in the present chapter. The sensitivity, specificity, and PPV of the common clinical presentations, signs, and

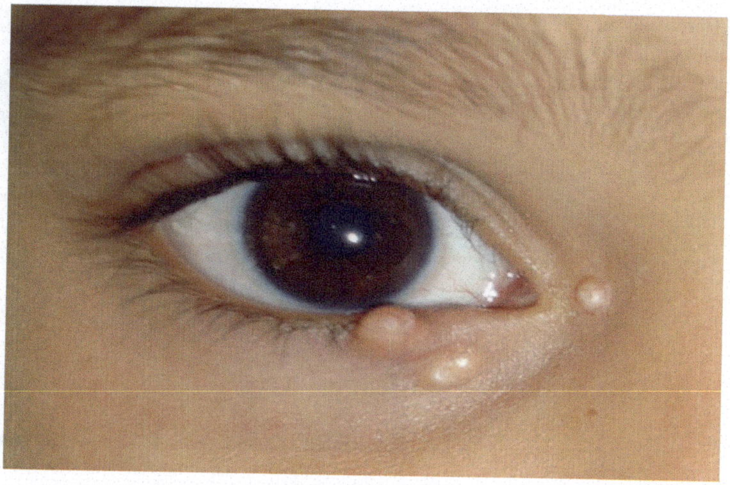

Fig. 7.2c Molluscum contagiosum. Note: Written permission obtained from the patient caretaker

Fig. 7.2d Herpes labialis. Note: Written permission obtained from the patient caretaker

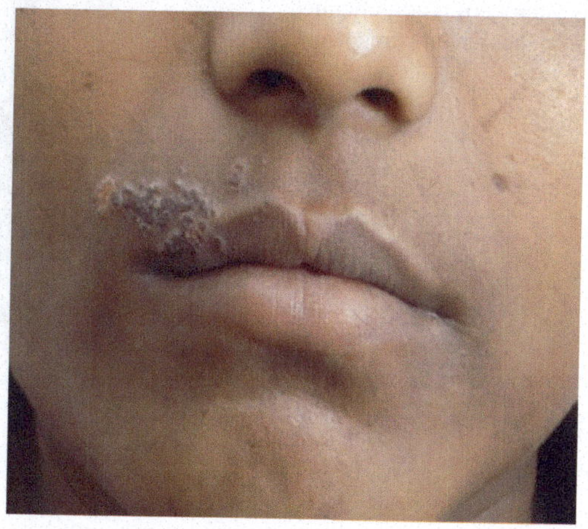

radiological/laboratory investigations were discussed. As per the resulted parameters, the history of chronic cough for >1 month, severe weight loss, history of contact with adults with chronic cough (TB), Mantoux test with induration of >5 mm, chest x-ray and non-response to conventional antibiotics are all parameters showed to be low to moderate sensitivity and specificity with the exception of severe weight loss of >-3SD. (sensitivity/specificity of 88.9% and 88.6%, respectively). The outcomes showed mere two patients (3.33%) died from disseminated TB and also they had developed an immune reconstitution inflammatory syndrome (IRIS). All patients received ATT and all were started on HAART therapy. The serial CD4 count after start of HAART had significantly improved ($p < 0.01$). TB is a communicable disease, spread primarily through droplets expelled by someone who has

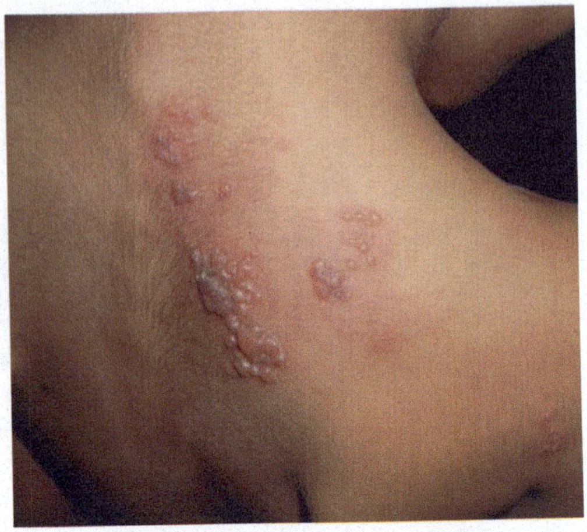

Fig. 7.2e Herpes zoster. Note: Written permission obtained from the patient caretaker

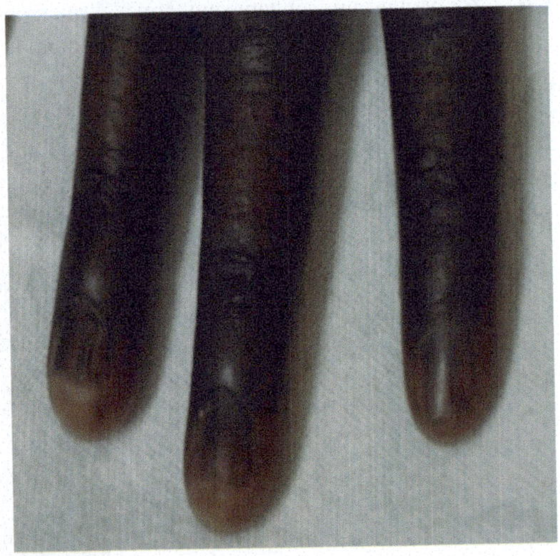

Fig. 7.2f Nail hyperpigmentation. Note: Written permission obtained from the patient caretaker

infectious pulmonary or laryngeal TB, when they cough or sneeze. It can occasionally be contracted by ingestion of contaminated unpasteurized cow's milk. The number/concentration of the organism expelled into the air during coughing or sneezing, the duration of exposure to infected persons, and the condition of the immune system of the host are the major factors that predict the transmission of TB to another person. Close contacts are at highest risk and children acquire this from infected adults. TB is equally a disease of poverty and easily acquired in overcrowded environment with low standard of living. Some studies among HIV patients have shown greater association between low CD4 cell counts and more susceptibility for TB, especially extrapulmonary forms. In the present chapter, all the TB co-infected children were in WHO stages III and IV disease with severe immune

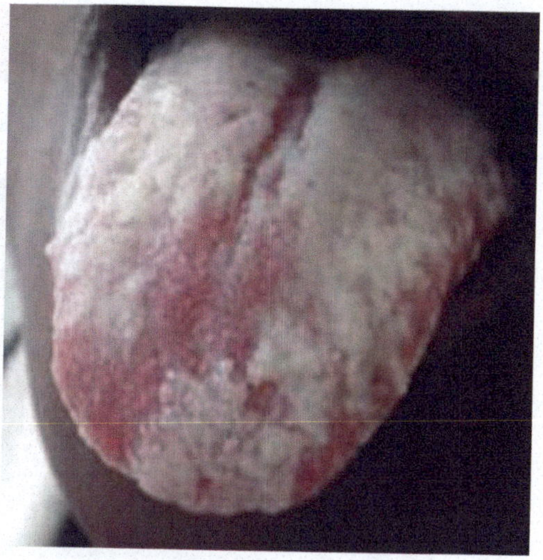

Fig. 7.2g Oral candidiasis. Note: Written permission obtained from the patient caretaker

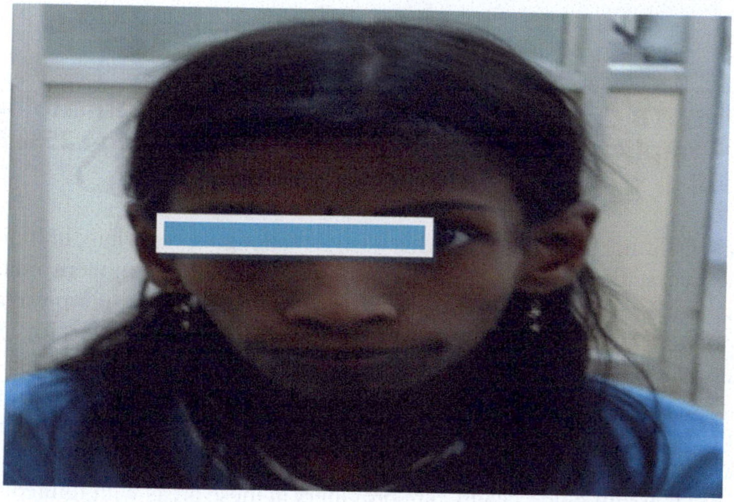

Fig. 7.2h Lipoatrophy. Note: Written permission obtained from the patient caretaker

suppression and very low CD4 count, at the time of inception of HAART. Some authors have reported that the association between low CD4 cell count and TB in HIV patients was statistically significant ($p < 0.01$) with HIV illness and mortality. Cohen et al. suggest that the inception of HAART with higher CD4 count can reduce the incidence of TB in children. The same findings were reported by (UNAIDS, 2001; Shah et al. 2013a; Sharma et al. 2000; Sharomi et al. 2008a; Sharomi et al. 2008b; Song et al. 2002; Tripathi et al. 2002; Tripathy et al. 1996; Shah et al. 2013b).

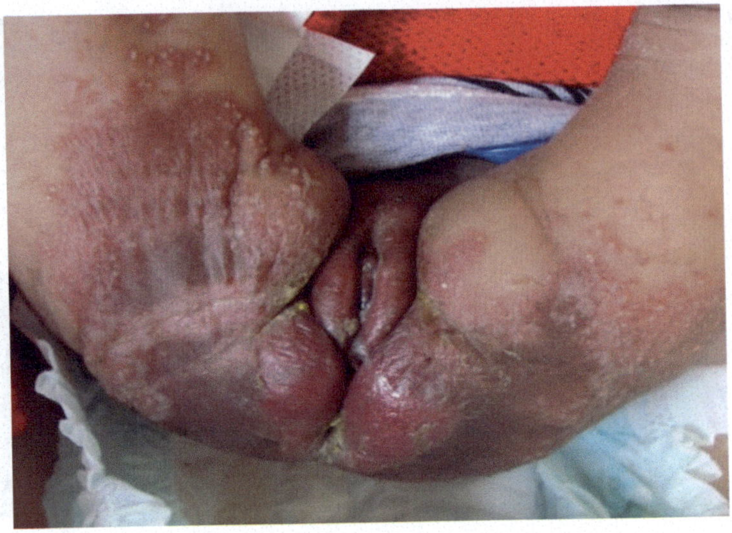

Fig. 7.2i Crural candidiasis on genital area. Note: Written permission obtained from the patient caretaker

7.6 HIV TB Co-infection Children Manifested Dermatological Complications at Low CD4 Count (CD4 Count <25% Micro/dl)

Diagnosis of TB in HIV children has been very challenging especially in India and as poor resource settings, because of non-availability of newer modern methods of diagnosis and overlap of TB and HIV symptoms and signs. In the present study, culture-proven methods and newer techniques were not available (Joyce 2015). Diagnosis was mainly based on combinations of older methods. These include history of contact with adult with chronic cough (80.10%), history of cough of greater than 1 month duration (82.60%), chest X-ray suggestive of pulmonary TB (95.1%), and Mantoux test of indurations (8.60%). The fitted model was to provide information that will guide health-care providers in these areas with limited facilities to predict HIV-infected children for risk of co-infection with TB (Wang et al. 2014; Wilkinson et al. 1998). Severe weight loss of greater than (>3SD) below the mean weight for age was found to have greater sensitivity and specificity, though with lower predictive value, and can be used to predict HIV-infected children for the risk of co-infection with TB (NACO, 2016). Many cases of IRIS associated with TB in adult HIV patients occur on commencement of HAART, and several have been reported in India. Little information is available on HIV-infected children. Immune reconstitution inflammatory syndrome (IRIS) is defined as paradoxical clinical deterioration after inception of HAART, the CD4 cell count recorded at the time of IRIS was (1256 ± 85.60 μ/Dl), and median duration was (IQR) 4–6 weeks, resulting from improving immune system interaction with organisms that have colonized the body during early stages of HIV TB co-infection (Central TB Division 2003; Escombe et al. 2008; Fernandes et al. 2002; Gakkhar et al. 2012; Harries et al. 2001) .

7.7 Summary

TB co-infection with HIV-infected children is very common. Severe weight loss and cough can be used as a clinical guide to identify HIV-infected children at risk of co-infection with TB who will require careful observation, further evaluation, and intervention. Our fitted model will help clinicians, policymakers, and researchers for predicting the accrual parameters for HIV TB co-infection, and also this model can allow for compilation and prediction of indicator variables of TB co-infection.

References

Bauer AL et al (2008) The effect of HIV-1 infection on latent tuberculosis. Math Mode Nat Phenom 3(Suppl 7):229–266

Central TB Division (2003) Directorate general of health services, RNTCP status report. TB India, New Delhi

Escombe AR et al (2008) The infectiousness of tuberculosis patients co-infected with HIV. PLoS Med 8(Suppl 9):189–191

Fernandes L, Lawande D, Mesquita AM (2002) Prevalence of HIV infection among tuberculosis patients in Goa. Indian J Tuberc 49:35–236

Gakkhar S, Chavda N (2012) A dynamical model for HIVTB co-infection. (Publisher Name,. J Appl Math Comput 218:9261–9270

Harries AD et al (2001) Deaths from tuberculosis in Sub-Saharan African countries with a high prevalence of HIV-1. Lancet 357(9267):1519–1529

Joyce KN (2015) Mathematical modeling of tuberculosis as an opportunistic respiratory co-infection in HIV/AIDS in the presence of protection. Appl Math Sci 9(Suppl 105):5215–5233. ID gov. https://www.aids.gov/hiv-aids-basics/. Retrieved 12/31/2015

Krischner D et al (1999) Dynamics of co-infection with M. tuberculosis and HIV-1. Theor Popul Biol 55:94–109

Kulshershtha R, Nigam M, Sarin S, Mathur A (1997) Prevalence of AIDS among tuberculosis patients in Lucknow. Indian J Med Microbiol 15:79–81

Kumarasamy N et al (2004) Incidence of immune reconstitution syndrome in HIV/tuberculosis-coinfected patients after initiation of generic antiretroviral therapy in India. J Acquir Immune Defic Syndr 37(5):1574–1576

Lange JMA et al (2004) What policymakers should know about drug resistance and adherence in the context of scaling-up treatment of HIV infection. AIDS 18(suppl 3):69–S74

Mahe D, Harries A, Haileyesus G et al (2005) Tuberculosis and HIV interaction in subsaharan africa: impact on patients and programmes; implications for policies. Trop Med Int Health 21 (Suppl 8):734–742

National AIDS Control Organization and Central TB Division (2016) New Delhi: treatment guidelines for TB in HIV infected. Ministry of Health and Family Welfare, Government of India, Delhi

Nita H, Shah JG et al (2014) Modelling of HIV-TB co-infection transmission dynamics. Am J Epidemiol Infect Dis 2(Suppl 1):1–7. 3

Paranjape RS, Tripathy SP, Menon PA, Mehendale SM, Khatavkar P, Joshi DR et al (1997) Increasing trend of HIV sero prevalence among pulmonary tuberculosis patients in Pune, India. Indian J Med Res 106:207–211

Pawlowski A et al (2012) Tuberculosis and HIV co-infection. PLoS Pathog 8(Suppl 2):1896–1898

Prasad JK, Saini RK, Kannaujia S, Sarin Suryakant R et al (2003a) Trend of HIV infection in patients with pulmonary tuberculosis in Lucknow area. Indian J Tuberc 39:41–45

Prasad R, Saini JK, Kannaujia RK, Sarin S, Suryakant, Kulshreshth R, Nag VL, Tripathi AK (2003b) Trend of HIV infection in patients with pulmonary tuberculosis in Lucknow area. Indian J Tuberc 50:39–41

Purohit SD, Gupta RC, Bhatara VK (1996) Pulmonary tuberculosis and HIV infection in Ajmer. Lung India 14:113–120

Quigley MA, Mwinga A, Hosp M et al (2001) Faussett, long-term effect of preventive therapy for tuberculosis in a cohort of HIV-infected zambian adults. AIDS 85:2137–2147

Rajasekharan S, Uma A, Jeyaganesh D, Senthamizhchlevan A, Sarin S, Gopinathan (2000) Trend of HIV infection in patients with tuberculosis in rural south India. Indian J Tuberc 47:223–226

Roeger WL, Zhilan F, Carlos CC (2009) Modeling TB and HIV co-infections. Math Biosci Eng 6 (Suppl 4):815–837. https://doi.org/10.3934/mbe.2009.6.815

Samuel NM, Alamelu C, Jagannath K, Rajan BP (1996) Detection of HIV infection in pulmonary tuberculosis patients. J Indian Med Assoc 94:331–333

Shah NH, Gupta Jyoti D (2013a) Mathematical modelling of pulmonary and extra-pulmonary tuberculosis. Int J Math Trends Technol 4(Suppl 9):158–162

Shah NH, Gupta Jyoti D (2013b) Modelling and analysis of HIV/AIDS menace using differential equations. J Adv Math 3(Suppl 2):190–200

Sharma SK, Saha PK, Dixit Y, Siddaramaiah NH, Seth P, Pandey JN (2000) HIV seropositivity among adults tuberculosis patients in Delhi. Indian J Chest Dis Allied Sci 42:157–l 60

Sharomi O et al (2008a) *M*athematical analysis of the transmission dynamics of HIV/TB co-infection in the presence of treatment. Math Biosci Eng 5(Suppl 1):145–174

Sharomi O, Podder C, Gumel A, Song B (2008b) Mathematical analysis of the transmission dynamics of HIV/TB confection in the presence of treatment. Math Biosci Eng 5 (Suppl):145–141

Song B, Castillo CC, Aparicio J (2002) Tuberculosis models with fast and slow dynamics: the role of close and casual contacts. J Math Biosci 31(Suppl 3):215–220

Tripathi S, Joshi DR, Mehendale SM, Menon P, Joshi AN, Ghorpade SV, Patil U, Paranjape RS (2002) Sentinel surveillance for HIV infection in tuberculosis patients in India. Indian J Tuberc 49:17–20

Tripathy SP, Joshi DR, Menon P, Paranjape RS Mehendale SM (1996) Sero prevalence of HIV -1 infection in tuberculosis patients at Pune (abstract) Xl, International conference on AIDS, Vancouver

UNAIDSAIDS epidemic update (2001)

Van den Driessche P, Watmough J (2002) Reproduction numbers and sub-threshold endemic equilibria for compartmental models of disease transmission. Math Biosci 8(Suppl 5):129–135

Wang XY, Bai YP, Yang JY, Zhang FQ (2014) Global stability of an epidemic model for HIV–TB co-infection with infection age. Int J Biomath 7(Suppl 4):1450043

Wilkinson D, Squire SB, Garner P et al (1998) Effect of preventive treatment for tuberculosis in adults infected with HIV: systematic review of randomized placebo controlled trials. BMJ 16 (Suppl 4):625–634

Bayesian Artificial Neural Network (ANN) Model Approach to AIDS Associated Illness

8

8.1 Introduction

AIDS associated illness (Stroke) is a major health problem and its impact is likely to increase in the future due to ongoing demographic transitional changes including ageing of population and health index observed worldwide (Baker et al. 2001). Data from the global burden of disease (GBD) 2015 study showed that although age standardized rates of stroke mortality have decreased globally over the past two decades, the absolute number of people affected by stroke worldwide increased significantly between 1990 and 2015 (Craig et al. 2001). Virtually no country in the world has seen a reduction in stroke burden in terms of absolute number of incidents and fatal strokes. The literature showed that various confounders viz age, gender, ethnicity and heredity have been identified as markers of risk of stroke (Hagan et al. 1992; Hammer et al. 2002; Huang et al. 2006; Jones et al. 2001; Jung and Wickrama 2008; Kaplan and Sieg 1993; Kennedy and Hagan 1996; Kleijnen and Helton 1999; Krantz et al. 2011; Kreuter and Muthen 2007; Lange et al. 2000; Lavine and West 1992; Levy 1993; Liu and Wu 2007; Lunn et al. 2003; Menezes et al. 2012; Mosterman et al. 1999; Mrawira et al. 1996; Muthen and Muthen 2004; Muthen and Shedden 1999). Although, these factors cannot be modified, their presence helps to identify those at greatest risk for enabling vigorous treatment of those risk factors that can be modified. However, age is the single most important risk factors for stroke. For each successive 10 years after age 55 the stroke rate more than doubles in both men and women worldwide (Muthen et al. 2002; Nagin and Land 1993; Nherera et al. 2011; Nie et al. 2002; Oakley and Hagan 2002; Perelson et al. 1996, 1997; Saltell and Sobol 1995; Singh and Valtorta 1995; Sobol et al. 1993; Srinivasan and Weidner 1999; U H and Zhang 2006; Varbanov et al. 2006; Wang et al. 2003; Watthayu and Peng 2004; Wojtek Przytula and Milford 2006). On the contrary, stroke treatment and prevention strategies have been very well documented, large volumes of stroke follow up data sets have been generated from the patient's side. However, in the light of up gradation of comprehensive treatment care and prevention health care services have started digitization of stroke data, resulting from

D. M. Basavarajaiah, B. Narasimha Murthy, *HIV Transmission*,
https://doi.org/10.1007/978-981-15-0151-7_8

increasingly widespread adoption of electronic health records and electroencephalogram EEG. Electronic activity of brain has greatly facilitated its analysis by varied type of estimation computational methods and thereby enabled large-scale secondary use thereof. This can be exploited to support public health activities; programme implementation such as pharmacovigilance and estimation of DALY (disability adjusted life year) etc. The safety of administered drugs is monitored to inform regularity well versed guidelines and decisions about sustained use. To that larger extent, electronic health records have emerged as potentially valuable data source, providing access to prospective, longitudinal observations of treatment response and drug use. In the context of policy intervention, mathematical and statistical modelling has tremendous potential in improving the quality and efficiency of health care delivery, tool for decision making by health care professionals. New innovative model based discoveries could be necessary to prevent and implementation of new health policy guidelines consideration with risk assessment of genetic interaction, behavioral health related quality life domain (BHQOL) characteristics and associated clinical determinants of stroke (Dempster et al. 1977; Wojtek Przytula and Milford 2013; Wu 2002; Wu and Ding 1999; Wu et al. 1998).

Many researchers are fitted predictive modelling for assessment of risk of stroke patients by using traditional frequentisitc statistical approach such as estimation of MLE's based on the assumed hypothesis (normality). In the vague of frequentisitc analysis entire data sets are repeatable process and various parameters, which are fixed in nature. Further more confidence interval are used to draw the significant inference, but in real life the clinician/policymakers do not have fully developed prior beliefs about clinical, biological, behavioral and drug interaction information, and also estimated parameters (traditional way) providing spurious decisions about the population without estimation of credibility intervals. However, in case of Bayesian approach, the decision is based on subjective basis and using prior beliefs to define a prior probability distribution on the probabilistic values of unknown parameters. Although, the parameters of interest are interpreted differently by adopting practical approach, from a frequentisitc view point, the parameters are fixed but unknown quantities and also random variables. Hence, Bayesian approaches will be afforded the convenience of basic probability computations is derived in accordance with credibility intervals and getting rid of nuisance distribution state (Baker et al. 2001; Craig et al. 2001; Currin et al. 1991; Chu et al. 2005; Dragic et al. 1996). Most importantly, Bayesian network model makes conditional inferences on the data observed (but does not consider hypothetical life data sets that were not observed). A Bayesian approach is very natural when constructing predictive emulators with the chosen statistical model treated as a prior distribution on the simulator outputs and prediction, with associated uncertainty quantification via posterior predictive distribution parametric state. The 'nascent' line of this research pressing to build predictive modelling of health care data for the automatic detection of risk, genetic and environmental interactions. Now day's health delivery practice for specific population such as patient suffering from chronic disability *eg* stroke, terminal illness, life threatened disease such as HIV etc. The elderly people are shifting towards the constant health monitoring 24 h/day or 24×7 per day at defined state.Health monitoring may be determined not only in hospital environment but at home as well, through establishment of modern patient tale-monitoring system. The reason for all better possibilities for managing chronic care, controlling health delivery cost, increased quality life domain and distinct possibility of predicting and thus avoiding serious complications. Therefore, the execution of a risk analysis is necessary to assure health information system safety and quality services (QOS), estimation of DALY's to know the credibility of risk as well as life span index. In this context, traditional statistical approach is not able predict the Bayesian probabilities and MLE's of long entries of continuous state variable function. In view of the existing analytical research gap, the present study aims to fit new probabilistic model by Bayesian emulator approach.

8.2 Probabilistic Diagnostic Gaussian Model for Risk Analysis

Self learning probabilistic diagnostic which can be implemented in medicine are reported by many authors years. This general approach towards creating self learning risk assessment can also be used in other disciplines (e.g., detect spam, credit and debit financial risk flow and biological science). In general case a risk assessment of real time medical massive data sets consists of pertinent data base, the comprehension skills and decision support by practical approach etc. This is the reason why these plausible interventions of the risk element probabilistic diagnostic model are discussed and simulated at greater accuracy and reduced error. Probabilistic diagnostic methods fitted based on the Gaussian simulator Bayesian method is discussed below. Let us assume that there are 'N' events mutually exclusive and Independent and identical nature, β_n is normally distributed with 'μ' and variance 'σ^2' variance $\beta_n \sim N(\mu, \sigma^2)$ which are excluded each other and are mutually independent finally in addition to we can hypothetically assumed that these events create the total system which means that probability of these events can meet the general condition or probability theory, the formulation and salient characteristics of the model is here with discussed below

$$P\left(\beta_n\right) = N\left(\mu, \sigma^2\right) = 1 \tag{8.1}$$

The event β_n is understood as occurrence of assumed that P (A_n > 0, *if* $(n = 1, 2, 3, \ldots, n)$.Further we assume that there are 'M' independent events A_m $= m = 1,2\ldots$Mi which do not exclude each $\left\{\sum_{i=1}^{m} A_m = m\right\}$ where the probability of this conjunction is determined as

$$p(A) = \prod_{I=1}^{N} P(A_m) = 1 \tag{8.2}$$

Events 'β_n' and 'A' are mutually exclusive dependent because nth unknown parameters comes in to being by defined symptoms of evaluation A_m, $m = 1$,

2, . . ., *M*. The unknown Bayesian parameters normally distributed with conjunction of dependent events.

$$
\begin{aligned}
p('\beta_n A) &= P(\beta_n).P(A/\beta_n) \\
&= P(A_i).P(\beta_n/A_i)\, N(\mu, \sigma^2) \\
\mu &= 0, \sigma^2 = 1 \\
\therefore &= P(A_i)P(\beta_n/A_i)\tilde{N}(0,1)
\end{aligned}
\tag{8.3}
$$

Where the conditional probability

$P(\beta_n/Ai)$ is obtained from the formula (solved by using 8.2 and 8.3 equation)
$P(\beta_n/Ai) = P(A_i)\ P(\beta_n/A_i)/P(A_i)\ i = 1, 2, \ldots, n$

As it was assumed that event A_m is not independent, so it can be written as

$$P(Ai/\beta_n) = \prod_{i=1}^{n} P(A_i/\beta_n)$$

Assumed the normalcy the equation becomes

$$P(\mathrm{Ai}/\beta_n) = p(\mathrm{Ai})P(\mathrm{Ai}/\beta_n)/\sum_{i=1}^{n} p(\mathrm{Ai}) + P(\mathrm{Ai}/\beta_n)\tilde{N}(\mu^2, \sigma)$$

The probability of nth risk assessment can be determined from the Bayesian matrix conditions that the conjunction of *Ai* symptoms comes in to being if the following probability is known. The emulator of each probability will tends to Gaussian approach (Table 8.1).

The expected value of probability or credibility has calculated

$$P(E_i) = \sum_{i=1}^{n} P(\beta_{n11})\ \mathrm{x}P(A_{11})x\sum_{i=1}^{n} P(\beta_{n\cdot})\ \mathrm{x}P(A_{1\cdot})/\sum_{i=1}^{n}\sum_{i1}^{n} P(\beta_n)\ \mathrm{x}P(A_n)$$

Therefore, the true credibility of genetic linkage was calculated by $\chi_{(n-p)\mathrm{df}}{}^2 = \sum_{i=1}^{n} \frac{(O_{\mathrm{ij}} - E_{\mathrm{ij}})^2}{E_{\mathrm{ij}}} \tilde{N}(\mu^2, \sigma)$.

Further, we continued to test risk credibility by seeing whether the observed data's summary statistics is inside of the Gaussian approach around the parameters tested by the estimation of Likelihood unknown parameters $\widehat{\theta}$ (Fig. 8.1).

The whole series of risk out comes $\widehat{\theta}$ $(x \in \theta)$ can be finite series of real Bayesian probability values, the extension random variable mutually exclusive and independent with MLE's $(\widehat{\theta})$. Therefore intuitive variation was estimated $\widehat{\theta} = [X_0, X_1]$ $\widehat{\theta} = P[X_0 \le \theta \le X_1]$, $\widehat{\theta} = (X - \frac{\delta X}{2} \le \theta \le X + \frac{\delta X}{2}) = F(X)\delta X; \int f(x)\delta x$, $f(x)$ is the probability Gaussian density function. An experiment approaches the Bayesian

Table 8.1 Bayesian matrix table for risk assessment (diagnosis test table)

	Ai						Row
β_n	$P(A_1)$	$P(A_2)$	$P(A_3)$	$P(A_4)$	$P(A_5)$	$P(A_n)$	Total
$P(\beta_1)$	$P(\beta_1)xP(A_1)$	$P(\beta_1)xP(A_2)$	$P(\beta_1)xP(A_3)$	$P(\beta_1)x\ P(A_4)$	$P(\beta_1)x\ P(A_5)$	$P(\beta_1)x\ P(A_n)$	$\sum_{i=1}^{n} P(\beta_n.)\ xP(A_{1.})$
$P(\beta_2)$	$P(\beta_2)x\ P(A_1)$	$P(\beta_2)x\ P(A_2)$	$P(\beta_2)x\ P(A_3)$	$P(\beta_2)x\ P(A_4)$	$P(\beta_2)x\ P(A_5)$	$P(\beta_2)x\ P(A_n)$	$\sum_{i=1}^{n} P(\beta_n)\ xP(A_1)$
$P(\beta_3)$	$P(\beta_3)\ xP(A_1)$	$P(\beta_3)x\ P(A_2)$	$P(\beta_3)x\ P(A_3)$	$P(\beta_3)x\ P(A_4)$	$P(\beta_3)x\ P(A_5)$	$P(\beta_3)x\ P(A_n)$	$\sum_{i=1}^{n} P(\beta_n)\ xP(A_1)$
$P(\beta_4)$	$P(\beta_4)x\ P(A_1)$	$P(\beta_4)x\ P(A_2)$	$P(\beta_4)x\ P(A_3)$	$P(\beta_4)x\ P(A_4)$	$P(\beta_4)x\ P(A_5)$	$P(\beta_4)x\ P(A_n)$	$\sum_{i=1}^{n} P(\beta_n)\ xP(A_1)$
$P(\beta_5)$	$P(\beta_5)\ xP(A_1)$	$P(\beta_5)x\ P(A_2)$	$P(\beta_5)x\ P(A_3)$	$P(\beta_5)x\ P(A_4)$	$P(\beta_5)x\ P(A_5)$	$P(\beta_5)x\ P(A_n)$	$\sum_{i=1}^{n} P(\beta_n)\ xP(A_1)$
$P(\beta_n)$	$P(\beta_n)\ xP(A_1)$	$P(\beta_n)x\ P(A_2)$	$P(\beta_n)x\ P(A_2)$	$P(\beta_n)x\ P(A_2)$	$P(\beta_n)x\ P(A_2)$	$P(\beta_n)x\ P(A_2)$	$\sum_{i=1}^{n} P(\beta_n)\ xP(A_1)$
Column Total	$\sum_{i=1}^{n} P(\beta_{n11})\ xP(A_{11})$	$\sum_{i=1}^{n} P(\beta_{n2})\ xP(A_{21})$	$\sum_{i=1}^{n} P(\beta_{n3})\ xP(A_1)$	$\sum_{i=1}^{n} P(\beta_n)\ xP(A_1)$	$\sum_{i=1}^{n} P(\beta_n)\ xP(A_1)$	$\sum_{i=1}^{n} P(\beta_n)\ xP(A_1)$	$\sum_{i=1}^{n} \sum_{i1}^{n} P(\beta_n)\ xP(A_n)$

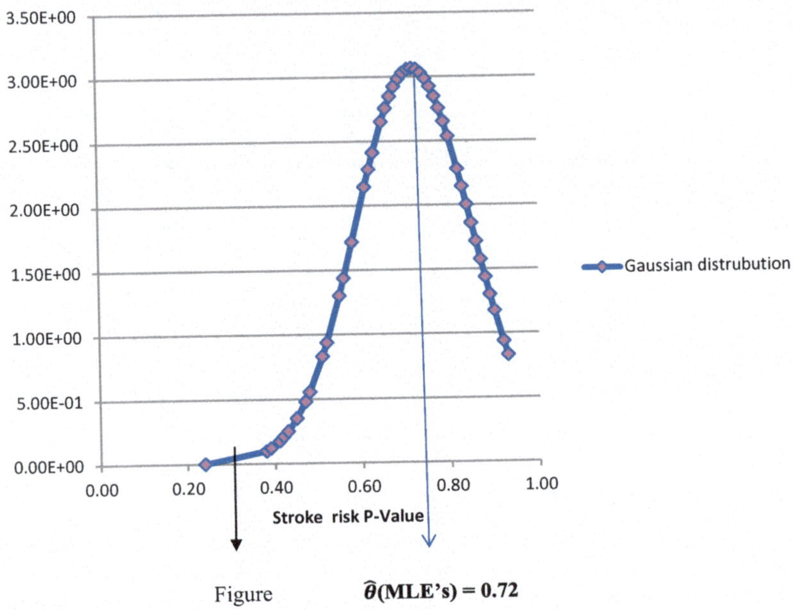

Fig. 8.1 Gaussian distribution probabilistic curve of stroke risk

trail with 'k' independent outcomes with MLE's $\widehat{\theta} = I = 1, 2, \ldots K \sum \theta_i 1 = 1$. Probability distribution of 'N' outcomes of the same experiment getting n_i occurrences of outcomes 'i' $\sum n_i = N$

$$M\left(\frac{N}{\theta}\right) = \frac{N!}{\pi\ n_i!} \prod_{i=1}^{K} \theta_i^{n_i} \tag{8.4}$$

From Eq. 1.4 Bayes probability outcomes is generated (without overlapping loop) Let we assumes that $\widehat{\theta} = \left(\widehat{\theta}_1, \widehat{\theta}_2, \widehat{\theta}_3, \widehat{\theta}_4 \ldots \widehat{\theta}_k\right)$ with constant values $\alpha_1, \alpha_2, \alpha_3. \ldots \alpha_k$ which gives different probability distribution over $\widehat{\theta}_i$ (MLE's) the density function of Bayesian risk probability'DALY' is accord to equated

$$f(\theta/x) = \prod_{i=1}^{n} \theta_i^{\alpha_i - 1} \delta \left(\sum_{i=1}^{n} \theta_i - 1\right) \tag{8.5}$$

8.3 Practical Component of DALY (Stroke)

Disability adjusted life year is measure of the overall burden of disease –it adds the years of life lost due to early death and years spent living with disability or ill health together. One important component of 'DALY' can be thought of as one lost of health life. The sum of thee 'DALY' across the population or the burden of diseases can be thought of as a measurement of the gap between current health status and an ideal health situation where the entire population lives to an advanced age, free of disease and disability. Following diagram depicted major diseases of 'DALY' (Fig. 8.2).

DALY's = YLD+YLL

(Years lived with disability=Years of life lost)

Years of life lost: Number of death at each age multiplied by the expected remaining years of life according to a global standard life expectancy

Years lost to disability: Number of indirect cases due to injury and illness is multiplied by the average duration of diseases and a Weightage factors reflecting the severity of diseases on scale from 0 and 1(0 perfect health and 1 dead from diseases).The estimated the net health effect,the 'QALIBRA' (Quality of life benefit risk assessment)

$$\text{DALY } Y_{a,s} = \left[P_{\text{eff}(a,s)} * (P_{\text{rec}} * \text{YLD}_{\text{rec}} * w + P_{\text{die}} * (\text{YLD}_{\text{die}} * w + \text{LE}_{a,s} - \text{CA} - \text{YLD}_{\text{die}}) + (1 - P_{\text{die}} - P_{\text{rec}}) * (\text{LE}_{a,s} - \text{CA} * w\right]$$

Where,

DALY $Y_{a,\,s}$ =Disability adjusted life years at age group a and sex's'
$P_{\text{eff}(a,\,s)}$= Probability of onset of the diseases at age and sex per year

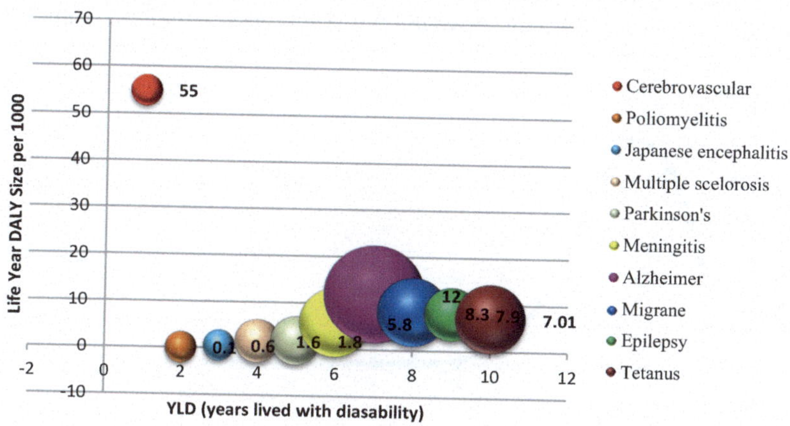

Fig. 8.2 distribution of disability with yearly lived

P_{rec}= Probability of recovery from the diseases
$P_{die=}$ Probability that the diseases cause death
YLD_{die}= Mean duration of disease for those who die
YLD_{rec} = Mean duration of disease for those who recover
CA= Current age of Individuals in year of disease onset.
$LE_{a,\ s}$= Normal life expectancy (i.e. expected year death) with 'w' disability weight for disease.

DALY is only quantitative indicators of burden of disease that reflects the total year lost (premature mortality) or some degree of disability (morbidity) during a period of time

Maximum likelihood estimation of DALY's = $\{Age\ at\ on\ set * e^{-r\theta}\}$, θ is parameter constant (MLE's) or number of years to be discounted, i.e. (45–35).The DALY age at 35 = 19.95 $* e^{-0.03x10}$ =14.50.Hence the total DALY lost=YLD +YLL=6.95+14.50=21.75

For practical approach we applying with a 3% discount rate, the YLL becomes

YLL = $\frac{N*(1-e^{-0.032})}{0.03}$, where, N is number of deaths=standard life expectancy at age of death and r= discount rate

YLD = $\frac{I*DW*(1-e^{-0.032})}{0.03}$, where I= number of incident cases, DW = disability weights, L = duration of disability and r = discount rate (Fig. 8.3, Tables 8.2 and 8.3).

The results indicate that Risk analysis of DALYs was learned case to serve as an advance method, specifically when simulating data from Bayesian emulators; the ability of the model are indicated in the (Table 8.1).Note that a Disability-adjusted life years combine years of potential life lost due to premature death has predicted in accordance with Bayesian risk analysis approach of DALY's. The results is being correlates life lost due to premature death event has been happened unfavoured between the age group 20 and above,the MLE's is less associated with DALY.

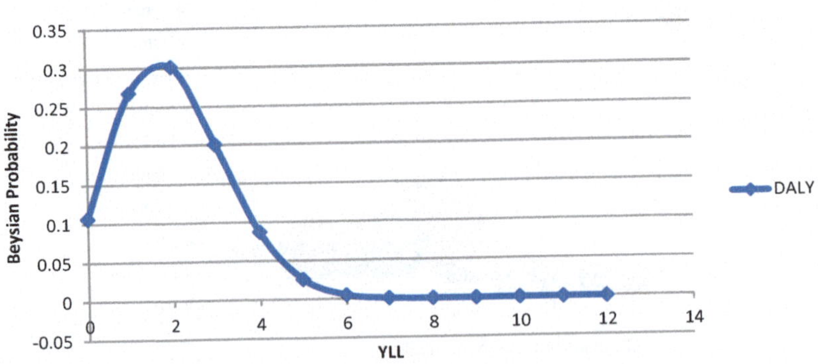

Fig. 8.3 Overview of potential life lost due to stroke (Population based)

Table 8.2 Disability-adjusted life years combine years of potential life lost due to premature death with years of productive life lost due to disability (age standardized)

Life lost due to premature death (PYLL)	Bayesian P-value	MLE's emulators $(\widehat{\theta})$
20 and above	0.13	0.88
15–19	0.27	0.97
10–14	0.76	5.85
5–9	0.82	8.11
Below 5	0.86	9.02

Model Statistically significant (AUC = 0.86–0.92, $P < 0.01$)

Table 8.3 Distribution of disability weighting classes

Disability weighting classes	Bayesian ANN's P-value
Limited ability to perform at least one activity in one of the following areas: recreation, education, procreation or occupation	0.033
Limited ability to perform most activities in one of the following areas: recreation, education, procreation or occupation	0.45
Limited ability to perform activities in two or more of the following areas: recreation, education, procreation or occupation	0.56
Limited ability to perform most activities in all of the following areas: recreation, education, procreation or occupation	0.66
Needs assistance with instrumental activities of DALY living such as meal preparation, shopping or housework	0.84
Needs assistance with activities of DALY living such as eating, personal hygiene or toilet use	0.93

Although, the patients profusely suffering from the illness due to co morbid conditions. Therefore, risk bearing of potential life lost due to premature death event has accrued 5–9 and 10–14 years after the event happened (stroke), were emulators statistically signifies the incidence of the happening of the event (Diagnosis test AUC = 0.92),original data extracted from Disability weighting classes (Table 8.4), data sets was simulated based on the Bayesian approach; Montecarlosimulation techniques method (Table 8.5).

Model uncertainty and risk assessment is essential to disease management and informed decision making has been drawn at population level. In this study we apply a continued test to risk credibility by seeing whether the observed data summary statistics is inside of the Gaussian approach around the parametric value, The 'MLE's' to calibrate a risk of stroke approaches with Bayesian trail with 'k' independent outcomes with MLE's $\widehat{\theta} = I = 1, 2, \ldots K \sum \theta_i 1 = 1$.In the covet of data scarcity in modelling of stroke follow up data lead to using boot strapping as a way to estimate the uncertainty of relations in Gaussian distribution approach. The idea of the model is as follows; parameters estimation can be used as a non parametric estimates of a statistics of interest, for which we can take the probabilistic risk of an event (stroke) as we can seen in Fig. 8.1. The intuition behind the normalcy

Table 8.4 Bayesian emulator estimation of DALYs and final result

	Bayesian emulator estimation (age standardized)			
Age class	YLLs	YLD's	DALY's	AUC
30–35	253	30.16	283.16	0.73
36–40	325	35.22	360.22	0.77
41–45	368	36.22	404.22	0.76
46–50	385	40.96	425.96	0.78
51–55	392	43.25	435.25	0.76
56–60	452	44.44	496.44	0.80
61–65	563	45.66	608.66	0.82
66–70	665	47.25	712.25	0.84
71–75	675	48.55	723.55	0.88
>76	886	49.50	935.5	0.92

Table 8.5 Distribution of co-morbidities

Co-morbidities	DALY score	MLE's $(\hat{\theta})$	Bayesian ANN's emulator P-value
Ataxia and dysarthria	80.20	10.21	0.66
Attention deficit hyperactivity disorder	56.34	4.28	0.52
Left and right hemiparesis	74.32	3.63	0.28
Psychosis	24.90	0.98	0.11
Valproate induced tremor	48.70	0.43	0.16

curve is that if we assume a generative probabilistic model, the actual data sets are traversed in real value. However, each of the estimation has some latency which is attached to it, so as better approximation to the real probability can be obtained from the 'Gaussian emulators'. The diagnosis and evaluation of the model and their performance will use standard matrices from classified matrices (Table 8.1). Classification and evaluation of Bayesian emulators is often based on measuring true positive (TP) cases and that are correctly classified as positive; false positive (FP), incorrectly classified as positive; and analogously for true/false negative (TN;FN). The true positive rate (TPR) is then defined as TP/(TP+FN) and the false positive rte FPR as FP/(FP+TN), plotting a curve of TP-FPR of different cut-off points results in an 'ROC' curve which is often summarized in a single number by computing the AUC.

8.4 Discussion

The increasing burden of stroke health transition is pushing the scientific community towards the development of computational tools to support decision making when defining health risk, such as estimation of MLE's of DALY (disable adjusted life year) at population level by taking into account the progression of stroke incidence and health care needs. To this end decision analysis is early paramount tool to assess the better outcomes, and increasingly using, simulation of MLEs to derive Bayesian simulators (Table 8.2) about decision making correlate with health outcomes in target population. The most reliable practical approach of this model outcome is represented by the Gaussian emulator method $G{\sim}N(\mu, \varepsilon)$. Model was fitted with time course of co morbidities with a probabilistic finite continuous state –time representation of different state function or events. According to the model, a entire stroke data sets is simulated by Gaussian approach, the value of emulators were determined based on 'Montecarlo simulation techniques'. Although, the emulators describes the state function of DALY (Bayesian emulator) with respect to different health indicators of stroke disability health score. Similarly, the temporal evaluation of the patients is then obtained by sampling, at each continuous state treatment follow up period, state of Bayesian risk p value will generated on his/her state in the previous time in accordance to a transition probability matrix. An annually 15 million people worldwide suffer a stroke, of these, 5 million die and another 5 million are left permanently disabled, placing a burden on family and community. Stroke is uncommon in people under 40 years; when does it occur, the main cause is high blood pressure. Stroke also occurs in about 15% of adults between age group 45–55 years associated with type I diabetes complications. The major risk factors are similar to those for coronary heart disease with high blood pressure and tobacco usage is the most significant modifiable risks. Atria fibrillation, heart failure and heart attack are other important risk factors. As per the literature, the incidence of stroke is declining in many developed countries, largely as result of better control of high blood pressure, and reduced levels of smoking. However, the absolute number of strokes continues to increase because of the ageing population. Between 1990 and 2016, there was a significant increase in prevalent cases, total deaths and DALYS's due to smoking, sedentary life style, elevated BMI 35–42 in younger adults aged 35–46 years. Deaths and DALY's rates increased in Indian context but a significant increase in absolute number of stroke deaths among younger adults was found to be detected new incidence of stroke. Asper the model the DALY's Bayesian emulator estimation (age standardized). Minimum DALY were attained in the age group 30–35 years (283.16 years,AUC 0.73,Bayesian probability is $P = 0.78$; followed 36–40 years (360.22,AUC;0.77; 41–45 years 404.22;AUC0.76; significantly increased DALY trend was observed in the age group 56–76 years age class intervals,the mean DALY was 935.50;AUC 0.92 (Table 8.4). The greater burden was due to ischemic stroke. While the trends in declined death and DALY rates in developing countries like India are encouraging, this is more aggressive approach towards primary prevention and increased access to adequate health care services for stroke is required to substantially narrow these disparities. The total health loss due to stroke as measured by DALY's risk analysis was similar for men and women for stroke both types in 2012–2016, with hemorrhagic higher than ischemic stroke, earing its inherent weakness in mind, DALY is still a very useful measure, because it is the first comprehensive attempt made to summarize the world's burden of injury, disease and premature death. It has initiated a debate and new research to find even better complex indicators for global comparisons. The DALY measures are useful to describe the burden across the world and to make projections for the future. At present, many countries are exploring the possibilities of using DALY as a measure of trends in disease burden and as tool for cost effectiveness studies and priority setting.

Summing of the results, the present study concludes that Bayesian predictive risk analysis model gives a good consistent result, replicated as an automated tool to predicting the DALY risk emulators of stroke. This can be particularly useful in developing countries for implementation of policy intervention. Furthermore, with a larger health record database the results will be more consistent and accurate.

8.5 Summary

For short of the target, many researchers has fitted innumerable predictive models for the assessment of stroke risk by using traditional frequentisitc Statistical approach, the edifice of fitted traditional frequentisitc models produce less consistent and inexact results, because the results were simulated based on the assumed hypothesis. In the precise of frequentisitc analysis, entire data sets are repeatable process; the parameters are fixed in nature, credibility of the parameters is undefined. Correspondingly, in case of Bayesian artificial neural network 'ANN' emulator approach, the decision of the population has been drawn on the subjective basis with prior beliefs (prior probability). In this impression, the traditional Statistical approach is incompetent to predict the unknown parameters of MLE's of long standing entries of continuous state variables 'x'. This uneven penuriousness research gap, the present study aims to derive the new probabilistic model (Bayesian 'ANN' emulator approach and disability adjustment life year score -DALY's) from the continuous state variables $x_1, x_2, x_3, \ldots, x_n$. Model formulation; we assumed 'N' events mutually exclusive, independent and identical (IID's) in nature, β_n is normally distributed with 'μ' and variance 'σ^2' variance $\beta_n \sim N(\mu, \sigma^2)$. The Bayesian risk probability was obtained with maximization of $f(\theta/x) = \prod_{i=1}^{n} \theta_i^{\alpha_i - 1} \delta \left(\sum_{i=1}^{n} \theta_i - 1 \right)$, MLE's and DALY's probability values were obtained from the Bayesian simulation techniques (Thompson-iteration method). As per the resulted findings of the model, the life lost due to premature death event has wafts between the age group $\geq$20 years and above, the MLE's is more associated with DALY's as wells as, patients amply suffering from the illness due to co- morbid conditions. The risk bearing of potential life is lost due to premature death (5–9 years and 10–14 years after the stroke incidence).The 'ANN 'emulators statistically signifies ($p < 0.01$) the higher incidence of stroke in developing countries. The entire summing of the results concludes that, the Bayesian predictive risk analysis ANN model is the best simulation model to produce consistent result for estimation of DALY's at greater accuracy and lesser time intervals ($R^2 = 0.96$). Particularly the present fitted models can be very useful in developing countries for implementation of policy interventions and reduction of high dimensional data sets with continuous state variables. In addition to that, the consistency and accuracy of the model can be enhanced with a larger health record database.

References

Baker RD et al (2001) Sensitivity analysis for health care models fitted to data by statistical methods. IMA J Manag Sci 12:1–17

Chang LC, Lander HS, Lue MT (1994) Bayes analysis for fault location in distributed systems. IEEE Trans Reliab 43(Suppl 3):457–469

Chaurasia S, Chakrabarti P, Chourasia N (2012) An application of classification techniques on breast cancer prognosis. Int J Comput Appl 59(Suppl 3):6–10

Chevret S, Roguin H, Ganne P, Lefrere JJ (1992) Prognostic value of an elevated CD8 lymphocyte count in HIV infection. Results of a prospective study of 152 asymptomatic HIV-positive individuals. AIDS 6:1349–1352

Chu H, Gange SJ, Yamashita TE, Hoover DR, Chmiel JS, Margolick JB, Jacobson LP (2005) Individual variation in CD4 cell count trajectory among human immunodeficiency Virusinfected men and women on long-term highly active antiretroviral therapy: an application using a Bayesian random change–point model. Am J Epidemiol 162:787

Craig PS, Goldstein M, Rougier JC, Seheul AH (2001) Bayesian forecasting for complex systems using computer simulators. J Am Stat Assoc 96:717–729

Currin C, Mitchell TJ, Morris M, Ylvisaker D (1991) Bayesian prediction of deterministic functions with applications to the design and analysis of computer experiments. J Am Stat Assoc 86:953–963

Dempster AP, Laird N, Rubin DB (1977) Maximum likelihood from incomplete data via the EM algorithm. J R Stat Soc Ser B 39:1–38

Diebolt J, Robert C (1990) Bayesian estimation of finite mixture distributions, part I: theoretical aspects. Technical Report 110, LSTA, University Paris VI, Paris

Diebolt J, Robert C (1994) Estimation of finite mixture distributions by Bayesian sampling. J Royal Stati Soc Ser B 56:363–375

Doguc O, Emmanuel Ramirez-Marquez J (2009) Using Bayesian approach for sensitivity analysis and fault diagnosis in complex systems. J Integr Des Process Sci 13(Suppl 1):33–48

Dragic T, Litwin V, Allaway GP, Martin SR, Huang Y, Nagashima KA, Cayanan C, Maddon PJ, Koup R, Moor JP, Paxton WA (1996) HIV-1 entry into CD4+ cells is mediated by the chemokine receptor CC-CKR-5. Nature 381:667–673

Embretson J, Zupancic M, Ribas J, Burke A, Raca P, Tenner-Racz K, Haase AT (1993) Massive covert infection of helper T lymphocytes and macrophages by HIV during the incubationperiod of AIDS. Nature 362:359–362

Fauci AS (1988) The human immunodeficiency virus; infectivity and mechanisms of pathogenesis. Science 239:617–622

Gelfand AE, Hills SE, Racine-Poon A, Smith AFM (1990) Illustration of Bayesian inference in normal data models using Gibbs sampling. J Am Stat Assoc 85:972–985

Gelman A, Rubin DB (1992) Inference from iterative simulation using multiple sequences. Stat Sci 7:457–511

Gray RH, Wawer MJ, Brookmeyer R, Sewankambo NK, Serwadda D, Wabwire-Mangen F, Lutalo T, Li X, van Cott T, Quinn TC, akai Project Team (2001) Probability of HIV-1 transmission per coital act in monogamous, heterosexual, HIV-1-discordant couples in Rakai, Uganda. Lancet 357:1149–1153

Grewal A, Stephan DA (2013) Diagnostics for personalized medicine: what will change in the era of large-scale genomics studies. J Personalized Med 10(Suppl 8):835–848

Guo X, Carlin BP (2004) Separate and joint modeling of longitudinal and event time data using standard computer packages. Am Stat 58:16–24
Hagan A et al (1991) Bayes-hermite quadrature. J Stat Plann Infer 91:245–260
Hagan A et al (1992) Some Bayesian numerical analysis In Bayesian Statistics Oxford University Press; 24: 345–363. 23
Hammer SM, Vaida F, Bennett KK, Holohan MK, Sheiner L, Eron JJ, Wheat LJ, Mitsuyasu RT, Gulick RM, Valentine FT, Aberg JA, Rogers MD, Karol CN, Saah AJ, Lewis RH, Bessen LJ, Brosgart C, DeGruttola V, Mellors JW, AIDS Clinical Trials Group 398 Study Team (2002) Dual vs single protease inhibitor therapy following antiretroviral treatment failure: a randomized trial. J Ame Med Assoc 288:169–180
Huang Y, Liu D, Wu H (2006) Hierarchical Bayesian methods for estimation of parameters in a longitudinal HIV dynamic system. Biometrics 62:413–423
Jones BL, Nagin DS, Roeder K (2001) A SAS procedure based on mixture models for estimating developmental trajectories. Sociol Methods Res 29:374–393
Jung T, Wickrama KAS (2008) An introduction to latent class growth analysis and growth mixture modeling. Soc Personal Psychol Compass 2:302–317
Kaplan D, Sieg S (1993) Role of the FAS/FAS ligand apoptotic pahtway in HIV-1 disease. J Mol Biol 72:6279–6282
Kennedy MC, Hagan A (1996) Bayesian calibration of computer models (with discussion). J R Stat Soc B 63:425–464
Kleijnen JP, Helton JC (1999) Statistical analyses of scatterplots to identify important factors in large-scale simulations review and comparison of techniques. Reliab Eng Syst Saf 65:147–185
Krantz EM, Hullsiek KH, Okullicz JF, Weintrob AC, Agan BK, Crum-Cianflone NE, Ferguson TM, Hale BR (2011) Elevated CD8 count during HAART are associated with HIV virologic treatment failure. J Acquir Immune Defic Syndr 57:369–403
Kreuter F, Muthen B (2007) Longitudinal modeling of population heterogeneity: methodological challenges to the analysis of empirically derived criminal trajectory profiles. Advances in latent variable mixture models. Information Age Publishing, Charlotte
Lange N, Carlin BP, Gelfand AE (2000) (1992). Hierarchical Bayes models for the progression of HIV infection using longitudinal CD4 T-cell numbers. J Am Stat Assoc 87:615–626
Lavine M, West M (1992) A Bayesian method for classification and discrimination. Can J Stat 20:451–461
Levy JA (1993) Pathogenesis of human immunodeficiency virus infection. Microbiol Rev 57:183–289
Liu W, Wu L (2007) Simultaneous inference for semiparametric nonlinear mixed-effects models with covariate measurement errors and missing responses. Biometrics 63:342–350
Lunn DJ, Thomas A, Best N, Spiegelhalter DJ (2003) WinBUGS–a Bayesian modelling framework: concepts, structure, and extensibility. Stat Comput 10:325–337
Menezes AC, Pinheiro Placido R, Pinheiro MC, Cavalcante TP (2012) Towards the applied hybrid model in decision making: support the early diagnosis of type 2 diabetes. In: 3rd international conference on information computing and applications (ICICA 2012), Lecture Notes in Computer Science; p. 648–655
Mosterman PJ et al (1999) Diagnosis of continuous valued systems in transient operating regions. IEEE Trans Syst Man Cybern Syst Hum 29(Suppl 6):554–564
Mrawira D, Welch WJ, Schonlau M, Haas R (1996) Sensitivity analysis of computer models: world bank HDM-III model. J Transp Eng 125:421–428
Muthen L, Muthen B (2004) Mplus (Version 3.1) [Computer software]. Muthen & Muthen, Los Angeles
Muthen B, Shedden K (1999) Finite mixture modeling with mixture outcomes using the EM' algorithm. Biometrics 55:463–469
Muthen B, Brown CH, Masyn K, Jo B, Khoo ST, Yang CC, Wang CP, Kellam SG, Carlin JB, Liao J (2002) General growth mixture modeling for randomized preventive interventions. Biostatistics 3:459–475

Nagin DS, Land KC (1993) Age, criminal careers, and population heterogeneity: specification and estimation of a nonparametric, mixed Poisson model. Criminology 31:327–362
Nherera L, Marks D, Minhas R, Thorogood M, Humphries SE (2011) Probabilistic cost-effectiveness analysis of cascade screening for familial hypercholesterolemia using alternative diagnostic and identification strategies. J Heart 97(Suppl 14):1175–1181
Nie Z, Phenix BN, Lum JJ, Alam A, Lynch DH, Beckett B, Krammer PH et al (2002) Badley AD. HIV-1 protease processes procaspase 8 to cause mitochondrial release of cytochrome c, caspase cleavage and nuclear fragmentation. Cell Death Differ 9:1172–1184
Oakley JE, Hagan A (2002) Bayesian inference for the uncertainty distribution of computer model outputs. Biometrika 89:769–784
Perelson AS, Neumann AU, Markowitz M, Leonard JM, Ho DD (1996) HIV-1 dynamics in vivo: virion clearance rate, infected cell life-span, and viral generation time. Science 271:1582–1586
Perelson AS, Essunger P, Cao Y, Vesanen M, Hurley A, Saksela K, Markowit M, Ho DD (1997) Decay characteristics of HIV–1–infected compartments during combination therapy. Nature 387:188–191
Saltell A, Sobol IM (1995) About the use of rank transformation in sensitivity analysis of model output. Reliab Eng Syst Saf 50:225–239
Singh M, Valtorta F (1995) Construction of Bayesian network structures form data: a brief survey and an efficient algorithm. Int J Approx Reason 12:111–131
Sobol IM et al (1993) Sensitivity analysis for nonlinear mathematical models. Math Modling Comput Exp Dermatol 1:407–414
Srinivasan V, Weidner J (1999) Mathematical modeling of electrochemical capacitors. J Electrochem Soc 14(Suppl 6):1650–1658
U H, Zhang JT (2006) Nonparametric regression methods for longitudinal data analysis. Wiley, Hoboken
Varbanov M, Espert L, Biard-Piechaczyk B (2006) Mechanisms of CD4 T-cell depletion trigged by HIV-1 viral infections. AIDS Rev 8:221–236
Wang H et al (2003) Fault diagnosis and fault tolerant control for non-gaussian stochastic systems with random parameters fault diagnosis and fault tolerance for mechatronic systems, vol 5. Springer-Verlag, Berlin, pp 59–84
Watthayu W, Peng Y (2004) A Bayesian network based framework for multi-criteria decision making, In: Proceedings of the 17th international conference on multiple criteria decision analysis
Wojtek Przytula K, Milford R (2006) An efficient framework for the conversion of fault trees to diagnostic Bayesian network models, In Proceedings of IEEE aerospace conference; 5: 1–14
Wojtek Przytula K, Milford R (2013) An efficient framework for the conversion of fault trees to diagnostic Bayesian network models. In Proceedings of IEEE Aerospace Conference, 1–14
Wu L (2002) A joint model for nonlinear mixed-effects models with censoring and covariates measured with error, with application to AIDS studies. J Am Stat Assoc 97:955–964
Wu H, Ding AA (1999) Population HIV–1 dynamics in vivo: applicable models and inferential tools for virological data from AIDS clinical trials. Biometrics 55:410–418
Wu H, Ding AA, De Gruttola V (1998) Estimation of HIV dynamic parameters. Stat Med 17:2463–2485

HIV Projection Models

9

9.1 Introduction

The HIV forecasting disease modelling is that it leads to clear statements of the assumptions about the biological and social mechanisms, which influence disease spread and dynamism. The model formulation process is more valuable for statistician, epidemiologists, mathematicians, and modelers, because it forces them to be precise about the relevant aspects of disease transmission, course of infectivity, recovery, treatment prognosis, and renewal of susceptibility (Newell et al. 1998; Wig et al. 2006). The statisticians need to formulate the models clearly and precisely using different clinical and biological parameters, which have been very well-understood in connection to the dynamics of HIV diseases, such as increase in CD4 count after inception of HAART, spectrum of HIV-TB co-infection, HCV and HBV co-infection, etc (Simwa et al. 2003). The complete statements of the assumptions have been crucial role for testing the geometric progression of HIV, so that the reasonableness of the parameters can be interpreted by the relevant conclusion. The matrix of the forecasting model will help physician, policymakers, young researcher, innovators, etc. A limited number of HIV forecasting modelling based-studies have been documented at global scenario. In this context, the present study aims to formulate the different forecasting models and also assess the quantitative conjectures and identify the trend of CD4 counts before inception of "HAART" therapy. A total 497 PLHIVs infected pre-ART and alive on ART cases were considered for the study with written consent. Retrospective cohort data, viz., baseline (start of ART treatment), first year, second year, third year, fourth year, and fifth year cohort data, was recorded systematically. As per the national ART guidelines, we have classified the CD4 count based on the mean and SD, namely, low CD4 count and medium CD4 count (threshold CD4 count <250 cells/microliter and >250 cells/microliter) (Detels et al. 2005). The collected data was compiled by using SPSS-16.50 version. Logistic regression forecasting model, Spearman rank correlation, and polynomial curve fitting models were used to draw the relevant conclusion about the population.

D. M. Basavarajaiah, B. Narasimha Murthy, *HIV Transmission*,
https://doi.org/10.1007/978-981-15-0151-7_9

9.2 Model Formulation

A retrospective secondary data was collected from the different government ART centers in Bangalore City. Logistic regression model was fitted to know the variation among CD4 count of PLHIVs and HIV-associated parameters. We have assumed "n" independent Bernoulli random variables of CD4 <250 μ/dL and CD4 >250 μ/dL with absolute values of $Y_1, Y_2 \ldots Y_n$, where "$i = 1,2\ldots n$", and (Xi_1, $Xi_2 \ldots Xi_P$, $Xi_{P+1} \ldots Xi_{P+q})_1$ be a (p + q) vector of explanatory variables and denoted $X = (X_1, X_2, X_3 \ldots X_n)_1$. Let ß $\Pi_i = \Pi(X_i) = \Pr(Y_i = 1/X_i)$ which is the event of probability for each observation of $i = 1, 2\ldots n$.

$\pi = (\pi_1, \pi_2, \pi_3, \ldots .\ \pi_n)$, and then the logistic regression model becomes logit $(\pi_i) = X\beta\phi$

$$\text{Logit}(\pi_i) = \log\left(\frac{\pi_i}{1-\pi_i}\right) = X_1\beta \tag{9.1}$$

$$\text{Logit}(\pi_i) = \text{Log}\left(\frac{\prod i}{1-\prod i}\right) = \text{X1i}\beta$$

where $(\beta = \beta_1, \beta_2, \beta_3 \ldots \beta_{p+q})$ is an unknown parameter vector; the joint probability of the observed y_o is a product of "n" Bernoulli ith function

$$\begin{aligned} \text{L}(\beta) &= \left\{\prod\nolimits_{\text{I}=1}^{\text{n}} \pi_i 0_i (1-\pi_i) 1 - y_{0\text{i}}\right\} \\ \text{L}(\beta) &= \left\{\frac{\text{Exp}\left(y_0, \text{X}_\beta\right)}{\prod\nolimits_{\text{i}=1}^{\text{n}}(1+\exp\text{X}_\text{i}, \beta)}\right\} \end{aligned} \tag{9.2}$$

The hypothesis was tested from unconditional likelihood method of estimation (for maximizing the likelihood function). As per the resulted model, our fitted model is in the form of Logit (P) = $\beta o + \beta_j X_j$; the parameters β_o, $\beta_1 \ldots \beta_k$ were typically estimated by using maximum likelihood theory, let "n" denote the sample size with X_{i1}, $X_{i2} \ldots X_{ky}$ variables for ith observations ($i = 1, 2, \ldots n$), and treating each Y_i as an outcome of the independent random variables with success of probability P_i, the equation becomes

$$\prod_{i=1}^{n} p_i^{\text{yi}}(1-\pi_i)(1-y_{0i})$$

$$\exp\left\{\frac{\sum_{\text{i}}\text{yi}\left(\beta_0 + \sum_{\text{j}}\beta\text{jX}_{\text{ij}}\right\}}{\pi_i\left(1+\exp\beta_0 + \sum_{\text{j}}\beta\text{jX}_{\text{ij}}\right.}\right.$$

The maximum likelihood estimates (MLEs) (β_1, $\beta_2 \ldots \beta_k$) showed parameters of estimation, and these were used to compute MLEs by using Newton-Raphson iteration method. The convergent of fitted model became

$$\mathrm{Log}\left(\frac{P}{1-P}\right) = \beta_o + \beta_1 X_1 + \beta_2 X_2 \ldots + \beta_k X_k \tag{9.3}$$

9.3 Baseline Characteristics

A total of 497 PLHIVs were considered for the study, out of which male comprises 295 (26%) and female was 202 (47%). The average age of the patient was 35.30 ± 6.19 years. CD4 count was recorded at follow-up period with different intervals, and the mean baseline CD4 count was 123.44 ± 71.98 μ/dL (*P* = 0.492). The average CD4 count at 6-month to 5-year follow-up was 348.56 ± 142.13 (*P* = 0.036) micro per dL, 405.87 ± 66.40 (*p* = 0.006) micro per dL, 430.61 ± 49.96 (*P* = 0.021) micro per dL, 464.53 ± 38.30 (*P* = 0.085) micro per dL, 498.50 ± 33.57(*P* = 0.011) micro per dL, and 505.27 ± 27.97 micro per dL (*P* = 0.003), respectively, presented in Table 9.1. A total of 51.0% PLHIVs received first-line HAART, and only 4 (0.80%) patients received second-line HAART; the mortality rate was found to be 40 (8.08%). The mean body weight was 63 kg (70.25 kg for men and 62.38 kg for women), and the mean hemoglobin was 13.8 g/dL (14.2 g/dL for men and 12.6 g/dL for women). The median CD4 count was 330 cells/micro dL, and median TLC was 1692 cells/L.

Table 9.1 Baseline characteristics of PLHIVs

Variable	Male Mean ± SD	Female Mean ± SD	Pool	P-value
Age (year)	36.24 ± 6.96 (295–59.35%)	32.26 ± 7.18 (202–40.64%)	35.30 ± 6.19 (497)	0.029
Baseline CD4	128.29 ± 82.62 (295)	116.36 ± 56.46 (202)	123.44 ± 71.98 (497)	0.492
CD4 at the end of 6 months	380.36 ± 135.20 (287)	302.01 ± 152.28 (196)	348.56 ± 142.13 (483)	0.036
CD4 at the end of 1-year cohort	428.86 ± 45.65 (285)	372.28 ± 96.73 (195)	405.87 ± 66.40 (480)	0.006
CD4 at the end of 2-year cohort	465.69 ± 39.40 (282)	379.36 ± 65.39 (193)	430.61 ± 49.96 (475)	0.021
CD4 at the end of 3-year cohort	502 ± 30.61 (278)	410.00 ± 49.50 (191)	464.53 ± 38.30 (469)	0.085
CD4 at the end of fourth year cohort	534.89 ± 28.33 (275)	445.00 ± 41.29 (187)	498.50 ± 33.57 (462)	0.011
CD4 at the end of fifth year cohort	542.16 ± 20.02 (272)	451.00 ± 36.98 (185)	505.25 ± 27.97 (457)	0.003

Significant $p < 0.01$

9.4 Logistic Regression Model

As per the fitted model, the actual predicted observed odds ratio of the baseline CD4 count was (OR) 0.35, 95% confidence interval (CI) 0.26–0.59, and $P < 0.0028$. Later initiation of ART was reported (OR 1.16; 95% CI 1.03–1.3; $P < 0.02$) and found to be statistically insignificant ($p > 0.05$). After 1-year completion of HAART, CD4 count will be directly proportional to the increase of immunological goal. The result showed that the CD4 count improved after 1-year completion of HAART (mean 405.87 ± 66.40 μ/dL ($P = 0.006$)). At the end of the fifth year cohort, the mean CD4 count was 505.25 ± 27.97 μ/dL ($P = 0.003$); it was clearly shown that the immunological factor (increase of CD4 count) was found to be inversely proportional to the declining trend of plasma RNA viral load.

The associated parameters for the increased trend of CD4 count were presented in Table 9.2. As per the fitted model, the age coefficient β was −0.053, and SE was 0.021 with 95% CI of 0.910–0.988. The CD4 count at baseline (inception of HAART) β was 1.92, and SE was 0.002 with 95% CI of 0.997–1.003, and type of regimen (NRTI+2NNRTI, NNRTI+2NRTI) β was 0.377, and SE was (0.296) with 95% CI of 0.817–2.603. In case of WHO clinical stage, β was −0.440, and SE was 0.190 with 95% CI of 0.44–0.935, and in the blood group, β was 1.280, and SE was 0.996 with 95% CI between 0.652 and 0.889. The age of the patient, type of regimen, WHO clinical stage and blood groups were found to be statistically significant ($p < 0.05$) when compared with other HIV-associated parameters, and low CD4 count was found to be more induced factor for the reduced rate of immunity of PLHIVs (IQR CD4 count up to 10–192 micro per dL).

Correlation matrix of HAART and concurrent parameters were analyzed by using Spearman rank correlation method presented in Table 9.3. In case of age parameters was negatively correlated with CD4 count ($r = -0.753$), CD4 count at inception of HAART ($r = -0.088$), regimen ($r = -0.386$), and WHO clinical stage ($r = -0.429$) were found to be negatively correlated with patient blood group. The CD4 count ($r = 0.70$) and WHO clinical stage (stage I, II, III, and IV) ($r = 0.082$) were positively associated with age of the patients, type of regimen, and advanced

Table 9.2 Association between CD4 count and age of the patients

Clinical parameters	B	S.E.	Wald	Sig.	Exp(B)	95.0% CI for Exp(B)	
					Lower	Upper	
Age	−0.053	0.021	6.438**	0.011	0.948	0.910	0.988
CD4 at baseline	1.92	0.002	.018 ns	0.892	1.000	0.997	1.003
CD4 at the end of the 5-year cohort	0.002	0.001	4.766**	0.029	1.002	1.000	1.003
Regimen	0.377	0.296	1.626**	0.202	1.458	0.817	2.603
WHO clinical stage	−0.440	0.190	5.358**	0.021	0.644	0.444	0.935
Blood group	1.280	0.996	1.653**	0.199	3.597	0.652	0.889

2 Log likelihood, Cox & Snell R Square-0.076, Nagelkerke R Square-0.103

Table 9.3 Correlation matrix of influenced parameters of HAART

Clinical parameters		Blood group	Age	CD4 baseline	CD4 present	Regimen	WHO clinical stage
01	Blood group	1.000					
02	Age	−0.753	1.000				
03	CD4 baseline	−0.088	−0.062	1.000			
04	CD4 at fifth year cohort	0.62**	0.70**	−0.266	1.000		
05	Regimen	−0.386	−0.047	−0.240	0.742*	1.000	
06	WHO clinical stage	−0.429	0.082*	0.490*	0.541*	0.000	1.000

Significant $p < 0.01$
*Significant at 1% level
**Significant at 5% level

WHO clinical staging ($r = 0.490$) that were found to be positively correlated with mean CD4 count at the end of the fifth year cohort period ($r = 0.742$).

9.5 Curve Fitting Estimation

An extent of long-term HIV therapy, the present study fitted various curve fitting polynomial models. The models estimated the trend and effectiveness of ART. The results depicted that the mean CD4 cell count after initiation of antiretroviral therapy (ART) was 310 ± 15.86 cells/mm^3. The mean baseline CD4 was 128 ± 82.62 cells/mm^3 (95% confidence interval [95% CI] 105–136) in case of males, and in females, it was 116.36 ± 56.46 cells/mm^3 (95% CI =96–102.50), respectively. Independent predictors of long-term CD4 cell reconstitution variables were analyzed by the linear and polynomial curve fitting method. Fifth- and fourth-degree polynomial equation was fitted with respect to gender (Figs. 9.1, 9.2, 9.3, and 9.4).

9.6 Logit Model Reflects the 2 × 2 Contingency Table

The present study demonstrated CD4 trend from odds ratio model, and the model expressed the ratio of the number of patients who acquired CD4 count (<250 to >250 μ/dL) with respect to the age group of the patients between 25 and 35 years. The formulation of the model was expressed by 2 × 2 contingency table method (Table 9.4):

$$\mathrm{OR} = \left(\frac{\mathrm{A} \times \mathrm{D}}{\mathrm{B} \times \mathrm{C}}\right)$$

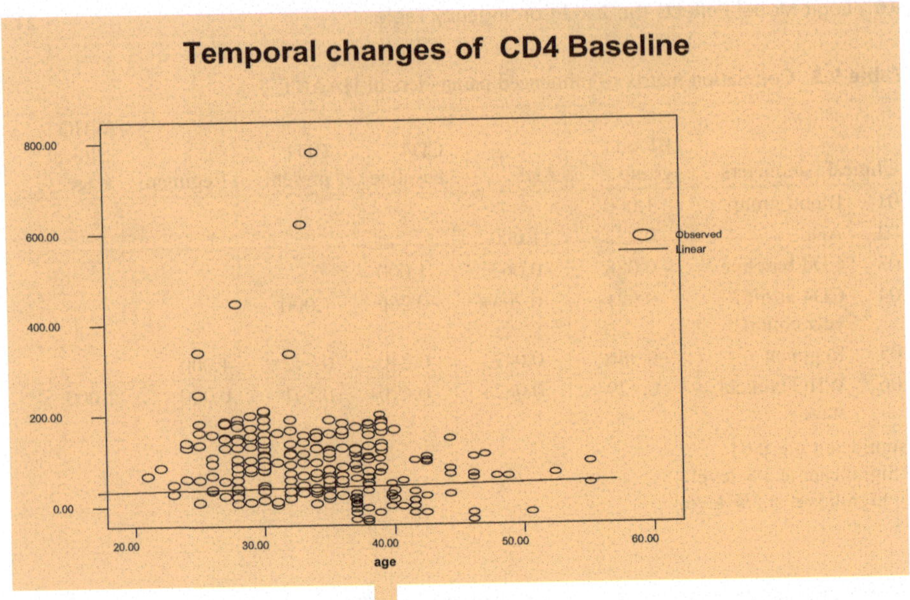

Fig. 9.1 Curve fitting linear trend (CD_4 count at baseline)

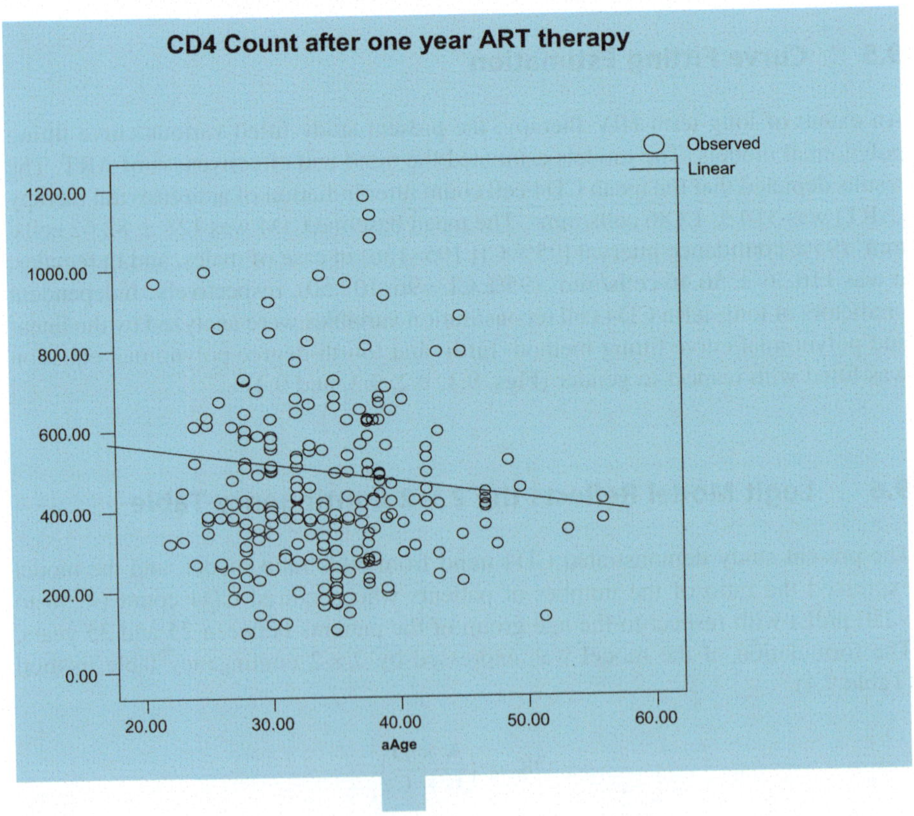

Fig. 9.2 Curve fitting linear trend (CD_4 count at the end of the cohort)

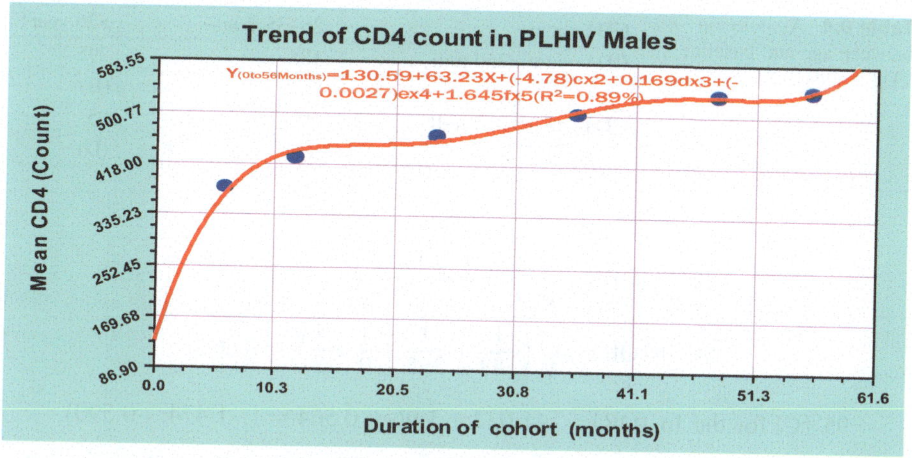

Fig. 9.3 Fifth-degree polynomial trend of CD_4 count in PLHIV males ($N = 295$)

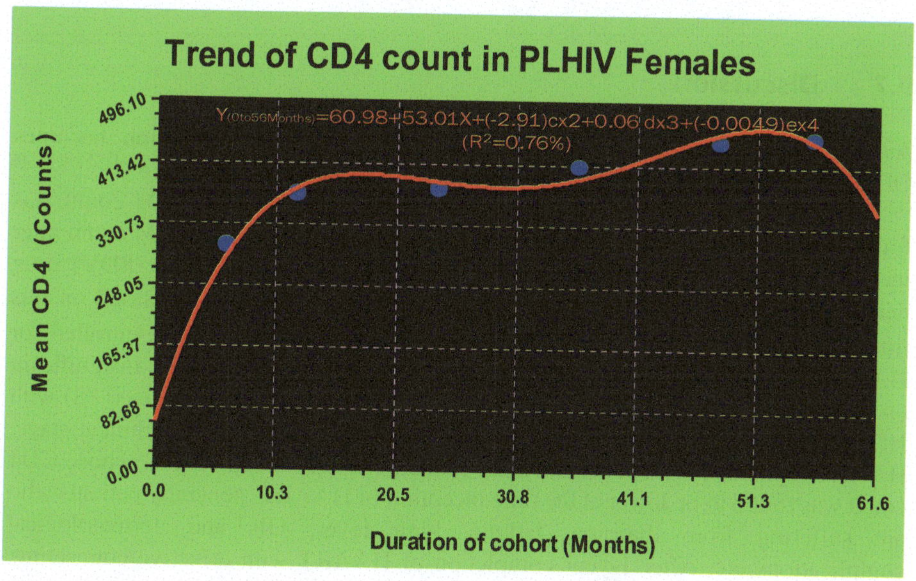

Fig. 9.4 Fifth-degree polynomial trend of CD_4 count in PLHIV females ($N = 202$)

$$\text{OR} = \left(\frac{188(A) \times 05(D)}{295(B) \times 09(C)}\right) = 0.35$$

The model determined that a total of 65% of patients were expressed above the age group of 36 years with baseline CD4 count <250 μ/dL. The standard dispersion of CD4 count and age group of the patients was calculated by following equation:

Table 9.4 Association between age and baseline CD4 counts

CD4 count	25–35 years	>36 years
CD4 count <250 μ/dL	188 (A)	295 (B)
CD4 count >250 μ/dL	09 (C)	05 (D)

$$\text{SE}\ \ln(\text{OR}) = \sqrt{\left(\frac{1}{a} + \frac{1}{b} + \frac{1}{c} + \frac{1}{d}\right)}$$

$$\text{SE}\ \ln(\text{OR}) = \sqrt{\left(\frac{1}{188} + \frac{1}{295} + \frac{1}{9} + \frac{1}{5}\right)} = 0.564$$

$$95\%\text{CI for the}\ \ln\ (\text{OR}) = -1.032 \pm 1.96 \times 0.564 = (-1.474, -0.590)$$

$$95\%\text{CI for OR} = (\text{e} - 1.474, \text{e} - 0.590) = (0.229, 0.554).$$

9.7 Discussion

As per the model formulation, the odds prediction model equation becomes ODDS $= e^{a\ +\ \text{bX}}$. The fitted model R^2 was 80.26% (ODDS $= e^{-.053\ +\ 1.28\ (1)} = e^{.37} = 1.458$). Over a period of time, the male and female CD4 count was found to be 45 μ/dL and 14.58 μ/dL, which were likely to improve CD4 count after inception of HAART. Due to adverse (ADV) and serious adverse (SDV) drug reactions, the demonstrated model was $\widehat{Y} = \frac{\text{ODDS}}{1+\text{ODDS}} = \frac{0.450}{1.458} = 0.30$. Based on this fitted model, a total of 30.80% and 59.0% of women and men were enrolled for HAART. The baseline CD4 count was found to be statistically insignificant ($p < 0.05$), and it was found to be negatively correlated ($r = -0.62$) (−0.88) with HIV clinically associated parameters, viz., age of the person, WHO clinical stage, HAART regimens, etc. As per the fitted model, the results opined that, whose CD4 count was found to be lower at the time inception of HAART, generally patients who are suffering from diarrhea, fatigue, high fever, OIs and dermatological complications etc. After 1-year completion of HAART with effective counseling, palliative care, and comprehensive supports, the CD4 count was positively correlated with clinically associated parameters ($r = 0.70$) presented in the table. Statistically, the variance of the estimated model was calculated by using MLE method. The main implications of our fitted model were designed to ensure maintaining a maximum efficiency, accuracy, and relevancy of the HIV data sets. However, our fitted model clearly demonstrated that the MLEs of the model -2 log likelihood was found to be 107.49 with very less expression of CoxSnell R^2. As per the above study, the results showed that the fitted model would be considered as user-friendly due to relative predictions, efficiency, sufficiency, and good accuracy. Further, the present fitted model will be very useful for the clinicians for taking clinical decisions about the population, and also it can be used to estimate/predict the future trend of different HIV biomarkers. The methods of "odds" ratio model will provide a very good estimation of slopes and their standard errors of statistics.

9.8 Estimation Models on CD4 Count and Plasma RNA Viral Load

Statistical modelling of HIV/AIDS infection is very useful to project the future trend of disease progression rate, AIDS counts, and healthcare needs; the present study objective is to stress the needs of modelling of AIDS, and a few approaches were discussed in this chapter. Modelling has been pro-founded from a long time; many authors studied the projection models and its application to AIDS progression. In this connection, the forecasting epidemic modelling is an active and expanding field in the present days. Different models were fitted based on the transmission mechanisms of AIDS, which can help medical and scientific fields to understand and anticipate its spreads, etc. AIDS is expected to place enormous demand on healthcare facilities and implementations of comprehensive care, supports, and treatment program by the policymakers. Therefore, the present study demonstrated various projection models. Many authors discuss the choice among alternative strategies, which play a crucial role in determining degree of uncertainties of AIDS projections. In developing countries, a statistical modelling will create separate algorithms or logical structure to organize existing information into a framework and suggests what new data is being collected from the patient records. Thus, the projection models will provide insight information into the system even when the data are lacking or missing (Detels et al. 2005; Detels et al. 2005; Czerwinski et al. 2007). Hence, the statistical model is very essential for understanding AIDS and its relationships with social, biological, environmental mechanisms, influencing the spread of HIV/AIDS and its progression at global level. The secondary data was collected from records at various ART centers in Bangalore City, Karnataka State. The inclusive and exclusive criteria rule was considered for the study. HIV-infected population below 18 years of age group was not taken into consideration. The CD4 T lymphocyte count was done by the flow cytometric techniques, and data was collected at different intervals, viz., baseline, 6-month, and 12-month follow-up periods. RNA viral load copies per cells at the intervals of <47 target were not detected, and 5000–10000 RNA copies per cells and >10,000–20,000 copies per cells were collected. The data was compiled by SPSS-16.50 version; the following statistical models were fitted to know the geometric progression of CD4 and virological suppression among PLHIVs.

9.9 Double Hit (Event) Model

There are several biological changes that were noticed at infection and onset of AIDS, though CD4 T cells are the key indicators and they will maintain the body's immune system, considered for the principal target for HIV progression rate. The distribution of RNA plasma was extracted from the database, and it was considered as type I HIV marker for deciding the progression rate of infection, and CD4 cells were shown to be severely depleted during the course of the epidemic stage. The statistical association between disease progression and loss of CD4 cells was discussed by Berman et al., Cox et al., and Farr et al.. Let the independent random variables X_1,X_2 be the time of onset of HIV/AIDS and X_2 be the development of disease progression. Y_1 and Y_2 CD4 Tlymhocyte count and plasma RNA viral load (5000–10,000 copies per/mL).

X_1: Time for Y_1 to reach a specified lower limit L_1 (event E1)
X_2: Time for Y_2 to reach a specified higher limit L_2 (event E1)
Z: Time for onset of AIDS (E1 $\cap$ E2)
$Z \approx X1 \cap X2$

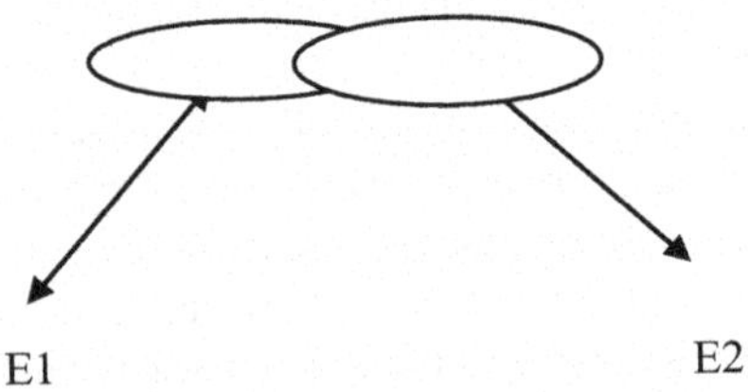

Due to parallel nature of the system, Z = max(X_1, X_2), then the immune failure AIDS on set distribution is.

$$\begin{aligned} \mathrm{Fz}(t) &= Pr(Z \le t) = 1 - Pr(Z > t) \\ &= 1 - Pr(X1 > t, X2 > t) \end{aligned}$$

$1 - \prod_{i=1}^{n}(1 - \mathrm{Fi}(t))$. Assuming that the event E_1 and E_2 are independent, here F_1(.),F_2(.) are the distribution functions of X_1 and X_2, respectively.

9.10 Compound Growth Rate (CGR) Model

A numerous studies were conducted pertaining to the medical and agricultural research for the formulation of growth models. The growth rate model is a very important analytical method to know the incremental changes of the selected biological variables, and earlier, this model was fitted by Vasanth Kumar et al. to know the price trend of timber species in Western Ghats. The important functional forms of the model that were employed to study the growth are linear, exponential, logarithmic forms, etc. However, many global studies highlighted the geometric forms for estimation of trend of selected variables. In this present model, we have formulated $Y = AB^t$, where Y is a variable under study, "A" is a constant, and "B" represents the regression coefficients, and further we have modified it in the form of 1 + CGR where "t" is time period. The compound growth rate model of RNA plasma (copies per/mL) is expressed in the following equation CGR $= \frac{b}{y} \times 100$, where Y = log values of plasma RNA viral load replica, A a = Constant, B b = coefficient of regression, $\overline{y}$ = Average multiplication of RNA replication at a time "t".

9.11 Exponential Smoothing Model

Exponential smoothing model was fitted it was originally developed by operational researcher in 1950s, and it has been extensively used in areas of short-range forecast or inventory control. Some empirical studies were conducted by Makridkis et al., and they found there is a little difference in the accuracy of forecasting between exponential techniques and Box-Jenkins. They have assumed that the time series data of CD_4 count will decompose at time "t" as Xi = μi + Ut, where μi is the mean CD4 count and U_t is the random error at time "t"; further mean CD4 count will not be constant over time, and it is not a realistic one in most of the cases. The current mean level was assigned exponentially with weighted moving average of the current and past observation of Xis, and the equation becomes $\mu t = \mathrm{aXt} + a(1-a)\mathrm{Xt}+1+a(1-a2)\mathrm{Xt}+2\ldots a\sum_{t=0}^{\infty}\frac{(1-a)}{X_{t-i}}$ equation (i).

The above equation will be simplified in the form of $\mu t = \mathrm{aXt} + (1-a)\mu t + 1\ldots$ Equation (ii).

Equation (ii) is known to be a simple exponential smoothing and showed forecasting numerals of mean CD4 counts at different intervals, viz., 6 months, 12 months, and 24 months. The weighted averages were assigned to the current observation and the previous baseline averages; the assigned weights were considered for extrapolation of smoothing constants. The raw data sequences were represented by (xi), and the output of the exponential smoothing algorithms was commonly written as (si), which may regarded as our best estimates of what is the next value of x will be generated from Equation (ii). When the sequence of observations begins at time t = 0, the simplest forms of exponential smoothing were given by the formula

$$s1 = \mathrm{xo}, \mathrm{St} = \propto \mathrm{xt} - 1 + (1-\propto)\mathrm{st} - 1, t > 1$$

where $\propto$is the smoothing factor and $0 < \propto < 1$.

$$S1 = X0$$

$$St = \propto Xt - 1 + (1-\propto)St - 1 = St - 1 + \propto (Xt - 1 - St - 1), t > 1$$

In other words, where $\propto$ is smoothing factor and $0 < \propto < 1$, the smoothing statistics St is a simple weighted average of the previous observation Xt – 1 and the previous statistics S_t-1.

9.12 Moving Average Model

The moving average (MA) model may be designated to remove the seasonal and random noise variation within a time series data of serial CD_4 count and plasma RNA viral load of PLHIVs. MA was routinely used for estimation of each newly generated series; it succeeded for removing most of the cyclic variations presented in the data series. Left out of the original series with noise data after early smoothing, the smoothing constant can remove seasonal and random variations in the data sets, and also an irregular component was estimated by the MA model (successor series retaining some combination of trend and cyclical behavior). The smoothing may leave a successor series, the data sets were plotted on new horizontal line against the time on the rotational axis, and the model would provide the greatest efficiency. If the data trend tends to linearity with presence of irregular trend and cyclic behavior, the model will not be suitable for estimation of accurate trend cycles.

9.13 Study Design

The design/methods and outcome measures of the study have been described previously [15]. Eligible patients were initiated therapy with the following drugs, which were administered twice daily: 300 mg of zidovudine plus 150 mg of lamivudine, 300 mg of abacavir, and 1200 mg of amprenavir. Alteration to this initial regimen was allowed for treatment-limiting toxicities or compliance issues, and the patients were followed up for the period of 12 months.

9.13.1 Ethics

Written consent was obtained from all eligible patients, and they provided signed informed consent prior to study enrollment. Prior permission has been taken from Karnataka State AIDS Prevention Society for the collection of secondary data sets.

9.13.2 Measurements and Evaluations

At initial enrollment for HIV care, the healthcare specialists recorded patient's medical history, risk factors of HIV acquisition, and symptoms and signs of OIs (with date of onset) and performed clinical examinations. Baseline blood sample examination was included for the study, and safety parameters and immunological and virological data sets were extracted from the institutional database. After enrollment, we have assessed clinical status and adverse drug reactions that were extracted from the patient's registration cards. The safety parameters, plasma HIV-1 RNA load and CD4, CD8, and CD8+/CD38++ T cell counts, were recorded at regular intervals. The cell-associated RNA levels were extracted from database of second-line HAART treatment. The CD4 counts and plasma RNA viral load data sets at different intervals were also extracted from pre-ART registry.

9.13.3 Patient Population and Baseline Characteristics

From January 2009 to July 2010, a total of 100 enrolled PLHIVs were started second-line ART. Demographic and baseline characteristics of the patients were shown in the table. The majority of the patients were men who had sex with men, and they were symptomatic during PHI (90% of patients; fever was reported in 66%, malaise 54%, lethargy 53%, headache 44%, myalgia 42%, skin rash 40%, and gastrointestinal symptoms 39%, and weight loss was observed in 37%). HAART treatment was initiated within 1–2 weeks of diagnosis (64% and 83% patients).

9.13.4 Baseline Plasma Viral Load and Immunological Parameters

The median HIV-1 load was 5.4 log copies/mL (range, 2.1–7.9 log copies/mL), and the median CD4 cell count was 514 cells/mm^3 (range, 162–1380 cells/mm^3) presented in Table 9.1. Plasma viremia was inversely correlated with CD4 cell count (Spearman's correlation, *r*p −0.41; *P*! 0.001). Patients with symptoms derived to have higher viral loads than did patients who did not have symptoms (5.5 log copies/mL vs. 4.9 log copies/mL; *P*p.13, by Mann-Whitney *U* test). More recent symptom onset was associated with higher viral load and lower CD4 cell count. Correlations of time since symptom onset with viral load and CD4 cell count were 0.35 (*P*! 0.001) and 0.17 (*P*p.052), respectively (Figs. 9.5 and 9.6).

Alpha (level): 1.01105 (actual), 1.01105 (adjusted)
Gamma (trend): -0.00905 (actual), 0.01000 (adjusted)

Accuracy Measures

MAPE: 40.14
MAD: 27.20
MSD: 1708.34

Row	Period	FORE1	LOWE1	UPPE1
1	3	126.428	−158.335	411.19
2	4	126.583	−311.620	564.78
3	5	126.737	−472.454	725.93
4	6	126.891	−636.075	889.86
5	7	127.046	−801.008	1055.10

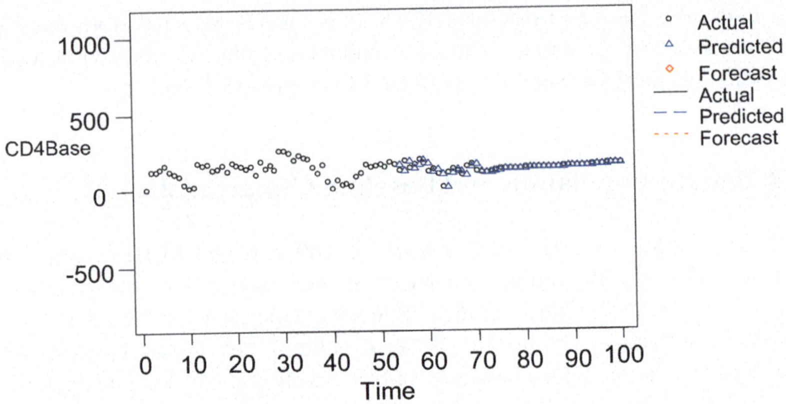

Fig. 9.5 Exponential model variation in baseline CD4 count in PLHIV

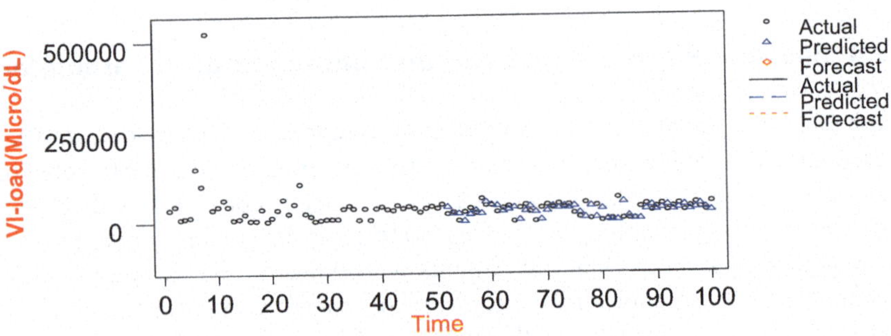

Fig. 9.6 Exponential model variation in baseline plasma RNA viral load in PLHIV

Smoothing Constants

Alpha (level): 0.822442
Gamma (trend): 0.014207

Accuracy Measures

MAPE: 1681
MAD: 27364
MSD: 4.26E+09

Row	Period	FORE2	LOWE2	UPPE2
1	3	40529.9	−7447	88,506
2	4	35642.9	−29,638	100,924
3	5	30756.0	−53,074	114,586
4	6	25869.1	−77,084	128,822
5	7	20982.2	−101,399	143,363

9.14 Model Discussion

Herein, we report the largest prospective therapeutic study of PHI. The majority of patients were men who have sex with men and were symptomatic during PHI. By week 48, 36% of the patients who had started receiving ART were either not receiving treatment or lost to follow-up, with an initial high rate of treatment change, which stabilized later during the study. The vast majority of patients who stopped receiving ART prematurely had undetectable HIV-1 loads when therapy was interrupted (Anderson et al. 1998). ART initiation was associated with decreases in HIV-1 load and cell-associated RNA and DNA levels and an improvement in immunological parameters. Baseline CD8+/CD38++ T cell count and cell-associated DNA level were independent predictors for achieving a viral load copies/mL. Toxicity was generally reversible. This study provides important information regarding the feasibility of starting quadruple ART in a large cohort of patients with PHI. Previous studies, which generally used three drugs, have shown treatment discontinuation rates of 19–50% at first year. A recent diagnosis of HIV infection, a rapid life-changing decision, clinical symptoms, and future rather than immediate administration of ART may compound the problems of treatment-related toxicity and high pill burden when comparing treatment discontinuation rates between patients with acute infection and those with chronic infection. Kulikov et al. (2003) revealed a higher number of patients stopping a similar ART regimen when they were treated during early infection, compared with those treated during chronic infection. Among newly infected patients, nonadherence and intolerance to adverse effects of therapy were the main reported reasons for stopping treatment. The availability of newer drugs with lower toxicities and pill counts may positively impact patients' adherence in future studies. Our results confirm those from previous smaller studies of PHI that reveal the possibility of achieving an undetectable HIV-1 load. The extent of virological control after ART initiation was further exemplified by the percentages of patients receiving ART at week 48 who had HIV-1 loads 50 copies/mL, 10 copies/mL, and 3 copies/mL, a median decrease in HIV-1 load of 5.4 log copies/mL, and an HIV-1 load of 0.7 log copies/mL. Even during a conservative intention-to-treat analysis (with missing data counted as "failure"), 64.0% of the patients had an HIV-1 load 50 copies/mL at week 48, a result comparable to that found during chronic infection [25]. Baseline parameters were helpful in forecasting virological outcome. Cell-associated HIV-1 RNA and DNA levels are indirect markers of treatment efficacy. Previous studies, including a study by Garrigue et al. [26], have revealed a median HIV-1 mRNA level of 1.7 log copies/million PBMCs and detectable mRNA levels after 12 months of ART in some aviremic patients with PHI who received ART and in all patients with chronic infection who received ART. We extend these results by revealing that plasma replication was dramatically decreased overall, because 33% of the patients had viral loads 3 copies/mL, and that the overall cell-associated RNA level decreased from 2.6 log copies/million PBMCs to 0.8 log copies/million PBMCs. When looking at cell-associated DNA level, which reflects the reservoir size, we found a median decrease of the cell-associated DNA level of 1.1 log copies/million PBMCs and a cell-associated DNA level of 1.6 log copies/million PBMCs at the end of the year. Previous studies of PHI have described a decrease of the cell-associated DNA level of 1.0 log after 18 months of ART, compared with the one half log decrease and absence of undetectable levels during chronic infection. Garrigue et al. reported that, after 1 year of ART, cell-associated DNA levels were 2.0 log copies/million PBMCs, with 1 of 22 patients having a cell-associated DNA level! 10 copies/million PBMCs; these findings contrast our figure of 6 patients (9.5%) with cell-associated DNA levels 3 copies/million PBMCs. Five of these six patients had a viral load of 10 copies/mL at the time of proviral measurement. These patients did not differ in terms of baseline CD4 cell count and HIV-1 load from those who had detectable cell-associated DNA levels. Our results suggested that the lower levels of cell-associated DNA are achievable with ART initiation during PHI than with ART initiation during chronic infection (Naresh et al. 2006). Our data also illustrate the changes in immune activation. Normalization of the CD8+/CD38++ T cell count occurred in 28 (27.7%) of 101 patients at week 48. These cell counts decreased initially in parallel with viral load and continued to decrease in patients achieving a viral load 50 copies/mL but not in patients with a viral load 3 copies/mL and could, therefore, represent a sensitive indicator of residual viral replication. Patients with an undetectable cell-associated RNA level at week 42 indeed had lower CD8+/CD38++ T cell counts at weeks 36 and 48, compared with those who had detectable cell-associated RNA level at week 42. The initial follow-up of six patients who had stopped treatment prematurely suggested that the CD8+/CD38++ T cell count tended to increase with subsequent viral load rebound (data not shown). Safety is an important factor to consider when initiating early treatment. Grade 3 or 4 clinical and laboratory severe adverse events occurred in a substantial proportion of patients but were generally reversible, as previously reported (Adegboye et al. 2012). The incidence of hypersensitivity to abacavir (3.0%) was comparable to that in other studies. The rate of severe adverse events in our study was compared with that in a previous study in which 17 of 39 patients with acute and chronic infection experienced 19 severe adverse events; significant depression accounted for 2 severe adverse events (Adegboye et al. 2012). In a French cohort study of PHI, 124 patients (51%) described having experienced at least 1 adverse event, and 19% of these events were reported as mood disorder (Adegboye et al. 2012; Agarwala et al. 2002). The 14 psychiatric severe adverse events in our study were not considered to be related to study medication. Strong past confounding factors were present in 11 of 13 patients, revealing the potential for serious psychiatric events during the immediate post-seroconversion phase in patients with a previous psychiatric history. In conclusion, we have described that the first year outcome of a large cohort of patients who initiated a protease inhibitor-based, 4-drug anti ART regimen during PHI. Our results are very encouraging for achieving a very low HIV-1 load, considering the virological parameters in patients receiving ART, undetectable cell-associated RNA and DNA levels. The fitted models will be able to predict accurate values and should maintain a greater accuracy, fewer SE, and reduced cost.

9.15 Summary

Statistical modelling of HIV/AIDS is a very useful information for projecting the future trend of disease progression, estimation of AIDS counts, and efficacy of "HAART" and for forecasting healthcare needs, etc. This chapter objective stresses the needs of modelling of AIDS, and a few approaches were discussed briefly. The projection models and its application to AIDS were described by using analytical approach. The forecasting epidemic modelling was fitted by different attributed data sets to describe HIV geometric progression, the present fitted model is an active and expanding practical insight for the researcher and policymakers, and the present CGR model was derived based on the transmission mechanism of AIDS, and this model will help medical and scientific field to understand HIV progression rate anticipated with its spread. The secondary data was collected from the patient records at various government tertiary care hospitals in Bangalore City, and the inclusion and exclusion criteria rule was considered for the study. Exclusion: PLHIVs below 18 years of age group were not taken into consideration. The CD4 T lymphocyte counts and plasma RNA viral load data sets were collected at different intervals, viz., treatment inception (baseline), 6-month, 12-month period, etc. The data was compiled by using SPSS-16.50 versions, and the compound growth rate, double hit, exponential smoothing, and moving average model was fitted to quantify the geometric progression of HIV despite CD4 count and virological suppression. As per the research findings, the risk of virological failure was triggered at very low CD4 counts ($<50 \times 10^6$ cells/μL) at inception of "HAART," and also it was found to be statistically significant ($p < 0.01$) when compared to inception of "HAART" at higher-level CD4 count $>250 \times 10^6$ cells/μL (hazard ratio (HR) 2.28, 95% confidence interval (CI) 0.95–2.01). The same research findings was seen in plasma RNA VL. If the "HAART" started at CD4 count >450–550 μ/dL, the HIV-associated complications were negatively related (VL $\geq$150,000 copies/mL when compared with a lower VL $\leq$ 10,000 copies/ml (HR 1.20, 95% CI 0.91–1.78). The CGR was numerically expressed at the rate of 8.96, and it was found to be statistically significant ($p \leq 0.001$) at inception of lower CD4 counts with more associated complications. The mean "CD4" count at inception of HAART was 156 $\pm$ 78.96 cells per μL (IQR 296–365). The greatest mean yearly CD4 count differences were seen during the study period (100 cells per μL increased trend were seen after 1-year HAART treatment). CD4 count trend was observed by exponential smoothing method and polynomial curve fitting, and the smoothing constant ($\alpha = 0.072$) MAPE was 227.40, respectively, with $R^2 = 0.75\%$. In patients for whom viral load (VL) suppression was expressed below the level <47 μ/dL, the VL detection was not possible; fitted forecasting model figures were easily generated by the compound growth and exponential smoothing constants. The normalization of CD4 counts among HIV-infected patients has to be maintained by achieving the viral load VL suppression with effective "HAART" that can be maintained for a longer period.

References

Adegboye ZA et al (2012) Reformulation of Runge-Kutta method into linear multistep method for error and convergence analysis. Pac J Sci Technol 13:238–243

Agarwala BD et al (2002) On two ODE models for HIV/AIDS development in Canada and a logistic SEIR model. Far East J Appl Math 6(1.) (2002):25–70

Anderson RM et al (1988) The role of mathematical models in the study of HIV transmission and the epidemiology of AIDS. J AIDS 1:241–256

Anderson RM, Medly GF, May RM, Johnson AM et al (1998) A preliminary study of the transmission dynamics of the human immunodeficiency virus (HIV), the causative agent of AIDS IMA. J Math Appl Med Biol 3(1986):229–263

Czerwinski IA et al (2007) Short-term forecasting of halibut CPUE: linear and non-linear univariate approaches. Fish Res 86:120–128

Detels R, Munoz A et al (2005) Patterns of the hazard of death after AIDS through the evolution of antiretroviral therapy. J AIDS 19(17):2009–2018

Kulikov GY et al (2003) Symmetric Runge-Kutta method and their stability. Russ J Numer Anal Math Model 18:13–41

Naresh R, Tripathi A, Omar S et al (2006) Modelling the spread of AIDS epidemic with vertical transmission J. Appl Math Comput 178:262–272

Newell ML et al (1998) Mechanism and timing of mother to child transmission of HIV-1. J AIDS 12:832–837

Sankar J et al (2011) Stochastic modeling approach for forecasting fish product export in Tamilnadu. J Recent Res Sci Technol 3(7):104–108

Simwa R, Pokhariyal GP et al. (2003) A dynamical model for stage-specific HIV incidences with application to sub-Saharan Africa. Department of Mathematics, University of Nairobi

Wig N et al (2006) The impact of HIV/AIDS on the quality of life: a cross-sectional study in North India. Indian J Med Sci 60(1):3–12

Simulation Modelling Techniques of HIV/AIDS

10

10.1 Introduction

AIDS incubation period as a key epidemiologic descriptor has been discussed in Chap. 1. A contrasting feature of HIV syndrome in relation to other infectious diseases is its incubation period which is a random variable and probably the longest one. An HIV infected exhibits disease symptoms after completion of this period and thereafter presents an AIDS case. The levels of CD_4 T lymphocyte immune cells and HIV RNA in the human body determine the progression of the infection. HIV spread mechanism and its manifestation to AIDS are random phenomena, and hence stochastic modelling is expected to be a better descriptor of the scenario. The present chapter (i) highlights some stochastic features of HIV spread, (ii) discusses the applicability of a few well-known probability models to cover the essence of immune system failure mechanism, (iii) proposes a model for time to AIDS onset, and (iv) examines the applicability of two standard stochastic models in the AIDS situation.

10.2 Rationality of the Stochastic Modelling

Many phenomena in life sciences are now studied not only as random but also as changing with time or space. For example, the growth of HIV-infected population over time may be considered to be a stochastic process. The growth of HIV in blood is a determining factor to confer seropositivity. Once this occurs, its progress to AIDS is characterized by several stages associated with depletion of CD_4^+ cells.

This forms a discrete-space continuous time stochastic process providing a basis for modelling of AIDS. Moreover, as AIDS epidemiological data become more extensive and on occasions deal with smaller-risk groups than those relevant for large areas, the elements of random variation become more prominent. McKendrick et al. were the first to give a stochastic treatment of an epidemic process. Excellent reviews on the current modelling work on AIDS have been provided by Anderson

D. M. Basavarajaiah, B. Narasimha Murthy, *HIV Transmission*,
https://doi.org/10.1007/978-981-15-0151-7_10

et al., Isham et al., Bailey et al., and Mollison et al. There are several advantages of stochastic modelling as compared to the deterministic approach. For instance, (i) the former provides more information, i.e., besides expected values, one can compute variances and covariances and assess the effects of various factors, (ii) stochastic models along with computers provide a wider choice in formulating the underlying assumptions and model structure, and (iii) Monte Carlo methods may be used to assess whether solutions of some non-linear difference equations are in fact measures of central tendency for random functions of the epidemic process.

10.3 Distribution of Time to Onset

The endemiology of AIDS is two-dimensional; one is the problem of seroprevalence where different transmission modes and HIV spread mechanisms are dealt with. The other is the progression of HIV infection to AIDS. In non-communicable diseases like cancer, the first problem does not arise. In HIV syndrome, from individual as well as societal viewpoints, the problem is more serious in terms of its control and management. Though the second problem is a consequence of the first, a study of progression of HIV infection to AIDS is all the more difficult. The distribution *F*(.) of time to onset *T* is one of the main parameters used for measuring the growth of the epidemic. For instance, Weibull, gamma, beta, and exponential distributions have had wide uses as *F*(.). If T follows a Weibull distribution with positive shape and scale parameters α and β, then the survival function of *T* takes the simple form

$$\mathbf{S(t) = P[T > t] = \mathit{exp}—(t/\beta)^{\alpha} \text{ for } t > O.}$$

On the other hand, if *T* follows a gamma distribution with positive index and scale parameters α and β, then the survival function takes the form

$$\mathbf{S(t) = \frac{1^{\infty}}{r(\alpha)\beta^{\alpha}} S_t{}^{\alpha-1} \mathit{exp}(-s/\beta) ds,}$$

where $t \geq 0$ and $r(\alpha)$ is a gamma function.

Suppose – is a positive integer such that *S*(*r*) is, for all practical purposes, equal to zero. Then a set of conditional survival probabilities defined by

$$\mathbf{P(t) = P[T > t \mid T > t - 1],} \tag{10.1}$$

for $1 < t < r$ plays a basic role in the stochastic population process to be described. Given a numerical implementation of *S*(*t*), the conditional survival probabilities in Eq. (10.1) may be computed by using the formula

$$P(t) = S(t)/S(t-1), \text{for } 1 < t < r \tag{10.2}$$

Three sets of estimates of the parameters for the Weibull distribution and one set for the gamma distribution have been used in the computer experiments reported in Mode et al. The gamma distribution specified by

$$F(t) = \frac{1}{r(\alpha)\beta^{\alpha}} S_{x=0} \frac{t}{\beta^{\alpha} X^{\alpha-1}} \cdot \exp(-\beta x) dx,$$

is one of the assumed models for *F*(.).

Here, α and β are, respectively, the shape and scale parameters of the distribution. The non-parametric Kaplan-Meier (KM) method is also widely used for estimation of *F*(.). It appears that there are no clear guidelines for choosing *F*(.). It is important to understand the nature of *T*, the causes for its variability, and their impact on the other factors which affect disease progression. It has been noted that *F*(.) is affected by treatment with antiviral drugs such as zidovudine and by prophylaxis of opportunistic diseases like tuberculosis. This has led to non-stationary incubation distribution.

10.4 Basic Concepts of Immune Failure

The variable *T* represents the lifetime of an HIV infected before AIDS onset. The following functions of *T* defined over the interval (o, ∞) are useful in further analysis. Let *f*(*t*) denote the pdf of *T*. Then the distribution function indicating system failure (AIDS onset) on or before time t is given by $F(t) = Pr(T < t) = S_o^t f(x).dx$. The probability of an infected individual not experiencing onset until time *t* is given by

$$S(t) = 1—F(t) = Pr(T > t) = S_t^{\infty} f(x).dx = \exp\left(S_o^t h(x) dx\right.$$

where the hazard function *h*(*t*) is defined by

$$h(t) = 1_t^{\Delta t \to 0} \frac{Pr(t < T < \Delta t + t > t)\ f(t)}{\Delta t} = S(t)$$

which specifies the instantaneous rate of immune failure at the time of t. In particular, *h*(*t*) Δt is the approximate probability of AIDS onset in $(t, t + \Delta t)$ given that there is no onset until *t*. The expressions for these functions for a few widely used distributions like exponential, Weibull, and gamma distributions are summarized in Table 10.1.

Table 10.1 Select lifetime distributions and their features

Function	Exponential	Weibull	Gamma
F(*t*)	1-e-λt	$1 - \exp[(-t/\lambda)\beta]$	R(t/1α, β)
f(*t*)	be-λt		

10.5 Uncertainties in Estimates

Estimating *F*(.) has been a subject of recent research. For some data sets (where the date of infection is known, e.g., blood transfusion cases), one can estimate this directly from longitudinal studies. For other data sets (where infection time is not known), some statistical modelling is necessary to account for date of infection. In the former case, the uncertainties may be due to short follow-up times, inadequate sample size, and incomplete follow-up or inaccurate date of infection. In the estimation of *F*(.) for seroconvert cohort (subjects who become infected during the follow-up period), the problems may be due to short follow-up times and small number of reported AIDS cases. To overcome this, Taylor et al. have used multiple imputation technique (a model-based scheme for analyzing data with missing values) for imputing time of AIDS diagnosis from the predictive distribution of the missing values given the observed data. Use of a data set from a 4-year multicentric AIDS cohort study with 4954 homosexual gay men recruited in 4 cities of the USA during 1984–1985 and KM estimation on 100 imputed data sets revealed the following main points:

(i) Less than 3% individuals develop AIDS within 2 years of infection, and for longer times, the hazard rate increases.
(ii) It is important to consider the effect of age of an individual and mode of transmission in estimation of *F*(.).
(iii) The median time to AIDS for the data is about 9.5 years.

There have been other estimates of incubation period. A widely used estimate obtained from Weibull regression has a median *T* of 10 years. Bacchetti et al. provide a non-parametric estimate of median T as between 10 and 11 years. These studies suggest that the probability of progression to AIDS within 2 years is <0.02, and it rises to between 0.25 and 0.35 within 7 years and to about 0.50 within 10 years. In fact, estimates of mean and median T have lengthened steadily since an early estimate of 4.5 years. This may be the result of:

(i) Use of antiviral drugs as mentioned above
(ii) Employing Weibull model which fits steadily an increasing hazard function

Tan et al. (1995) used a general stochastic model to characterize *F*(.) by generating Monte Carlo data under different conditions and compared fitting of data by KM method, expectation-maximization (EM) algorithm, linear spline, and Bacchetti method for estimating *F*(.). They concluded that EM algorithm and generalized log logistic distribution provide satisfactory fits.

10.6 Need for Precise Time to Onset

The estimate of T depends upon the method and the efficiency of estimation, amount of data used, age and immunity level of the infected, use of drugs, and cause of infection. In blood transfusion, due to heavy viral inflow directly into the blood, the onset will be early. This is more so in repeated transfusions to the same individual. These uncertainties affect the precision of the estimate, which accounts for large discrepancies between observed and estimated AIDS counts. A popular method based on infection density and *F*(.) for projecting AIDS counts is back calculation. In the absence of these inputs, Srivenkataramana et al. have proposed a workable alternative to back calculation based on seropositivity rate, which is generally available.

10.7 A Staged Markov Model

A staged Markov model which was successful in the studies of cancer has been used to estimate the mean length of T for AIDS from a cohort of 603 HIV infected who have been followed through various stages of infection. The model partitions the infection period into five progression stages, (i) infected but antibody negative, (ii) antibody positive but asymptomatic, (iii) pre-AIDS symptoms, (iv) clinical AIDS which have transient states, and (v) death due to AIDS (an absorbing state), and obtains the estimates as under the mean (median) waiting times in each stage of infection which are stage (i) 2.2 (1.5) months, (ii) 52.6 (36.5) months, (iii) 62.9 (43.6) months, and (iv) 23.6 (16.3) months. The mean incubation period is 9.8 years with a 95% CI of 8.4 and 11.2 years. The model is described with the following notations:-

$\lambda_i(>0)$ ($I = 1,2,3,4$): transition intensities, where λ_i dt + o (dt) is the probability that an infected individual in stage i will make a transition to stage (i + 1) in time interval (t, t + dt) for $t > o$. Then Pr [an individual in stage i at time t_o will be in stage $k \geq i$ at time (t_o + t)] is

$$P_{\mathrm{ik}}(\mathrm{t}) = (-1)^{k-i}\,\lambda_i \ldots .\lambda_{k-I} \sum_{I}^{\mathbf{k}} e^{-\lambda}{}_{j^{-t}}/\left(\lambda_j - \lambda_{\mathrm{u}}{}^{\mathbf{k}}_{I=i} \atop \mathbf{I}=\mathbf{j} \right);1$$

$$= 1, 2, 3, 4, 5 \tag{10.3}$$

and from state i to absorbing state is

$$P_{i5}(t) = (-1)^{5-i}\,\lambda_i \ldots \lambda_4 \sum_{\mathbf{j-i}}^{4} \left(1 - e^{-\lambda_j t}\right)/\lambda_j \quad \left(\lambda_j - \lambda_u{}^{k}{}_{\mathbf{u}\,=\,\mathbf{i}} \atop \mathbf{u} = \mathbf{j}\right) \tag{10.4}$$

The pdf of T is $f(t) = \lambda_3 P_{13}(t)$ and the cdf is $F(t) = P(T < t) = S^t{}_o f(t)\,dt$.

Then the hazard function for developing AIDS is $h(t) = f(t)/(1 - F(t))$. This follows from the assumption that waiting time in stage i is exponentially distributed with mean $\mu_i = 1/\lambda_i$ $(i = 1, 2, 3, 4, 5)$. The expected length of the AIDS incubation period is $E(T) = \mu 1 + \mu 2 + \mu 3$ and $V(T) = \mu 12 + \mu 22 + \mu 32$. Further, the mean time to death and its variance from state i are $E(Ti) = \Sigma\, \mu_j$ and $V(T_i) = \Sigma\, \mu_j{}^2$; $I = 1, 2, 3$. The survival function for individuals from state i is $S_{Ti}(t) = P(T_i > t) = 1 - P_{15}(t)$.

10.8 Double Hit Model

There are several biological changes between infection and onset of AIDS. Though $CD_4{}^+$ cells of the human immune system are the principal target for HIV, the concentration of HIV RNA in plasma is also considered as a HIV laboratory marker in deciding progression of infection. $CD_4{}^+$ cells get severely depleted during the course of the epidemic. The statistical association between disease progression and loss of $CD_4{}^+$ cells has been discussed by Lange et al., Taylor et al., Fahay et al., and Phillips et al. Data from multicentric AIDS cohort study suggest that for patients with $CD_4{}^+ > 500/mm^3$ who have RNA < 10,000 copies/nil, the risk of AIDS in the subsequent 2–4 years is practically non-existent. A mathematical modelling approach = estimated that a patient with $CD_4{}^+ > 500/mm3$ and RNA of 1,00,000 copies/nil has at least 2.8 years before progressing to AIDS. Thus reaching certain defined levels determines the onset of AIDS.

10.9 Independent X_1 and X_2

In view of two markers of AIDS onset, the human immune system can be considered to have parallel components (say C_1, C_2) since there is no onset as long as the markers do not reach specified levels. Since AIDS onset requires changes in two types of body cells, a double hit model can be considered here. The theory can be developed with the following variables:

Y_1 and Y_2: Respectively denote CD cell and HIV RNA counts
X_1: Time for Y_1 to reach a specified lower limit L_1 (event E_1)
X_2: Time for Y_2 to reach a specified higher limit L_2 (event E_2)
Z: Time for onset of AIDS (event $E_1 \cap E_2$)
Due to parallel nature of the system, clearly, $Z = \max(X_1, X_2)$.

Then, the immune failure (AIDS onset) distribution is given by

$$\mathbf{F}_z(\mathrm{t}) = \mathbf{P_r}(\mathbf{Z} \leq \mathrm{t}) = \mathbf{1} - \mathbf{P_r}(\mathbf{Z} > t) = \mathbf{1} - \mathbf{P_r}(\mathbf{X}_1 > \mathrm{t}, \mathbf{X}_2 > \mathrm{t})$$

$$= \mathbf{1} - \left(\mathbf{1} - \mathbf{F}_{\mathbf{i}} \quad (\mathbf{t}) \atop \mathbf{i} - \mathbf{1} \right),$$

assuming that the events E_1 and E_2 are independent. Here $F_1(.)$ and $F_2(.)$ are distribution functions of X_1 and X_2, respectively. As both the events denote failures, we first take them to have a common distribution, say $F(t)$, so that $F_z(t) = 1 — [1\text{-}F(t)]^2$.

10.10 Illustration

Let us consider exponential distribution for X_1 and X_2 with parameters λ_1 and λ_2. That is, $\mathbf{F_i(t) = 1 - \ exp\ (-\lambda_i t),\ for\ i = 1,2.}$

Then

$$\begin{aligned} \mathrm{Fz}(t) &= 1 - \ \exp\,(\lambda_i t)^2_{i.1} \\ &= 1 - [\exp\ (-\mu t)] \text{ where } \mu = (\lambda_1 + \lambda_2). \end{aligned}$$

Estimation of μ

In longitudinal studies of the HIV infected, periodical measurements are made on the two markers. This provides data on (Y_1, Y_2). Since X_1 is the time for Y_1 to fall below L_1 for the first time and X_2 is the time for Y_2 to exceed L_2 for the first time, the recordings (Y_1, Y_2) lead to data on (X_1, X_2). Let Y_1 be available for n1-infected and Y_2 for n_2-infected persons. This is the ideal case where the two markers are individually observed. In this case, μ can be estimated by estimating λ_1 and λ_2 separately as $\lambda_2 = n_2 / \Sigma X_{2i}$. And an estimate of μ is

$$\mu = \lambda_1 + \lambda_2$$

In the absence of longitudinal data on Y_1 and Y_2, one may only have information on the AIDS onset time Z. For example, this is the case when facility for measuring Y_1 and Y_2 is not available, but AIDS onset can be diagnosed. This produces information on Z. Then, from standard theory, the

$$\text{MLE's of } \mu \text{ is } \mu = n / \sum_1^n Z_i$$

where n is the sample size.

The literature on AIDS shows use of all the three distributions (exponential, Weibull, and gamma) for X_1 and X_2. There is no clear-cut guideline for making a specific choice in the AIDS situation. The relevant theoretical results are in Johnson et al. (1980). The practical suitability of these models is worth investigating. In the above discussion, it is assumed that the events E_1 and E_2 are independent. Alternatively, if E_1 and E_2 are dependent (which is likely), we may adopt the following approach using a Bivariate distribution.

10.11 Dependent X_1 and X_2

In a parallel system, instead of assuming independence of components, it is more realistic to consider them as following a bivariate distribution. This has an inbuilt allowance for dependence. In the AIDS context, failure of one component may imply an unchanged form of the distribution of the other but with a possible change in failure rate. This leads to the following formulation. We consider bivariate extension of exponential failure distribution for the above purpose. The estimation of failure rates using information matrix has been considered by Freund et al. and Kale et al. Consider AIDS onset system with two components (C_1, C_2) such that the failure time distributions of C_1 and C_2 are both exponential with failure rates $\lambda 1$ and λ_2, respectively. If C_1 fails first, the system continues to work until C_2 fails, but the failure time distribution of C_2 is now exponential with failure rate $\lambda_1{}^2$ ($> \lambda_2$). Similarly if C_2 fails first, then the onset does not occur until C_1 fails, but the failure time distribution of C_1 is now exponential with failure rate $\lambda_1{}^1$ ($>\lambda_1$).

The joint pdf of (X, X2) is given by

$$\begin{aligned}\mathbf{log\ f} &= \mathbf{I_A(x_1, x_2)}\left[log\ \boldsymbol{\lambda_1\lambda_2{}^1}\text{—}log\ \boldsymbol{\lambda_1{}^1\lambda_2}\right] + log\ \boldsymbol{\lambda_1{}^1\lambda_2} - \boldsymbol{\lambda_1{}^1}\mathbf{x_1} - \left(\boldsymbol{\lambda_1} + \boldsymbol{\lambda_2} - \boldsymbol{\lambda_1{}^1}\right)\mathbf{x_2} \\ &+ \left(\boldsymbol{\lambda_1{}^1} + \boldsymbol{\lambda_2{}^1} - \boldsymbol{\lambda_1} - \boldsymbol{\lambda_2}\right)(\mathbf{x_1} - \mathbf{x2})\ \mathbf{I_A}(\mathbf{x_1} - \mathbf{x_2})\end{aligned} \tag{10.5}$$

where $A = \{x_1, x_2 | 0 < x_1 < x_2\}$ and $I_A(x_1, x_2)$ are the indicator function of the set A. This pdf depending on $\theta = (\lambda_1, \lambda_2, \lambda_1{}^1, \lambda_2{}^1)$ belongs to a four-parameter exponential family with Fisher information matrix:

$$\mathbf{I(\theta)} = diag\ \begin{matrix} \mathbf{1} & \mathbf{1} & \boldsymbol{\lambda 2} & \boldsymbol{\lambda 1} \\ \boldsymbol{\lambda_1(\lambda_1 + \lambda_2)} & \boldsymbol{\lambda_2(\lambda_1 + \lambda_2)} & \boldsymbol{(\lambda_1{}^1)^2(\lambda_1 + \lambda_2)} & \boldsymbol{(\lambda_2{}^1)^2(\lambda_1 + \lambda_2)} \end{matrix}$$

pdf (probability density function) divided, one for ($0<x_1<x_2$) and the other for ($0<x_2<x_1$)

The minimal sufficient statistic is four dimensional and is given by

$\Sigma I_A(x_1, x_2) = n_1$, the number of observations with $x_1 < x_2$, i.e., where C_1 failed first, together with Σx_1, Σx_2, $\Sigma(x_1 - x_2)\, I_A(x_1, x_2)$. The MLEs for a random sample of size n on f ($x_1, x_2, \lambda_1, \lambda_2, \lambda_1{}^1, \lambda_2{}^1$) are given by

The estimated MLEs are consistently distributed asymptotically with normal $(\lambda_1, \lambda_2, \lambda_1{}^1, \lambda_2{}^1)$ and variance-covariance matrix $I^{-1}(\theta)/n$ given by

Freund introduced the above bivariate exponential distribution and obtained the MLEs but not their asymptotic variance-covariance matrix, and they did not note that pdf in Eq. (10.12) is a four-parameter exponential family. The asymptotic distribution of MLE has been derived by Hanagal et al. They use it to propose test of hypotheses for symmetry—H_o: $\lambda_1 = \lambda_2$ and $\lambda_1{}^1 = \lambda_2{}^1$. They have also given a test for Ho: $\lambda_1 = \lambda_1{}^1$ and $\lambda_1 = \lambda_2{}^1$ which is equivalent to independence of X_1 and X_2 in the Freund model and which leads to the model discussed above. In that it was assumed that the time for HIV RNA count to reach a specified upper limit L_2 is independent of the time required for $CD_4{}^+$ immune cell count to reach a specified lower limit L_1. However, the appropriateness in the application of these two cases discussed in the context of AIDS onset is another important issue to be investigated through more and more clinical studies.

10.12 Discussion

The HIV spread mechanism and manifestation of virus into AIDS differ significantly from several other communicable diseases. In the bulk of literature on AIDS, the time from infection to seroconversion (window period) is ignored as it is very short and lasts only for a few weeks and all HIV infected are assumed to be seropositives. However, Sathiyamoorthy et al. use shock models and a cumulative damage process to discuss the impact of accumulating damages on the immune system. They derive mean time to seroconversion and its variance and deduce that an increase in the number of contacts tends to shorten the window period. Also, interval-censored time-to-event data arise when the event time is only known to lie within a window. For example, in a cohort study with follow-up, seroconversion for HIV may only be known to have occurred between a negative blood test and a later positive one. Left truncation caused by exclusion of subjects who had already experienced an event before recruitment is another complication. A novel approach to this problem has been attempted by Bacchetti and Quale, who extended smooth nonparametric modelling to time-to-event data where the event may be known only to lie within a window of time. Maximum penalized likelihood is used to fit a discrete proportional hazard model that also models the baseline hazard, and left truncation and time-varying covariates are accommodated. The method is illustrated on a well-known interval-censored data set on time of HIV infection in a multicenter study of hemophiliacs. Since HIV infection and its manifestation to AIDS exhibit randomness, a stochastic modelling is desirable. Progression of HIV infection is negatively correlated with the count of $CD_4{}^+$ immune cells in the body, which depletes gradually after infection. Prominent failure time (or survival time) models such as exponential, Weibull, or gamma may be assumed to measure the changes in immune cells. However, a choice is difficult to make, and it may be restricted by data availability. The main purpose of using statistical models for transmission dynamics of HIV is to focus attention on the important epidemiologic parameters such as incubation period that need to be measured to predict future trends in AIDS counts.

10.13 Model for Probability of Infection

Mode et al. describe a model for probability of infection in a male homosexual population with the following notations:

N: Number of sexual partners (individuals) during the time interval (*t*-1, *t*)
C: Number of sexual contacts per partner

Both N and C are random variables with P(*N* = *n*) = f(*n*) and P(C = *c*) = g(*c*) as their pmf's (*n* = 0,1, 2,. . . ..,*M* and *c* = 1, 2,. . . ., *K*) where M and K are positive integers.

The probability-generating functions (pgf) of *N* and *C* are

$$\mathbf{F(s) = E\left[S^N\right] = \sum_{n=0}^{M} f(n)s^n \text{ and}}$$

$$\mathbf{G(s) = E[sc] = \sum_{c=1}^{k} g(c)s^c, \text{ for } 0 < s < 1.}$$

Let *p* and *q* (= 1—*p*) be the probabilities of being infected and escaping infection per sexual contact and G (*q*) be the probability that a susceptible individual escapes infection during (*t*-1, *t*) per infected sexual partner. Suppose that at time (*t*-1), the target population contains I-infected and S-susceptible individuals. Then 1/(*I* + *S*) is the probability that a susceptible individual meets a partner infected with HIV during (*t*-1, *t*). If it is assumed that AIDS patients, though they are infective, are no longer sexually active, then the conditional probability per sexual partner that a susceptible individual is infected during (*t*-1, *t*) is *P*(*t*) = [*I*/(*I* + *S*)] [1 – *G*(*q*)]. Further if it is assumed that sexual contacts among partners are stochastically independent, then *Q* (*t*) = *F*[*q*(*t*)] is the conditional probability that a susceptible individual escapes infection during (*t*-1, *t*), where *q*(*t*) = 1-*p*(*t*). Therefore, *P*(*t*) = 1 - *Q*(*t*) is the conditional probability that a susceptible individual becomes HIV infected during (*t*-1, *t*). This probability will be useful to estimate the number of new HIV infections in a given interval of time, say during a particular year.

10.14 Choice for the Distributions of N and C

The authors suggest the use of distributions like two-parameter negative binomial, binomial, and Poisson for the generating functions of N and C. But Anderson found that although the negative binomial did provide a fair fit to the number of sexual partners per month among homosexual males, the distribution did not pass a x^2 test of goodness of it. Therefore, the choice of binomial family with parameters (M,θ) with a generating function of the form *F*(*s*) = (θ^1+*s* θ)M; 0 < θ < 1; θ^1 = 1 — θ for the distribution of N can be made. In this case, E(N) $= F^{1}(s)_{s=1} =$ Mθ. Since the number of contacts is random and generally varies for different pairs of partners, the generating function of C can be taken as a member of Poisson family. Also, for a variety of reasons, the exact number of contacts during the interval (t-1, t) may not be known for individual partners, but known only to exceed a certain number. This gives rise to left truncation of the distribution. If λ is the parameter (mean) of Poisson distribution, then the generating function of C is $P(s) = \exp[\lambda(s-1)]$.

10.15 Estimation of Parameters

Then $E(C) = P^{1}(s)_{s=1} = \lambda$, the average number of contacts per partner which can be estimated on the basis of a sample. The methods available for fixing the truncation point C_o are the following: (i) assessing the value from the previous (similar) studies, (ii) estimating the value by using the present data, and (iii) estimating the values using simulated data. For Indian setup, C_o may be taken to be equal to 12 times a month, as obtained from the large-scale sexual behaviour study.

10.16 Modelling of HIV Transmission

The spread of HIV in a heterogeneous population with different mixing pattern is a phenomenon of interest and importance. We examine below the applicability of stochastic model for the diffusion of news and rumors which is a special case of the pure birth process, to understand the HIV spread phenomenon among homosexuals. There are many similarities between these two phenomena. In news diffusion model, information is transmitted by the members of the group from a source either at an initial point in time or continuously. The source may be a television, a newspaper, a hoarding, or a group of people introduced into the population from outside. Persons who receive information may become spreaders themselves by transmitting information to others whom they meet. Similar is the situation in homosexual population in the context of HIV spread.

The system which we study may be described as follows: There is a closed population of N homosexuals who are at risk of HIV infection. This represents the set of all adults of the same sex in a given region. The virus is transmitted to the members of this group from a source at some point in time or through homosexual transmission. The sources of infection considered are infected needle, infected blood, and other contaminated material. Persons who receive the virus from the source may become spreaders by transmitting the infection to others in the population with whom they mix. The virus spread continues until all in the population are HIV infected. From practical viewpoint, the characteristic of interest is the total number of HIV infected at any time t. In this type of HIV transmission, the stochastic element enters at two points. Whether or not a given person gets infected depends on (i) the person coming into contact with the source or a spreader and (ii) on the infection being transmitted when contact is established. Here neither (i) nor (ii) is a sure event, and hence the HIV spread is a stochastic phenomenon. We consider the model with three different cases with respect to the mixing of members in a pair.

10.17 Case (A): Perfect Mixing

In this the assumptions of the model are that (i) all members are equally exposed to the source and (ii) all pairs of members have equal likelihood of acquiring infection. Assumption (i) is not crucial unless the intensity of transmission from source is large compared to the intensity of transmission between the members in a pair. The second assumption is unlikely to hold for human populations in the context of HIV. We later examine the effect of relaxing assumption (ii). First we define two random variables as follows:

N (t): size of the homosexual population at time t which is closed for migration
H (t): number of persons HIV infected at time t
t_H: time taken for the number infected to reach level H
Consider two events as follows:
E_s: transmission of infection from the source to any member of the population
E_P: transmission of infection by a spreader

Assume that the probabilities of these events are proportional to the length of time intervals.

Thus,

$$\boldsymbol{P\{\text{Es in } (t,t+\delta t)\} = \alpha.\delta t, (\alpha > 0) \text{and } P\left(E_p\text{in } (t,t+\delta t)\right\} = \beta.\delta t, (\beta > 0)},$$

where α and β are the intensities of transmission from the source and between the individuals in a pair, respectively. It is also assumed that all transmissions are independent of each other. The system is said to be in state H when exactly H persons have received the virus. Here the stochastic process is $P\ \{H \rightarrow (H+1)\}$ in $(t,\ t+\eth t) = \lambda_H\ \eth t\ (\lambda_H > 0)$. The infection rate, λ_H, is treated as a parameter of the model. When the total number infected is H, there are $(N - H)$ persons not yet infected. Thus the total contribution to λ_H from the source is

$$(N - H)\alpha.\ \eth t \tag{10.6}$$

Also, of all the possible pairs that could be formed in the given population, there are $H(N - H)$ pairs which consist of one infected and one susceptible. Therefore, the total probability associated with these pairs for $H \rightarrow (H+1)$ is

$$\boldsymbol{H(N—H)\beta.}\ \eth t \tag{10.7}$$

Combining the two contributions, we get

$$\lambda_H = (N - H)\ (\alpha + \beta H);(H = 0, 1, 2, \ldots, N - 1) \tag{10.8}$$

Thus, in epidemic theory, the source consists of one or more persons who spread the virus. If one person starts the epidemic, we have to put $\alpha = \beta$, and then Eq. (10.13) reduces to

$$\lambda_H = \beta(H + 1)(N - H);(H = 0, 1, 2, \ldots, N - 1) \tag{10.9}$$

Analysis of the model: Assuming Poisson law for infections to take place, the expressions for the distribution of $H\ (T)$ are given by

$$P\ (H\ (t) = 0) = e^{-\lambda o t}$$

$$P(H(t) = H) = \lambda_{i\,i=0}^{H-1} \sum_{i=0}^{H} \frac{e^{-\lambda_1^t}}{(\lambda_j - \lambda_i)};(H = 0, 1, 2, \ldots\ldots\ldots, N - 1)$$

Since λ_i can be found from Eq. (10.13) in terms of α, β, and N, the problem is solved in principle. The feature of the distribution, which is of particular interest, is the mean, H(t).

The plotting of $H(t)$ for a given population as a function of t gives the expected development in the HIV infection process. If we plot the derivative of $H(t)$, we get the rate at which the HIV infection spreads. This may be called the "HIV epidemic curve," which gives a clear picture of the growth of the epidemic. The expressions for $H(t)$ and its derivative are obtained by Haskey et al. and are reported in Bailey et al. At time t, if r susceptible are let uninfected, then changing time scale to $t = \beta t$ instead of t for simplicity, the stochastic mean is

$$H(t) = \sum_{r=1} nCr \left\{ (n - 2r1)^2 \delta + 2 - (n - 2r + 1) \sum_{u-r}^{n-r} u^{-1} \right\} e - r^{(n-r+)t}$$

where $n = N\text{-}H$ and r runs to n/2 if n is even and up to $(n + 1)/2$ if n is odd.

10.18 Case B: Imperfect Mixing

The assumption that all pairs of members have equal probability of virus transmission may not be fully justified in human populations. Therefore it is of interest to investigate the effect of relaxing this assumption. As an extreme case, suppose that there is no contact at all among members of the population. The diffusion is thus entirely attributable to the source. This case is covered by the above model and is obtained by setting $\beta = 0$. Then we have the pure birth process, and the distribution of $H\ (T)$ turns out to be binomial with

$$P\{H(t) = H\} = (N)(1 - e^{\alpha - t})^H e^{-\alpha t n};n = 0, 1, \ldots\ldots\ldots, N$$

Here $H(t)$ reduces to $N(1\text{-}e^{-\alpha t})$ and the epidemic curve becomes $\frac{dH(t)}{dt} = N.\, \alpha e^{-\alpha t}$. In this, unlike in case A, the rate of spread declines continuously with time instead of first rising to a maximum.

10.18.1 Duration of the Epidemic

The time taken for a proportion P of the population to get infected is obtained as $E(t_H) = \frac{1}{\alpha}\sum^{i=1} \frac{1}{N-i+1}$; considering the fact that t_Hs are partial sums of the t's.

If N is large and $P = H/N$ is not near 1, we get, $E(t_H) = -(1/\alpha) \log_e(1 - P)$. It may be noted that expected time taken to reach a given proportion does not depend on N unlike in case A where P will be reached faster for a large N.

10.19 Case C: Spreaders Active for a Random Time

In the pure birth process model in the context of epidemic theory, it is assumed that the spreaders of infection continue to do so indefinitely. As a consequence of this, all members of the population will eventually get infected. But, in HIV transmission, the infected after knowing their status or after onset of AIDS symptoms, generally stop the risk-prone activities and may cease to be spreaders. The other reasons for this include (a) social isolation, as there is a social stigma associated with the disease, (b) disinterest in spreading, and (c) death due to AIDS. A comprehensive model considering all possibilities is difficult to develop. Thus the model proposed here considers only reason (iii) and assumes that the spreaders are active only for a random period of time T. As this period is reported to be increasing steadily over time starting with mean T of 4.5 years, the number of new infections will be larger in the course of time. Thus T may be assumed to follow exponential distribution with mean μ^{-1}, where μ is the rate of infected who cease to be spreaders. The description of the model is as follows: The population of size N consists of infected persons and susceptible. At any time t, let i the number actively spreading HIV and s the number of susceptible. Then, $N - (i + s)$ is the number of persons who are infected but have ceased to be spreaders. Since N is fixed, the state of the process at any time t is defined by the values of any two of these variables. For example, the system is in state (i,s) if $i(t) = i$ and $s(t) = s$. Our interest is to know the development of the process in the course of time. In order to do this, we consider the joint probability distribution of i and s, viz.,

$$Pr\{i(t) = i, s(t) = s\} = P_{i,s}(t)\cdot$$

From the state (i, s), two transitions are possible during the interval $(t, t + \eth t)$. They are:

(i) (i,s) → $[(i + 1), (s\text{-}1)]$ with probability $s(\alpha + \beta i)\, \eth t$ for $s = 1,2,\ldots N$; $I = 0, 1, \ldots, N\text{-}1$ such that $0 \le (i\text{-}s) \le N$

(ii) $(i,s) \rightarrow [(i\text{-}1),s]$, with probability $i\mu\eth$ t

Transition (i) takes place when spreader mixes with a susceptible, and transition (ii) occurs when a spreader ceases to spread the virus. Using these transition probabilities and relating the joint probability at time (t + ðt) to that at t, the following bivariate differential-difference equations for $P_{((i,s)}(t)$ are obtained:

$$P^1{}_{(i,s)}(t) = - s\,\{s(\alpha + \beta i) + \mu i\}\; P_{(i,s)}(t) + (s+1)(\alpha + \beta\,(i-1))\; P_{s+1,i-1}(t)$$
$$+ (i + 1\_\mu P_{s,i+1)}(t)$$
$$P^1{}_{N,o}(t) = N\alpha P_N, \mathrm{o}(t) \tag{10.10}$$

And $P_{(N,o)}$ (0) = 1, where P^1 denotes the derivative.

Now, the problem is to solve the set of Eq. (10.4). Here if t = 0, there is no retirement for the spreaders. If $\beta = 0$ or $\mu = \infty$, retirement is irrelevant as no one is ever actively spreading the virus and $i(t)$ = 0, always. When $\mu = \infty$, the model reduces to pure birth process with $\beta = 0$. Although the system is difficult to solve, it is easy to find the limiting values of the probabilities $P_{(i,s)}(t)$ as $t \rightarrow \infty$. That is, after a long period, the spread of HIV stops either because everyone is infected or all the spreaders have ceased to be active. In either case, $i(\infty)$, the final number of spreaders, is zero with probability 1. Consequently, $P_{(i,s)}(\infty) = 0$ if $i > 0$.

When $i = 0$, $P_{(so)}$ (∞) will be the probability distribution of the terminal number of susceptible. This can be obtained using embedded random walk over the lattice point (s, i), which is Markovian since the transition probabilities depend only on the present state of the system.

When the system is in state (s, i), the two transitions which it can make and their associated probabilities are:

(i) **(i,s) → (i+1), s-1) = s/(S+ ƒ)**
(ii) **(i,s) → (s, i-1),** = ƒ/ƒ **(S+** ƒ)where f is the relative removal rate.

$$f = \frac{\text{average time taken for a randomly chosen pair to meet}}{\text{average length of time for which a spreader is active}}$$

A large value of ƒ indicates that the spreaders cease their activity relatively rapidly and a small value implies the reverse situation.

10.20 Discussion

Modelling should take care of data requirements to know the prevalence of infected people in different population groups by suggesting special studies. We must focus attention on persons with high-risk behavior such as homosexuals. Thus stochastic modelling is handy to study the HIV spread mechanism in a homosexual group. The virus spread phenomenon in homosexuals resembles the diffusion process of news described in Bartholomew et al. as an extension of pure birth process. Section 10.3 modifies this model to suit a homosexual population and considers three cases. Out of these, case C is particularly relevant to the AIDS situation, since HIV spreaders are active for a random period of time, that is, up to diagnosis as an AIDS case. After this, the spread activity is very likely to stop.

Case A of perfect mixing assumes equal exposure of all members to the source and also that all pairs have same probability of infection. On the other hand, case B examines the extreme situation of infection only from the source and no infection derived from the spreaders. The ground reality is an intermediate situation of infections directly from the source and also from the spreaders. Accordingly the assumptions will have to be modified and the probability expressions derived. In this setup, the probabilities from cases A and B can serve as upper and lower bounds for the actual infection probability. One way could be on the lines similar to the estimation of probability of HIV infection in the context of heterosexual contact, described by Basavarajaiah et al., by evaluating the effective number of pairs giving rise to the new infection.

10.21 HIV Disease Progression

The features presented below are an adaptation of the model discussed by Lagokos et al. for study of mortality of patients with cancer epidemic which was reported in Johnson et al. The different states in disease progression are common for the progression of cancer and HIV infection. Lagokos considered three states in the case of former. They are presence of cancer, growth of tumor (which is called progression), and death. A similar situation exists in the progression of HIV infection also. Hence this model may be tried for progression of HIV infection to AIDS and then to AIDS death. To estimate the parameters involved in the fitted model, a longitudinal clinical study of HIV infected may be conducted on the basis of a sample.

Progression of HIV infection is negatively correlated with the count of CD_4^+ immune cells in the body, which depletes gradually after infection. Three states can be identified with the disease progression: state of infection only (S_o), state of AIDS onset (S_1), and state of death of an infective person (S_2) (absorbing state). For a few individuals, transition takes place from S_o to S_2 without reaching S_1.

10.22 The Model

The notation for the states and time factors are as follows:

Let:

S_o: State of presence of HIV infection only

S_1: State of onset of AIDS

S_2: State of death (absorbing state).
T_1: Time for progression to AIDS
T_2: Time for death without AIDS onset
T_3: Time for death after AIDS onset

The two events, progression and death, are competing, since death without AIDS onset is observed if death occurs first; or progression is observed if it occurs before death.

Let $S_{12}(t_1, t_2) = P_r(T_1 > t_1, T_2 > t_2)$ be the joint survival function of T_1 and T_2 and let

$$h_i(t) = \frac{\eth \mathrm{LogS}_{12}(t_1, t_2)}{\eth t_i} \quad t1 = t2 = t; i = 1, 2 \text{ be the crude hazard rates/}$$

To evaluate the probabilities of reaching each state, we first define the following random variables:

$$I = \begin{cases} 0 \text{ if } T_2 < T_1 (\text{death occurs first}) \\ 1 \text{ if } T_2 < T_1 (\text{onset occurs first}) \end{cases}$$

And $Y = \min(T_1, T_2)$.
If T denotes the time at death, then clearly,

$$T = \begin{cases} T_2 & \text{if } T_2 < T_1 \\ T_1 + T_3 & \text{if } T_1 < T_2 \end{cases}$$

The probabilities of an individual reaching the different states have been evaluated in Johnson et al. To illustrate the model, the authors consider exponential distribution for the times T_1, T_2, and T_3. We now discuss the applicability of exponential and the two other familiar models, viz., Weibull and gamma, for these times.

10.22.1 Probability distribution model and parameters estimation of HIV DATA

Various distributions(descrete and continuous) are fitted with real datasets of HIV transmission. Normally the distributions assume random variable with varied scale and shape parameters which can give building blocks of other variables estimated stocastically. The entire section deeply describes the theoritical and practical applicability for the estimation of HIV transmission likelihood.The reader is advised to orbitarily assume structured and unstructured datasets considering scale and shape parameters for model setups.

10.23 Applicability of Probability Models

Several parametric models have been used for modelling immune failure process. Foremost among them are exponential, Weibull, gamma, and lognormal distributions. Theoretical motivation for particular models can be found in Kotz et al. Shooman examines aging and failure process but overlooks the threshold parameter $\mu \geq$ o (guarantee time) before which failure cannot occur. For example, inclusion of this parameter in exponential distribution converts $f(t) = \lambda \exp(-\lambda t)$, $t \geq 0$, into $f(t) = \lambda \exp[-\lambda(t - \mu)]$ $t \geq \mu$. Such a density may also be considered for the distribution of time to onset provided μ is known. Exponential model was the first one to be widely used in the study of lifetimes, e.g., Davis et al. and Feigl Zelen et al. This is a special case of both Weibull and gamma distributions. Weibull model is flexible and appears to be the widely used lifetime distribution in biomedical applications. However, the assumption of a constant $h(t)$ here is very restrictive. The simple expressions for $f(t)$ partly account for the popularity of the model. But it would be convenient to use $X = \log T$ rather than T, in which case, X has an extreme value distribution. It would be difficult to work with gamma model because its survival and hazard functions are not expressible in a simple closed form. The goodness of fit techniques as discussed in Lawless 1982), Chapter 3, was used for validating the chosen model. However, it is desirable to avoid strong assumptions in the model.

The time for transition from one state to another is also random which obeys a certain probability law. Prominent failure time models such as exponential, Weibull, or gamma may be assumed for the transition time. However, a choice is difficult to make, and it may be restricted by data availability. The applicability of these models for the states of HIV infection progression is discussed, and transition probabilities of different states along with the density and survival functions are obtained. An illustration of the model is included which assume exponential law for the time variables. Survey design, analysis in the study of longitudinal data, and stages in the progression of HIV infection are a few of the areas for statistical research in the years to come.

10.24 Application of Statistical Inference

Statistical inference helps in better understanding of the dynamics of HIV and its progression to AIDS in the presence of uncertainties. As the endemic is relatively new and data availability is meager, it is necessary to estimate several parameters from limited data. To cope up with future healthcare needs, it is imperative for health administration to take certain decisions well in advance, which makes good prediction quite important. In estimation, the unknown value of the population parameter is assessed through a sample from the population. A prediction is based on an equation, which describes a functional relation among variables to project the dependent variable into sampled observations.

10.25 AIDS Projection by Using Large Massive Data Sets

In AIDS study, our interest is in understanding the current state and predicting future path. Issues that are essential to management of the HIV endemic have generated numerous statistical challenges such as estimation of $F(.)$, choice of $I(.)$, dealing with confidentiality, and analysis of incomplete data as discussed in previous chapter. Further, there are large discrepancies between observed and estimated number of HIV/AIDS cases. Given the magnitude of the endemic and the vast geographical area with dense population, in India, the projection of AIDS cases is of critical importance. However, available data are inadequate for assessing the size and progression of the endemic. An apex database at national level, a focus of the next chapter, linked to regional centers would be of help.

10.25.1 Accuracy of Projection

Future counts of HIV and AIDS will be reliable and accurate if the projection methods are based not only on present estimates but also on past incidence of HIV. Past pattern of HIV helps us to know the future path of the endemic better. Thus, there is a need to apply a method which back calculates the past trend of the infection.

10.25.2 Applicability of Classical Methods

The following are some well-known prediction techniques which can be considered in AIDS context under certain assumptions.

10.25.3 Extrapolation

In this, the value of dependent variable y, say the number of AIDS cases, is estimated for a given value of x, the independent variable, say the number of HIV seropositives or the number of persons exposed to the risk of infection, which lies outside the existing range of x values. The fitted curve is extrapolated to a future time point. This classical method presumes a polynomial relation between y and x.

10.25.4 Time Series Analysis

In forecasting AIDS as a time series, one has to consider the questions:

(a) How regular are the past trends? What is the chance that these patterns continue?
(b) Are the past data on HIV infection accurate and reliable?
(c) Are future counts dependent at least partially on the present observable counts?

AIDS is beginning to spread, and in the absence of an effective cure, the present trend is likely to continue for some more time. Future counts are necessarily based on present incidence. Though the first two questions above are answered in the affirmative, the third one is not. This is due to sensitivity associated with AIDS and lack of adequate diagnostic facilities, which have led to large-scale underreporting. If the available data are corrected suitably, then they can be subjected to time series analysis. Forecasting with time series AIDS data may be needed for long or short terms. The former is necessary in view of long incubation period, while for specific healthcare needs, short-term projections are apt. One such statistical method is described in the next section.

10.26 Model Regression Method

Regression models describe the relation among random variables such as the number infected with HIV, incubation time, and AIDS counts. The first two variables influence the third one. The coefficients in the model are estimated from the sample data by least squares method. The fitted model forms a basis for prediction. But the assumption that the present regression environment continues is crucial for the effectiveness of regression as a projection tool, which is doubtful in AIDS scenario.

10.27 Traditional Methods for AIDS Projection

This is a relatively new and widely used technique for projecting AIDS counts. The method uses historical data on AIDS and is highly sensitive to data variations. The details of back calculation and its variants are explained in Sect. 10.6. The projection techniques are all based on true HIV/AIDS counts and therefore call for data correction before use. Two methods are outlined in the following section for this purpose.

10.28 Methods of Counts

Generally, the uncertainties in incubation period, non-availability of proper testing facilities, and reporting delays render the recorded AIDS counts as underestimates and not the true incidence. Heisterkemp et al. (1989) propose a method to correct reported AIDS counts as follows:

Let

n_{ij} = Total AIDS cases reported during period I for diagnosis period j, where $1 \leq j \leq I \leq t$, t being the number of period under observation. It is assumed that n_{ij} are independently Poisson distributed with parameter θ_{ij} and all the reported cases are diagnosed.

P_k = Proportion of cases reported (k: number of periods between diagnosis and report) such as the $\Sigma P_k = 1$.
$n._j$ = Cumulative reported incidence for each period of diagnosis.
$N._j$ = Actual number of diagnosed AIDS cases which are not observable due to reporting delays.

The parameters θ_{ij} are then defined by

$$\boldsymbol{\theta_{ij} = N._j P_k} \tag{10.11}$$

with $k = 1 - j$ and $P_k > 0$.

Maximization of log likelihood of Eq. (5.1) results in the equations

$$\mathbf{N._j = \sum_{1=j}^{t} n._j / \sum_{0}^{t-j} P_{k,} j = 1, 2 \ldots, t} \tag{10.12}$$

$$\mathbf{P_k = \sum_{i=1}^{t-k} n_{ij+k.j} / \sum_{i=1}^{t+k} N_{.i,}, k = 0, 2 \ldots, (t-1)} \tag{10.13}$$

Solutions to Eqs. (10.12) and (10.13) can be obtained using an iterative proportional fitting algorithm of Bishop and Fienberg et al. It can be shown that Eqs. (10.12) and (10.13) are conditional solutions to the problem of estimating the size of a multinomial population. Downs et al. and Morgan and Curran et al. have used similar estimators for the actual number of AIDS cases and subsequently fitted a curve by regression technique to the estimates. Healey et al. (1988) have used estimators for Ni by fitting an exponential model to the reported data up to a few years prior to time of report and, after correcting recently reported data with this model, again fitted an exponential curve.

10.29 Smoothing of Exponential Trend

The trend in AIDS data estimated by moving averages can be improved by assigning weights in geometric progression to yearly reported AIDS cases. Here larger weights are assigned to recent observations. The number of HIV positives can be taken as weights since the endemic is relatively young and there will be very few HIV positives in the very beginning of the spread than in recent years. If the weights assigned are 1, (1-w) 1-w)^2, …., (1-w)^{n}-1 to "n" observations x_1, x_2, …., x_n ($0 < w < 1$), then the weighted averages for the current year t and the succeeding year are given by

$$x_t = \frac{x_t + (1-w)x_{t-1} + (1-w)^2 x_{t-2} + (1-2)^{n-1} x_{t-n+1}}{1 + (1-w)(1-w)^2 + \ldots\ldots + (1-w)^{n-1}}$$

and

$$x_{t+1} = \frac{x_{t+1} + (1-w)x_t + (1-w)^{n-1}x_{t-n+2}}{1 + (1-w)^2 + \ldots\ldots + (1-w)^{n-1}}$$

Taking n to be large, ignoring higher powers of w and (1-w), and after some algebraic manipulation, the following relation between x_{t+1}, the forecast for the next period, and x_t, the forecast for the current period, can be established:

$$x_{t+1} w.x_{t+1} + (1-w)\, x_t \tag{10.14}$$

Thus the new forecast = [w (observed value) + (1-w) (old forecast)]. Here, x_{t+1} is the smoothed forecast, w is the smoothing coefficient, and (1-w)/w is the trend factor. The forecast for the first period is usually taken from some previous forecast, if available, or is often assumed.

10.30 Minimizing Forecast Error

To tackle the situation in which the trend is upward but the forecast is low or conversely, a factor is added to make forecast value closer to the actual value. Equation (10.4) may be written as $x_{t+1} = w(x_{t+1} - + x_t) + x_t$. By induction, $x_t = wx_t$ $(-w)$ and $x_{t-1} = w(x_t - x_{t-1}) + x_{t-1}$, where the quantity $(x_t - x_{t-1})$ is the error. The trend coefficient (θ_t) which is required for preparing the forecast is calculated by the formula θ_t = [w (change in smoothed value) + (1—w) (preceding trend coefficient)]. Then the forecast F_t is obtained by the relation F_t = smoothed value + trend factor., and the error of this forecast is, $E_t = - x_t — F_t$. As there is an upward trend in the actual number of AIDS cases, the forecasts resulting from the single-parameter exponential smoothing are consistently low. To overcome this, a second smoothing constant, say the HIV seropositivity rate, may be chosen for the trend itself.

Back calculation (abbreviated as BC in this chapter) is the main method used to reconstruct the past pattern of HIV infections, and it is widely used to predict the AIDS cases apart from knowing the present infection status. This method is especially suited for diseases with long incubation period such as AIDS. The method depends on three key components:

(i) A model for distribution of infections
(ii) Assumed incubation period distribution
(iii) Observed counts over time

10.31 Convolution Equation at Population Level

If X is chronological time of infection, T length of incubation period, and Z chronological time of diagnosis of AIDS, then for each case, $X + T = Z$ is the relation which links the variables. Assuming independence of X and T, the distribution of Z is thus the convolution of the distribution of X and T. If the distribution of T is known, then we can deconvolute the distribution of Z to obtain an estimate of the distribution of X. This, together with an estimate of the current cumulative number of infected individuals, is the basis of BC due to Brookmeyer, who subsequently use this information to predict future AIDS counts arising from those infected prior to the time of analysis. The method may be outlined with the following notations:

T_0: Beginning time of the epidemic (in India, $T0 = 1986$)
$T_0, T_1, T_2, \ldots\ldots, T_L$: Calendar dates
$(T_{j-1}, T_j), j = 1, 2, 3, \ldots\ldots L$: Non-overlapping intervals
X_j: Number of AIDS diagnoses in jth interval
X_{L+1}: Number infected before T_L but not yet diagnosed

Schematic Presentation of Available Data ($X_1, \ldots, X_L$) for BC to Estimate X_{L+1}:

Let $N = \sum_{1}^{L+1} X_j$ (X_{L+1} & N are unknown).

The vector of counts of AIDS, $X = [X_1, X_2, \ldots\ldots\ldots, X_L, X_{L+1}]$, has a multinomial distribution with unknown sample size N and cell probabilities

$$P = [P_1, P_2, \ldots\ldots, P_L, P_{L+1}] = [P_1, P_2, \ldots\ldots, P_L, 1 - P*],$$

where $p* = \sum_{1}^{L} P_j$.

If P_j: P_r (susceptible individual infected before year T_L and diagnosed in the jth interval), then

$$P_j = {}^{T_j}{}_{T_0} I(S)\left[F\left(T_j - S/S\right) - F\left(T_{j-1} - S/S\right)\mathrm{ds}\right. \quad (10.15)$$

If we treat $I(S)$ as the expected number of infections that have occurred by time S, then the right side of (5.5) is equal to $E(X_j)$, where $I(S)$ is the infection curve which represents the pdf of infection at time S for N individuals. This is also called the epidemic density, that is, density of infection times among individuals infected before T_L, and it integrates to 1 over (T_o, T_L). In other words, infections occur in chronological order according to an arrival process that yields an infection curve $I(.)$. The expected total number of infections that have occurred by chronological time S is ${}^{s}{}_{T_0} I(u)$ du.

Let $F(.)$ denote the incubation distribution, i.e., $F(t) = \Pr$ (AIDS diagnosis occurs within time t). Since this sometimes depends on the time of infection, we let $F(.|S)$, and we set $F(t|S) = 0, t \leq 0$, and all S. If AIDS diagnosis counts are available for a series of L intervals, then we have a vector $[X_1, X_2, \ldots\ldots, X_L]$ where expectation of each component satisfies (5.5) above. The basic idea of BC is to use external information on $F(.)$, together with observed $[X_1, X_2, \ldots\ldots, X_L]$ to estimate $I(.)$ through a form of deconvolution. The density $I(S)$ is assumed to come from a parametric family with unknown parameter θ. The log likelihood is maximized to obtain joint estimates of N and θ. An EM algorithm for incomplete data can be used for this purpose. Once the estimate of *I*(*S*) is obtained, a short-term projection of cumulative AIDS incidence up to the year T_{L+1} is given by

$$\sum_{1}^{L} \mathbf{X_j} + \mathbf{N^{TL}}_{\mathbf{To}}\mathbf{I(S;\theta)}\ \{\mathbf{F[T_{L+1} - S] - F[T_L - S]}\}\ \mathbf{ds} \tag{10.16}$$

This is an MLE, and it gives a lower bound for the AIDS counts under the assumption that no new infection occurs after T_L. Estimate of AIDS cases in a future interval $[T_A, T_B]$ is given by

$$\mathbf{X_{AB}} = {}^{\mathbf{TB}}{}_{\mathbf{TA}}\mathbf{I(S)\{F[T_B - S|S] - F[T_A - S|S]\}ds} \tag{10.17}$$

The first component of Eq. (10.16) represents the cumulative number of AIDS cases by time T_L, and the second component is an estimate of the number of persons infected before T_L who will be diagnosed in $[T_L, T_{L+1}]$. The parametric model *I*(*S*, θ) needs to be chosen with care. One approach is to assume a step function considering the growth of the infections to be in the recent past. In order to incorporate the new infections after T_L, the following modification can be made. Let the expected number of infections in the interval (T_L, T_{L+1}) be P(S) ds and the expected number of cases who were infected in $[T_L, T_{L+1}]$ and diagnosed before

$$\mathbf{T_{L+1}be\ \ P(S)\ FT_{L+1} - S|S]\ ds} \tag{10.18}$$

where *P*(*S*) is the intensity of occurrence of new infections according to a non-homogeneous Poisson process. The future infection rate, *P*(*S*), is unknown. Gail and Brookmeyer (1988) offer compartmental model approach for obtaining insight into *P*(*S*). However, such approaches depend on a number of critical parameters which are highly uncertain such as changing levels of high-risk behaviors. One ad hoc approach to account for new infections in short-term projections of AIDS cases is to extrapolate the current infection rate into the future.

10.32 Advanced Modelling Techniques with Respect to Non-parametric

The initial BC model depends on assumed parametric probability distributions for infection density, *I*(.), and T. Generally, some or all of these model parameters are unknown and require estimation. Sometimes this becomes difficult in the absence of necessary data. Also, parametric models tend to have limited potential for representing more elaborate feature of the infection process. Here, the use of non-parametric methods which do not assume any particular probability distribution for the population is handy. Becker et al. have suggested a method, which gives the data more opportunity to determine the shape of the estimated intensity function and uses modified EM algorithm that incorporates smoothing of estimated parameters at each step of the iterative algorithm. Also, the method is easy to implement on a computer since the computations are based on explicit formulae. The EM algorithm is a technique for obtaining MLEs in situations where only incomplete data are observed but where it is possible to define a set of "complete data" for which MLEs exist. The authors have taken the "complete data" to include information on the time of infection of each case.

10.33 Regression Approach

Rosenberg et al. present a regression approach to BC of flexible linear models of HIV infection curve. These models include step functions and splines. Because expected AIDS incidence can be expressed as a linear function of unknown parameters, regression methods may be used to obtain parameter and covariance estimates for a variety of interesting quantities such as the expected number infected in previous time intervals and AIDS incidence in future intervals. These ideas are used to show that estimates based on MLE are equivalent to those based on quasi-likelihood and on Poisson regression.

10.34 Assessment of MSE

Rosenberg et al. have simulated multinomial AIDS counts that spanned a period corresponding to previous application of BC and assessed MSE for several back-calculated estimators of HIV prevalence and short-term predictions. Estimators were based on flexible model selection procedures that chose the best fitting model of the infection curve from a family of possible step function models. A four-step model of width 4 or 4.5 years and having the smallest Pearson x^2 offered a favorable trade of between bias and variance when compared with models with three steps, which had substantially larger MSE in some epidemic situations. In this, $F(.)$ was modelled using the Weibull curve, 1-exp (−0.002 to 2316) which was derived from hemophilic cohort. Percentage root MSE of an estimator θ given by PRMSE $(\theta) = 100/\theta \sqrt{} V(\theta) + \{E(\theta) - \theta\}^2$ has also been calculated to assess the performance of different estimators.

10.35 Stage-Specific Models

Due to the heterogeneity in the population structure and the complexity in projecting HIV/AIDS counts for an entire risk population, we can divide a projection model into several stages of infection. The events may be defined as follows: non-susceptibility (E_1), susceptibility (E_2), infectivity (E_3), AIDS progression (E_4), and death due to AIDS (E_5). For an individual, these events can occur in the stated order. Estimation of the number of persons in a community experiencing these events at any given time point would be useful to plan and implement intervention measures. In turn this will check the number of persons progressing from one stage to the next. An approach similar to this has been suggested by Longini et al. They extend BC to provide estimates in the following stages assuming a time-dependent Markov process for transition: infected but antibody negative (stage I), antibody positive but asymptomatic (stage II), pre-AIDS symptomatic (stage III), and clinical AIDS (stage IV). They have applied stage-wise estimation for San Francisco City Clinic Cohort (SFCC) data. This is a group of 6705 homosexual and bisexual men recruited in 1978–1980 in San Francisco for a study of prevalence, incidence, and prevention of hepatitis B. The estimated mean waiting times are modelled.

Prior to this work, Longini et al. have estimated mean (median) waiting times in each stage of infection. They are stage I 2.2 (1.5) months, stage II 52.6 (36.5) months, stage III 62.9 (43.6) months, and stage IV 23.6 (16.3) months. The mean incubation period is estimated as 9.8 years with a 95% confidence interval between 8 and 12 years.

10.36 Age-Specific Model

It is a fact that persons in their prime age are at greater risk of HIV infection. Rosenberg et al. extend the use of back calculation (BC) to estimate past incidence of HIV infection in different age groups from age-specific AIDS counts. In this approach, the F(.) used to back-calculate HIV infection rates depends on the age at infection, because younger age is associated with slower progression. Becker et al. and Marschner et al. describe the first BC model to incorporate age. The effect of age on progression is estimated from a joint analysis of natural history data from several cohort studies of gay and bisexual men. Application of the method to AIDS incidence data for the USA reveals that persons under age 25 account for an increasing proportion of new HIV infections as the endemic spreads.

10.37 Cause-Wise Projection

On the basis of certain assumptions, organizations such as WHO, UNESCO, IHO, and NACO have projected HIV and AIDS cases using classical methods including the widely used component cohort approach. But all these projections are the cumulative numbers from all the four modes of spread and hence will be of limited use for planning healthcare needs and devising effective intervention strategies for the causes of infection separately. Policy decisions would be more appropriate and meaningful if they deal with individual sources of infection since different conditions persist in the spread of the virus under different modes. Also, the infections due to perinatal transmission are relatively less dangerous and not likely to cause further spread of virus since the infected child may not reach adulthood. Cause-wise projection is important for the following reasons:

(i) Virus spread mechanism is different for different sources.
(ii) Types of data required and their availability may vary with the cause.
(iii) Date of infection is known only in a few modes of spread. For example, in transfusion-associated infection cases, the date of transfusion can be retrospectively taken as the date of infection, and for perinatal, the date of birth may correspond to the infection date.
(iv) Incubation period may vary with the cause of infection.
(v) Intervention strategies will generally vary from one cause of spread to another.
(vi) Due to involvement of a number of parameters and variables, modelling the disease taking all the causes together will be difficult. A sub-model may be built for the causes separately. An aggregative model is then obtained by pooling the results.
(vii) Separate set of assumptions can be made depending upon the probability of infection, mixing pattern, etc. for the causes.
(viii) Cause-wise projections are likely to be more precise.

10.38 Possible Overlapping

It is possible that a few are exposed to risk from more than one mode of spread. These results in possibility of overlap if cause-wise projected estimates are aggregated. This situation may be presented in set notation as follows:

Let the set A_i ($i = 1, 2, 3, 4$) denote the set of all persons who are exposed to the risk from cause i. We note that set A4 does not overlap with any of the other sets as children are not exposed to cause 1, 2, or 3. But sets A_1, A_2, and A_3 may overlap. Thus the number of susceptible who is likely to be infected due to at least one of the causes 1, 2, and 3 is estimated by the expression

$$\begin{aligned} N(A_1' \mathrm{U}\, A_2' \mathrm{U}\, A_3) &= \{n(A_1) + n(A_2) + n(A_3)\} \\ &\quad - \{n(A_1 \cap A_2) + n(A_1 \cap A_3) + n(A_2 \cap A_3)\} \\ &\quad + \{n(A_1 \cap A_2 \cap A_3)\} \\ &= \{a\} - \{b\} + \{c\}, \text{say} \end{aligned} \tag{10.19}$$

Out of the three terms in (b), the first and the last are likely to be small, while the second may be considerable since causes 1 and 3, viz., unprotected hetero-/homosexuality and use of contaminated needles and syringes, are highly related. Term $\{c\}$ cannot exceed the smallest of the three terms in (b). To avoid overlaps, one may reorient the data recording system in the HIV testing centers to allow a direct estimation of the different proportions.

10.39 Estimation of Survival Function

In a sample study of incubation times of a group of infected, only those who develop AIDS prior to the end of the study period are included, and infected individuals who are yet to develop AIDS are excluded. This type of data is therefore right truncated. A model to estimate the survival function for such data is the following. Let t_i the chronological time at which the *i*th individual is infected; and T_i the time between infection and onset of AIDS. Then sampling consists of observing (t_i, T_i) for patients over a period (0 to t), and estimation proceeds by reversing the time axis. Let $R_i = (t\text{-}T_i)$. The R_i are then left truncated in that only individuals with values of $t \leq R_i$ are included in the sample. Using a method discussed by Klein and Moeschberger, the product limit estimator of Pr $(R > t \mid R \geq 0)$ can be constructed. In the original time scale, this is an estimator of Pr $(T < t \mid T \leq t)$.

10.39.1 Factors Affecting HIV Data Sets

Use of Auxiliary Data

Marschner et al. discusses BC by using the time of first HIV-positive test as auxiliary data, which provides extra information about T. Such data may have significantly improve HIV incidence estimates. The other information that may be considered are risk group-specific and age-specific AIDS incidence. Becker and Marschener et al. opine that this can improve the precision of estimation. However, the performance of the methods needs to be assessed as such data become available.

10.39.2 Effect of Treatment

Solomon et al. have extended BC method to incorporate distributional changes due to a treatment effect such as zidovudine (AZT), which is a vaccine to prolong the life of AIDS patient by a few months. It was found that the widespread availability and use of this drug was associated with the rate of diagnosis of new AIDS cases. This method has been applied to some Australian AIDS data.

10.39.3 AIDS Algorithmic Model

Marschner et al. modified EM algorithm proposed by Becker et al. for the estimation of past HIV incidence. Let λ_i the expected number of new infections in the interval i and $f(i, t\text{-}i) =$ Pr (individual infected in the interval I is diagnosed in the interval t $(t \geq i)$) and Y_i the observed number of AIDS diagnoses in interval t, $\mu_t = E(Y)$. Then the basic convolution equation is given by

$$\mu_t = \sum_{i-0}^{t} \lambda_i f_{i,t-i}$$

Let $F_{t,\ T-t} = \sum_{j=o}^{T-t} f_{t.j}$ be the cdf for the $F(.)$ for individuals infected in interval t.

The index T denotes the last observed interval, and N_t denotes the number of new infections in interval t. Then the expected step is given by λ^{old} which is the vector of expected values for the number of new infections as estimated in the previous step. The maximization step is simply given by the expression $\Phi_t = n_t$. The new values are smoothed in order to get a fresh set of estimates for the HIV incidence:

$$\lambda_t^{\text{new}} = \sum_{i=0}^{2} W_i \Phi_{t\_i-1,} \text{where } W_i \text{are weights for smoothing, } \left(\sum_{0}^{2} W_i = 1\right)$$

The iterations are continued until the following criterion is met.

10.39.4 Uncertainties in Back Calculation

Back calculation methods are subject to a few major systematic uncertainties. These include inaccuracy of AIDS incidence counts, misspecification of $F(.)$, and improper choice of parametric model for $I(.)$.

10.40 Window Period

This period is random and generally very long. Its distribution is to be estimated carefully. This is very difficult because the time of infection in the risk groups is usually unknown except in the transfusion-associated HIV cases where the time of infection is retrospectively ascertained from the date of transfusion. BC is very sensitive to the choice of T. There have been numerous estimates of T from many sources. This factor should be incorporated into the calculation method to make it more efficient. The evidence of different incubation in different population groups is an additional source of uncertainly. Further, it is possible that transfusion-associated cases have shorter period because a large dose of virus may weaken the immune system quickly. If this period is underestimated, the estimated AIDS cases are a lower bound for the size of the endemic.

10.41 Over-projection of AIDS Counts

The diagnosed AIDS counts are generally incomplete owing to reporting delays which represents the difference between date of diagnosis and its reporting to the national surveillance center. This causes underreporting. Rosenberg et al. have examined a few possible scenarios in which extent of underreporting changes over time. Less than 10% of cases are reported in the month of diagnosis, about 50% within 2 months, 85% within 1 year, and 95% within 2 years. There is evidence that length of reporting delay varies across geographic regions. Thus the reporting delay data are right truncated. Reporting delay and its estimation have been discussed by Harris, Brookmeyer and Gail, and Sellero et al.

10.42 Choice of Infection Density

The assumed parametric model for $I(.)$ may be incorrect. Step functions, logistic growth, and Poisson process are some of the models considered. A standard assumption is that the unobserved times of infection for different individuals are independent. This follows from a stronger assumption that infections occur according to a non-homogeneous Poisson process with intensity function $I(.)$. These assumptions may be sometimes violated. An excellent review in this regard is found in Isham. Further, BC does not account for AIDS-related cases (ARCs), whose percentage is significant.

10.43 Back Calculation Methods for Global HIV Data Set

Back calculation is difficult to apply to Indian AIDS data for several reasons. Due to sensitivity of the presence of the syndrome, response may not be reliable. The present data recording and compilation system is inefficient and so is the present surveillance mechanism for the counts. The number of surveillance centers is highly inadequate. Lack of HIV testing laboratories in rural parts results in a considerable number of cases going undetected. The problem of reporting delay causes underreporting. In India, there is virtually no information on T, and hence we depend on external data. Studies on T for different risk groups are non-existent. Likewise estimate of mean or median incubation period is not available. Further, non-recording of exact dates of infection in different groups makes estimation difficult. The dates of diagnosis and report for each case, which are necessary to estimate reporting delay, are not being recorded. Therefore some alternative statistical treatment for reported number of AIDS cases must be evolved.

In India, the endemic is less than 15 years old, the existing data do not involve all the incubation distribution features, and there is scope for adjusting the scale of the distribution function $F(.)$. Many researchers use 15–20% as an estimate of underreporting for projecting actual AIDS cases rather than merely reported cases. Projections of the course of the endemic must rely more on HIV seroprevalence surveys rather than on AIDS incidence data. However, such surveys do not exist in India. In a vast country like India, there may be several undetected/undiagnosed cases of AIDS in the remote corners. The other influencing factors for this may be poverty, fear of society, and lack of clinical diagnostic facilities. Thus, due to incompleteness of observed counts, BC may not produce acceptable estimates.

10.44 Alternative Method to Evaluate HIV Infections

The BC method needs information on (a) HIV infection density, (b) incubation distribution, and (c) AIDS counts. Here (a) and (b) are parameters and reliable estimates for these are unlikely to be available in several countries. For example, this is the case with India. Further, the data recording system on AIDS counts is inefficient. Thus BC, though theoretically well founded, cannot yet be applied in the Indian setup. The other drawback is that it does not hint or gives picture of intervention and policy parameters. As a viable alternative, we propose below a method of projection, centered around the HIV seropositivity rate ($r(t)$), the motivation being the availability of such information.

10.45 Seropositivity Rate as Key Parameter

The rate $r(t)$ is the number infected per 1000 high-risk group individuals tested for virus infection. This includes commercial sex workers and their clients, visitors of STD clinics, and IVDUs. However, usually the age group (15–49) is considered as a major risk group. A nationwide estimate of $r(t)$ is difficult to obtain. Alternatively, this is computed by pooling data on seropositivity from different STD clinics in the country (NACO report, 1999–2000), and it is taken as an overall estimate r (t). Table 10.2 displays this information for India during the period 1989–2000.

It is common to use $r(t)$ for projecting infections among adults in the country. The proposed method for this needs projections of (i) population and (ii) seropositivity rate. For the former, standard techniques can be adopted, and for the latter we can use the past data that exhibits the reported values (denoted by letter A) which suggest an exponential trend in $r(t)$. Accordingly, the model $r(t) = \alpha . t^{\beta}$ was fitted to give

Table 10.2 Staging of AIDS/HIV

	Mean waiting time (years)	
Stage	Without treatment (mean incubation period taken as 9.8 years)	With treatment (mean incubation period taken as 15 years)
Pre-antibody	0.2	0.2
Asymptomatic	4.4	4.4
Pre-AIDS symptoms	5.2	10.4
AIDS	2.0	2.6

expected values (shown by letter B). A high correlation of 0.983 between A and B is noted. It is desirable to validate the fitted model before using it for projection. This may be done applying one of the standard validation techniques (Montgomery and Peck, earlier chapters). We use dissection of $r(t)$ series for validation as outlined later.

10.46 Projection Formula

The rate $r(t)$ is applied to the size of the risk group (N(t)) to give the number of infections, $M(t)$. Thus we have

$$\mathbf{M(t) = N(t).r(t)} \tag{10.21}$$

No standard technique to estimate $N(t)$ is available at the present. In India this is further complicated by the large population with high density. An upper bound on $N(t)$ is clearly the set of all adults. Denote the size of this group by $N_u(t)$. This leads to the estimated upper bound

$$\mathbf{M_u(t) = N_u(t).r(t)} \tag{10.22}$$

It is clear that the gap between $N(t)$ and $N_u(t)$ reduces with increasing infection risk. Similar is the comparison between M(t) and $M_u(T)$. A fine-tuning of this method can be done by considering sex and urban-rural divide for the following reasons:

(i) The risk behavior percentage is higher for males as compared to females due to the differences in the nature of their activities and sexual mobility. As a result, men and women are not exposed to equal risks.
(ii) The rural population is less exposed to HIV infection as compared to its urban counterpart, and as a consequence, the urban incidence is higher. An experts' group in Kuala Lumpur has also noted these differentials. This motivates the following:

10.46.1 Stratification

Stratum no. (h)	Composition	Estimated size of the risk group, Nh(t)
	Urban male (UM)	N1(t)
	Urban female (UF)	N2(t)
	Rural male (RM)	N3(t)
	Rural female (RF)	N4(t)

Applying structure (10.12) separately to each stratum, we get

$$M_{\mathrm{uh}}(t) = N_{\mathrm{uh}}(t)\, r_h(t);\ h = 1, 2, 3, 4 \tag{10.23}$$

An overall estimate $M_u(t)$ is now obtained by summing over the strata. This approach needs estimation of $r(t)$ stratum-wise which implies that the data recording system in STD clinics is to be suitably designed. Otherwise, if a common $r(t)$ is used for the strata, a ratio of 2:1 may be applied to split $M_u(t)$ between men and women and a ratio of 3:1 for an urban-rural division, as per the recommendation of the experts' group.

10.47 State-Wise Projections

In a diverse country like India, a state-wise projection of infections is highly desirable for the following reasons:

(a) Infections are not uniformly distributed over the states.
   There is a large variation in the HIV-related population characteristics among the states.
(b) The data are available state-wise.
   Separate projection allows effective intervention strategies depending on the local conditions.
(c) An aggregation over states produces a national estimate as a corollary.

The state-wise strata sizes of the population can be obtained from census reports. Though the adults are at greater risk of HIV infection, the exposure may not be the same for all the ages in the range 15–49 years. Thus stratification by age or marital status may further improve the projection.

10.48 Validation of Projected r(t)

The HIV seropositivity data for 2000–2001 (Table 10.3) exhibit an exponential trend. Hence a model of the form $r(t) = \alpha.t^{\beta}$ is fitted for projection purpose. Dissection of time series is used for validating the fitted model. This is done by first considering data for a base period of 10 years (2000–2010) and obtaining predicted value as well as a 95% projection interval for the next year. This procedure is repeated by extending the base by a year at a time until 2011. It is noted that the predicted interval includes the corresponding observed value in all the cases. This validates the projections. The details are shown in Table 10.4.

Table 10.3 Seropositivity rate (per thousand) in India

Year	2000	2001	2002	2003	2004	2005	2006	2007	2008	2009	2010
r(t)	6.9	6.2	7.5	13.2	14.5	17.0	22.0	24.0	26.0	28.00	30.0

Source: NACO Reports, 2000–2010

Table 10.4 Projection of $r(t)$ values and their validation

Base period	Year of projection	Projected value	95% projection interval	Observed value
2000–2010	1998	23.0	(21.1, 42.7)	26.0
2011–2021	1999	32.5	(23.2, 45.5)	27.0
1989–1999	2000	34.5	(24.6, 48.3)	29.0
1989–2000	2001	36.5	(26.1, 51.0)	–

Table 10.5 HIV projections in India (figures in millions)

Year	Projected adult population	Projected $r(t)$	Number of HIV infected			% infected among adults
			M	F	T	
2000	5112	34.4[a]	117	58	175	3.4
2001	5260	37.78	130	68	198	3.7
2002	5413	41.10	149	75	224	4.1
2008	6231	61.60	256	128	384	6.2
2012	6626	75.70	334	167	501	7.6
2016	6913	90.30	416	209	625	9.1

[a]Accurate estimation of HIV adult population infected at baseline

10.49 Illustration

The proposed projection method is applied to the Indian data on $r(t)$ with the projected 1991 census population in the background. Country-level projections are made for selected years beginning with 2000 (Table 10.5).

The reported $r(t)$ for the year 2000 was 27 lakhs and the total HIV infected was 138 lakhs.

The Indian data show adult HIV incidence of 3–4% which is quite alarming. This also agrees with the projections made by a few other agencies. Projection of HIV and AIDS counts has to be done with a clear understanding of the present virus spread mechanism and the likely changes that may take place in the future.

10.50 Discussion

In epidemiology, the standard errors for rates (or derivatives of functions) and ratios of rates are generally based on the assumption that the counts like HIV positives have either binomial or Poisson distribution. In a large group, the individual chances of acquiring infection in a short period are quite small so that there is some plausibility to the assumption that acquiring infection is like a series of Bernoulli trials, where the total infections can be approximated by the Poisson distribution. However, when estimating seropositivity rate, we are not dealing with perfectly homogeneous group of people, and the rates are seldom completely stable over the relevant time periods, so that the Bernoulli assumption will be violated to some extent. One consequence of this is a greater variance associated with the counts than would be the case with binomial and Poisson distributions. This is sometimes dealt with by using models incorporating "overdispersion". The Indian data show adult HIV incidence of 3–4% which is quite alarming. This also agrees with the projections made by a few other agencies. Projection of HIV and AIDS counts has to be done with a clear understanding of the present virus spread mechanism and the likely changes that may take place in future. In epidemiology, the standard errors for rates (or derivatives of functions) and ratios of rates are generally based on the assumption that the counts like HIV positives have either binomial or Poisson distribution. In a large group, the individual chances of acquiring infection in a short period are quite small so that there is some plausibility to the assumption that acquiring infection is like a series of Bernoulli trials, where the total infections can be approximated by the Poisson distribution. However, when estimating seropositivity rate we are not dealing with perfectly homogenous group of people, and the rates are seldom completely stable over the relevant time periods, so that the Bernoulli assumption will be violated to some extent. One consequence of this is a greater variance associated with the counts than would be the case with binomial and Poisson distributions. This is sometimes dealt with by using models incorporating 'over dispersion'. Apart from incurability, the other disturbing feature of AIDS is non-availability of relevant, adequate, and timely data to the users. The present AIDS data reporting and compilation system in different states of India appears to be inefficient and incompatible. This chapter (i) stresses the need for collecting a variety of statistical information from appropriate sources, (ii) examines the existing three-tier surveillance system for HIV and AIDS and points out its limitations, and (iii) proposes a workable computer network that supported HIV/AIDS national database model for India incorporating the concepts of data warehousing and data mining. The model can replace the present three-tier system by an effective two-tier system which streamlines the flow of AIDS-related data. The features of this model are aimed to reduce data incompatibility, inaccuracy, and time delay. It is well accepted that reliable and timely data are the basic material in any system of analysis. As a consequence, the quality of the final results can never be better than that of the data input, in which the operation of the GIGO principle is short. We present below a proposal for improving the AIDS information system in India.

10.51 Data Versus Information

Data refer to known facts, texts, graphics, images, and sounds that could be recorded and stored on computer media. For example, in HIV/AIDS database (hereafter referred to as HA db), information on HIV/AIDS is a critical resource and the backbone of any decision-making process to control the HIV spread. With the present information explosion, getting right information on AIDS in right amount at appropriate time is not an easy job. Data should estimate the current status, predict future AIDS scenario in a region, and forecast healthcare needs of the society with reasonable accuracy. There must be an effective mechanism to share the data to answer the following crucial questions regarding variation in HIV transmissibility and incubation time and time interval between infection and transmission. Information on AIDS has become a requirement for survival rather than just a desirable goal to improve efficiency.

10.52 AIDS Data Management

Some health planning decisions are complex and can have a significant impact, particularly those concerning human lives. Three levels of decisions can be recognized. These are (i) operational decisions which govern the daily activities of the AIDS control organization, (ii) control decisions which determine the way the organization executes its designated mission of managing HIV spread (tactical decisions), and (iii) planning decisions which develop and design organization mission such as implementation of intervention strategies (strategic decisions). Wise decisions can be made only when enough updated data are available at the time of decision-making. The decision process becomes complex when many persons provide, update, or use the data. This is the case with AIDS. Manual gathering and updating of information results in delay.

10.53 Decision-Making on DBM

The large circle labeled "data" represents the overall data sources of an organization, for example, db on HIV. The small circle represents individual items of data, for example, records of HIV patients. These can be considered as raw data. They are aggregated in various ways to form information, based on which the optimum decisions are to be made. The results of decisions are actions, which in turn generate more data, which can be incorporated into the next decision cycle.

10.54 AIDS Data Management

AIDS data are meager and therefore expensive. They must be managed to produce needful information. AIDS data handling includes measurement, collection, transcription, validation, organization, storage, aggregation, updating, retrieval, and protection. Data on AIDS are to be (i) represented and stored so that they can be accessed later, (ii) organized so that they can be selectively and efficiently accessed, (iii) processed and presented so that they support the user environment effectively, and (iv) protected and managed so that they retain their value.

10.55 HIV/AIDS Surveillance in India

The spread of HIV is now rampant in all parts of the country. The epidemic shifts from the high-risk population to bridge population (clients of CSWs, STD patients, and drug users) and then to the general population. It has begun to shift toward women and young people with a vertical transmission and pediatric HIV. Low levels of infection in a country with large population like India can translate into large number of new infections. Currently the estimated infection in general population is at least 1%, and among adults, it is 3%. The second phase of the National AIDS Control Programme has become effective from the year 1999 with twin objectives: controlling HIV spread and strengthening long-term capacity to respond to HIV/AIDS. The total outlay for this phase is Rs. 11,550 million (NACO 2001). The Government of India with the funding support from World Bank has set up a National AIDS Control Organization (NACO) in 1992 at New Delhi and opened AIDS cells at the state-level health ministries, which are now converted into AIDS prevention societies. These are responsible for day-to-day monitoring and supervision of the programs in the states. These societies have a few local surveillance centers situated in major hospitals. In addition, a few other hospitals in district headquarters are asked to set up zonal blood testing centers. Rural areas have been neglected though they constitute the major portion. As the interval between HIV infection and AIDS is on an average 10 years, it is not AIDS cases but the estimated number of HIV infected which provides a more accurate picture of the growth of the epidemic. As HIV infection and AIDS are considered as two different stages of the epidemic, monitoring the trends of these two stages is to be done separately.

10.56 HIV Surveillance

HIV surveillance in India has undergone several stages. In the first stage, in 1985, ICMR started screening blood samples from high-risk groups and conducted the serological surveillance through NIMHANS. The objective of HIV surveillance during 1994 was to assess the geographical spread of HIV infection and to determine the major modes of spread. Testing facilities were available in only 71 centers in the country. These facilities were extended later. In 1989, screening was intensified resulting in mandatory screening of blood before transfusion. If the initial test is found positive, the sample is sent to a reference laboratory for confirmation.

In the beginning of the 1990s, the objective was redefined to include monitoring of HIV infection trend. This was achieved by annual cross-sectional survey of the same risk group in the same place over a few years by unlinked anonymous testing following ELISA and rapid test procedures. Later in 1994 it was decided to adopt sentinel surveillance methodology and take up 220 sites which were increased to 185 in 2002 and to 232 sites in the year 2006 covering various risk groups including mothers attending antenatal clinics. Each sentinel site monitors regular round of surveillance every year with a meager sample of size 250 for high-risk groups and 400 for low-risk groups. Based on the analysis of data collected from the sites, the HIV prevalence in the states is broadly classified into three groups, viz., high, moderate, and low. The zonal testing centers scattered over the country have links with other blood banks and receive samples for testing. However, these facilities are highly insufficient to meet the growing requirements. Moreover, the population is concentrated more in about 6 lakhs villages than in the urban centers. Information on AIDS reaches state AIDS societies periodically. Summarized reports in the prescribed format are being sent to the NACO at monthly intervals. These data are now considered inadequate for the changing priorities as these are often cumulative and pooled and are not very responsive to rapidly changing trends in infection rates.

10.57 AIDS Surveillance

Though HIV estimate ranges from 4 to 10 million, only 18,000 AIDS cases were reported to NACO as of year 2001. This small number, due to significant underreporting, does not reflect the true situation in the country. The specific objectives of AIDS surveillance are (i) to ensure reporting of AIDS cases as per the standard AIDS definition, (ii) to improve skills of physicians for diagnosis of AIDS cases, and (iii) to monitor the clinical profile of AIDS cases in terms of opportunistic diseases. The union government has been informed by some state governments that the national strategies developed by NACO are not appropriate for their states since they do not take cognizance of region-specific problems and that there is a need for more proactive surveillance policy. This policy should not wait for the HIV victims to come to the centers but rather reach out to the vulnerable groups without violation of their privacy. This is because some urban areas do not have concentrated population of CSWs in known localities like in Mumbai and Kolkata. The zonal testing centers suffer from several drawbacks. There is no system for evaluating the HIV test kits or to regulate their distribution to various centers, and there is a shortage of kits at several centers, while some others have an excess. The quality of test is often in doubt. Thus, there are many limitations in the present three-tier AIDS data management (three tiers being zones, states, and the country). It is difficult to gather RAT (relevant, accurate, and timely) data with the surveillance in its present form. The next section discusses the need for AIDS database in the country.

10.58 Need for AIDS Database

India is large in size, densely populated, and diverse in culture. HIV scenario is different in various parts of the country, due to different traditions, customs, and practices. AIDS-related data are available differently at different places. Data collection, their accuracy, and HIV reporting system depend upon the local surveillance mechanisms. This gives rise to loss of compatibility among the data available from different sources. Moreover, collection of the same data by different persons for different purposes at different points of time and their storage is a wasteful exercise. Similarly, there are many bottlenecks from data users' point of view. If all of them have access to the same source, then close scrutiny and uniformity are possible. This is feasible only when there is a national database. Such a DBMS using advanced electronic technology is the need of the day. The advantages of such a db are the following: program and data independence, reduction of redundancy and inconsistency of data, improved data sharing among various users, enforcing of certain data standards, application of security features, maintaining of confidentiality of data by means of centralized storage and control, enhanced data accessibility, and responsiveness. Computer networking presents a powerful method to integrate any data system. It facilitates integration and flow of data from one area to another at a fast pace. In India, the fully computerized railway ticket booking is a good example of a successful application of electronic networking. Wide area network (WAN) can be adopted for HA db organization as the computers will be spread further apart due to large geographical area. The database model suggested in the following section incorporates some features of data warehousing and data mining.

10.59 Model for HIV/AIDS Database in India

In view of several limitations in the existing surveillance system on AIDS in the country, an electronic networking db model is suggested as an alternative. This model exhibits the following features. Use of Internet and Internet application helps multiple AIDS data providers as well as their users spread across the country to update and use the latest data simultaneously. Internet also helps multiple users to communicate easily. All users get the same information, even though they are spread across the globe. Computers can be connected to the Internet through Public Switched Transmission Link lines. Enterprise networks consist of a group of computers having a proxy server which is connected to the Internet, and every computer communicates with others over the Internet through proxy server.

10.60 Database Design

Database gives us methods to capture the static and dynamic attributes of real entities. For example, if we want to capture the attributes of a HIV-seropositive patient, then we can scan photograph and get details like name, age, sex, blood group, address, profession, and risk behavior. The design of database determines the extent of information to be collected and represented in the db in order to be useful for application. The relational database model is the most popular model, which can be used for the organization of AIDS database. In this, relationship among entities is maintained since it has (i) a large user base; (ii) ability to apply data managing tools; (iii) good track record as data managing tool; (iv) use of popular commercial databases such as Oracle, Sybase, and MS SQL server; (v) effectiveness with one-to-many relationships between tables, expressed using data constraints like primary and foreign keys, and (iv) simplicity and generality in most kind of data processing. The relational database model views all the data in the form of tables and uses them to organize the data elements. Each table corresponds to an application entity. For example, a state in India is an entity, and each row represents an instance of that entity, for example, a different state. The other entities in a major hospital environment may be a department, a physician, a testing laboratory, a patient, or a test. Figure 7.3 shows the interrelations of these entities. Relations link rows from two tables, say one for HIV and other for AIDS by using row identifiers (keys). Structured Query Language (SQL) can serve as uniform interface for users providing a collection of standard expressions for storing and retrieving data.

10.61 Data Security

Data on the AIDS patients can be classified as sensitive and nonsensitive. Patient's name, address, infection status, risk behavior, and other contact details which identify the patient fall under sensitive data, while patient's region, occupation, age, marital status, etc. fall under nonsensitive data. The former can be made available to only those who submit written assurance that they will use them only for research and planning and will not misuse them. Restrictive data availability can be ensured through passwords. Nonsensitive data can be freely made available.

10.62 Agreement

To facilitate collaboration among the researchers, the db should furnish a standard agreement which would be signed by both the users and providers of data, covering the following aspects:

(i) List of all users and their affiliations.
(ii) Prior approval from the providers before adding new names to the users' list.
(iii) Non-release of data to persons outside the agreement.
(iv) Non-disclosure of identification of individuals by name.
(v) Cite the providers as authors and give proper acknowledgment.
(vi) Disposal of all user copies of raw data outside the database after use.
(vii) Agreement to abide by any other privacy law.

10.63 AIDS Control Center (ACC) and Its Objectives

ACC is an important component of the proposed HA db. It is required to set up ACC in all taluk headquarters and metropolitan cities. Each ACC should have the following three wings: (i) HIV testing laboratory, (ii) investigators' cells, and (iii) computer lab with necessary staff. HIV positivity of the visiting persons will have to be tested and the same to be confirmed by using test procedures including Western blot technique. Investigators are to collect necessary data from the HIV-positive persons and also from those found HIV negative through structured questionnaire (see Questionnaire Appendix 1). Randomized response technique may be adopted to tackle sensitivity in the questions. The data so collected are to be fed into the computer immediately so that they reach the national database. These data will update the existing data at the national center. This results in an effective functioning of data mechanism in two tiers. One can ensure that right data is entered by the data feeders by validating it through JavaScript and VBScript at the time of input. Data constraints can be imposed while creating the db which help to maintain uniformity of data and avoid duplication. Primary and foreign key constraints may be employed for this purpose. The former constraint is used when a particular data like the patient name appears only once and does not allow repetition. The latter constraint is used when two or more tables have a common column among them, for example, the patient name is to appear in all the tables but entered only once. The data so entered will be stored in the Oracle db through IIS (Internet Information Server) web server.

Any number of data feeders can update the db at a point of time from any region. The data users can view the latest data from the server as ASP pages which will be created instantly when such a request is made through the ASP pages from the Internet Explorer to the web server. Thus, there is no delay in getting the updated information. Data can be stored locally at the state level as well as at New Delhi center. The software recommended for creation and organization of HA db database is the following:

Database:	Oracle 9i
Web server:	IIS
Web tech.:	Microsoft ASP 3.0
Server-side scripting:	VBScript
Client-side scripting:	JavaScript
Web browser:	Internet Explorer 5.5

10.64 Flow of Data into the Database

HIV/AIDS surveillance in a country should start from grassroots level. Whenever a physician suspects an infection, he/she should be immediately referred to the nearest ACC for HIV test. If the test results are positive, the individual should be informed of this to avoid further involvement in high-risk activities. The investigators of the ACC should record the required information in a prescribed format, and the case must be monitored continuously till death. The health inspectors should be assigned the job of counseling the patient as well as his/her family members repeatedly so that the illness will not be considered as a sin or crime. Immediately after the death of the patient, the cause of death and the opportunistic infections, if any, should be recorded in the case file maintained at the ACC.

10.65 AIDS Data Flow

10.65.1 Record

The proposed db should contain one record for each reported case with the following information, viz., name, sex, age, nationality, marital status, employment, details of the spouse, number of children, area of residence, educational level, working status, nature of job, dates of HIV positivity test, diagnosis and report, opportunistic diseases at the time of diagnosis, and date of death.

10.65.2 Database Structure

The major components identified for the db are:

Data providers: AIDS data can be classified as primary or secondary. ACC is the major source of primary data. As the secondary data are available from different sources, they are to be first authenticated before updating the existing db.

Database staff: The chief of the staff (data administrator) is responsible for overall functioning of the db at the national level.

Users of data: There will be two types of AIDS data users: (i) national data users and (ii) state-level users. These include concerned health departments, health policymakers, NGOs, and researchers. The data on HIV-infected people are stored centrally so that they can be used for welfare and health plans for the affected people. Nonsensitive data such as age, occupation, place of residence, educational qualification, aggregate numbers of HIV infection, and AIDS cases can be made available for all the visitors of the proposed HA db website.

10.65.3 Database Questionnaire

The following is an example of database questionnaire to assist the user to identify the provider:

1. Institution/organization:
2. General description of study:

3. Purpose of study:
4. Duration of study in months:
5. Start and end dates:
6. Number of persons investigated Males ____ Females ____ Total ____
7. Criteria for selection of participants:
8. Location and allocation of investigators:
9. List of publications generated (if any)
10. Copies of all questionnaires:
11. Description of raw data requirements and format:
12. Funding sources:
13. Persons/organizations to contact for further information; restrictions that may apply to use the data:
14. Information on state/local laws that govern the use of data:
15. A copy of the raw data:

For detailed information, each user would have to contact a provider, and the burden of supplying the data would fall on the provider after reaching the agreement.

10.66 Information on Code Assignment

The following is a list of codes that may be used for composite attributes of HIV/AIDS patients.

1. Place code:	village—digits	District—2 digits
Breakup:	Taluk—digits	State—2 digits
2. Gender:	Male—M	Female—F
3. Infection status:	HIV negative—0	AIDS cases—2
	HIV positive—1	ARC—3
4. Risk activity:	Contact with CSW—1	Blood donor—4
	Multipartner sex—2	Blood recipient—5
	Drug abuse-3	Infected mother-6
5. HIV transmission mode	Sexual TM1	BT TM3
	Drug abuse TM2	Perinatal TM4
6. Opportunistic infection	TB—1	PCP—2

In view of multidisciplinary nature of the HIV syndrome, there are a variety of data surrounding it. But, due to the sensitivity associated with the disease and poor data recording system, especially in India, availability of relevant, accurate, and timely data is restricted. This silent killer disease is quite different from other life-threatening diseases in many respects. The complications in its spread are a phenomenon by itself. As a result there is no uniformity in the spread in different parts of the country, and there is large discrepancy between the reported and expected numbers of HIV positives and AIDS cases. The present data on AIDS are highly inadequate to meet the changing priorities. There is no uniformity in the data and their recording system and compatibility among the states. There appears to be no national agenda as of now to look into these related problems. In this background, it is felt that the present electronic facilities will allow full-fledged HA db in the country which is expected to fulfill many needs. For this, an effective and workable structured model for the national database on HIV syndrome is proposed. The use of computer networking; Internet techniques; setting up of AIDS control centers, one each for the taluk headquarters; and dealing with sensitive data are the special features of the proposed model. A significant aspect of the model is that it advocates the start of the surveillance right from the village level. This assigns greater responsibility of monitoring to the physicians in rural areas. They are to be instructed to direct the suspected HIV-infected persons to the nearest ACC and to follow up the cases. Also, the model stresses the need for taking special care in handling sensitive data on AIDS in the view of promulgation of right of information act and the special acts on human rights. There should be an agreement between the provider and user of such data. The staff of ACC at taluk level may be restricted to four (two lab technicians, one data enumerator, and a computer professional). With internal and foreign funding for AIDS prevention activities, the proposed model is cost-wise feasible. The suggested two-tier system of data flow directly from the ACCs to the center at New Delhi avoids intermediate delay and storage problems. Also, all the users will have access to the same data. Some variant of this model can be considered for implementation.

10.67 Empirical Analysis

The thrust of this chapter is to apply the HIV seropositivity rate as a key parameter for making projections. This presents a feasible method for projection when the input for sophisticated methods like back calculation is not available. The purpose is twofold. The first is to illustrate the projection formula as proposed in Chap. 5. The other purpose is to produce optimistic, moderate, and pessimistic infection scenarios for India and her states for the near future using past data. The latter part of this chapter is a numerical portrayal using secondary data. A few summary results are obtained using software. Some graphs are also displayed to provide a glance of the endemic trend. In the initial stages of AIDS spread, some countries speculated that AIDS would not be a major problem on their door steps. Though the pandemic is moving through the beginning of third decade, its full impact is not yet felt. India has now been identified by WHO as one of the most AIDS-prone countries in South East Asia, the others being Thailand where six people below the age group of 25 a gets infected with HIV every minute across the world, and the rate of infection for girls beats that of boys in many places. By the end of 1999, a total of 13.2 million children had lost their parents to AIDS. In India, the endemic started in the mid-1986 only to catch up with more vigor. A series of national- and state-specific scenarios were presented by Antony et al. which provide bounds on the estimates of adult HIV infections. To estimate the total burden of HIV infection and to monitor the trends in the country, some efforts have been made in the past by WHO, UNAIDS, and IHO

Table 10.6 HIV estimates: Indian and world scenarios

Year of projection	HIV+	AIDS cases	AIDS deaths
World scenario			
1999 (WHO)	> 40 m	10 m	> 10 m
2000 (UNAIDS)	36.5 m	NA	4 m children
Indian scenario (NACO)			
1998	> 10 m	10,000	–
2000	4 m	25,000	–

Table 10.7 Estimates for the year 2000 for India

	Scenario		
Particulars	Best	Moderate	Worst
HIV infections	20 m	30 m	50 m
AIDS deaths/day	6000	7500	10,000
Orphans/day	12,000	15,000	20,000

Source: Indian Health Organization (2001), a report

using the data generated by NACO through sentinel surveillance and other publications (Tables 10.6, 10.7 and 10.8).

Here, the study variables *Y*, *r*, and *X* may be taken as dependent on time t in the sense of forming time series. Also *X*, the materialized number of HIV infections (AIDS cases), depends on *Y*. The seropositivity rate r indicates the general level of HIV infection among the adults. Theoretically both *Y* and r indicate HIV prevalence. However, an advantage with r is that it is a rate. When this is not known for a particular year, one may use the rate for the previous year as an approximation. Likewise, a national rate can be used to approximate the rate for a region. There is a difference in computational aspect too. While r is computed as a ratio for a group of persons tested, *Y* is taken as the number of cases reported. The latter may be seriously in error due to underreporting. The relation between *X* and t can be viewed only as a time series and employed for projection purposes assuming that the present dependence structure continues in the future.

10.68 Compilation

The relation among the above four variables is analyzed by computing (i) pairwise correlations for the variables, (ii) simple regressions, and (iii) a multiple regression using Minitab software. Also, an exponential curve is fitted to the number of AIDS cases as dependent upon the HIV positives (Fig. 8.2). For the data in Table 10.3, the plane of regression of *X* on r and *Y* is given by $X = -4.67 + 0.194.\ Y = 0.003$ r with $100R^2 = 72\%$. The exponential fit is obtained as $X = 0.1815\ e^{0.2271Y}$. The implications of past Indian data are displayed by projecting the HIV scenario for

Table 10.8 AIDS data for India

Year	HIV positives (Y)	Seropositivity rate (r)	AIDS cases (X)
2005	0.18	1.2	0.06
2006	5.0	2.5	0.05
2007	9.0	4.0	0.03
2008	15.0	4.9	0.20
2009	26.0	5.2	0.26
2010	35.7	5.5	0.48
2011	57.1	11.2	1.82
2012	54.4	14.0	3.70
2013	71.8	16.0	3.60
2014	65.9	21.0	10.9
2015	160.3	23.0	10.9
2016	191.8	25.0	19.9
2017	83.0	26.0	15.4
2018	220.0	27.0	32.8
2019	230.0	29.0	67.6
Total	1225.2		167.30

NACO report, 2018

select years during 2002–2016. Three different scenarios are obtained by using (i) actual, (ii) projected, and (iii) expected HIV antenatal rates. In each case, the projected census population is taken as the background.

10.68.1 Correlation and Regression

The computed matrix of pairwise correlation is as follows:

$$\begin{array}{cccc} & Y & r & X \\ Y & [1.00 & - & -] \\ r & [0.89 & 1.00 & -] \\ X & [0.85 & 0.75 & 1.00] \end{array}$$

The pairwise correlations are noted to be high. The coefficient of determination ($100\ r^2$) for the pairs (X, Y) and (X, r) are 72% and 56%, respectively (Table 10.9).

For the last two cases, a log linear model is employed. Also, only short-term projections are meaningful in view of uncertainties.

10.68.2 HIV Infections in India

We apply below the projection methods proposed in later chapter for estimating adult HIV infections in India. The utility of the antenatal rate in this context is also

Table 10.9 Simple regressions

Regression	Fitted model	Projection (in '00) for year 2005	
		Value	95% CI
Y on t	$Y = 45.6 + 15.9\ t$	272.6	[172, 373]
r on t	$r = -3.38 + 2.22\ t$	41.0	[35.7, 46.3]
X on t	$\text{Log}(X) = -1.69 + 0.24\ t$	1380.4	[295, 6309]
X on r	$\text{Log}(X) = -1.28 + 0.106\ r$	–	–

illustrated. The background population size is derived by projecting the 1991 census count. Sexwise projection and urban-rural breakup are also attempted using the following ratio (experts' group, Kuala Lumpur, 1999): urban-rural differential of 3:1 and the male to female infection ratio of 2:1.

Projection methods: Two projection methodologies are suggested—(i) the sero-positivity rate r is applied to the size of the adult population M, to evaluate the number of infections among adults, and (ii) the antenatal rate of infection (s_t) is taken as indicator of infection level in the general population. Accordingly, this is applied to the size of the total population (N_t) to assess the total infections in the country. These respectively lead to the following computational formulae:

$$n(t) = M_t.r_t \tag{10.23}$$

$$n * (t) = N_t.s_t \tag{10.24}$$

An Upper Bound

Statistical bounds on the unknown quantities are difficult to obtain here. Conventionally, a margin of 20% on the estimates is placed to indicate an upper bound on the burden of HIV infections. This is due to the apprehension that the future size of population might be higher than projected. Moreover, overestimation is a less serious error as regards the planning of healthcare.

Three national- and state-level scenarios are produced and referred to as best, moderate, and worst scenario according to the estimated infected as of the end of year 2002. For obtaining future scenarios, the population count is first projected. An optimistic scenario can be arrived by assuming no increase in r (best scenario). On the other hand, if r is also projected, we obtain a moderate scenario accounting for increases both in population and r. Finally, if the antenatal rate is applied to the entire population (rather than r), we obtain a pessimistic scenario (worst scenario). The results are presented next. (Table 10.10)

Considering all the scenarios, the table reveals a possible range of [10.3, 21.3] million for HIV infections in the country. Application of this criterion leads to the following breakup of Indian states.

Table 10.10 Projected HIV scenarios

Scenario	Estimated HIV infected (in million
A: Best scenario	
National estimate (adults) based on actual r = 27	13.8
National estimate based on average rate of HIV infection 1%	10.3
B: Moderate scenario	
National estimate (adults) based on projected $r = 33$	16.9
State-specific national estimate based on expected antenatal rates	17.4
National estimate based on average antenatal rate of 1.5%	15.3
C: Worst scenario	
National estimate based on antenatal rate 2%	20.1
State-specific national estimate based on actual antenatal rates and actual female/male infection ratio	21.3

Category	No. of states	Estimated HIV infectious (M)		
		M	F	T
High prevalence (antenatal rate = 2%)	12	65	32	97
Low prevalence (antenatal rate < 2%)	24	69	34	103

Considering the fast growth of infections in the general population and non-availability of effective vaccine, the antenatal rate can be expected to rise. Taking the increase to be 0.5 for every 2 years, we get the following scenario (Table 10.11).

The precision of the estimates could be improved by the following:

(i) Making the AIDS data reporting system more effective
(ii) Using auxiliary data such as the past infections, prevalence of sexual and other opportunistic diseases, and number of deaths due to AIDS
(iii) Using new statistical methodology importing not only the available data but also the dynamics of HIV spread mechanism

Other Aspects

Based on published information, we now give a brief age-wise, mode-wise, and state-specific HIV-related numerical portrayal. Some key information on HIV infections in India is also provided (Tables 10.12 and 10.13).

From the above table, it can be concluded that AIDS mostly kills persons in their prime and productive ages (Table 10.14).

The incidence of HIV is noted to be the highest in Mumbai City, known to be a stronghold of HIV spread, in all the four major risk groups. HIV seropositivity is associated with several other disorders. This is supported by the diagnosis carried out at NIMHANS, Bangalore, during 1989–2000. Out of 30,190 serum bottles tested for the presence of HIV, 1691 were found to be HIV positive. The associated disorders are given in the following table (Table 10.15).

Table 10.11 Projected HIV infected based on expected antenatal rates

	Years						
	2004	2005	2008	2010	2012	2014	2016
Antenatal rate (in %)	3.0	3.5	4.0	4.5	5.0	5.5	6.0
Total HIV infections (million)	31.7	38.2	45.1	53.0	59.7	67.6	75.8

Table 10.12 A breakup by HIV transmission

Mode	TM1	TM2	TM3	TM4	Not available
Percentage of infection	82.6	4.2	4.0	1.5	7.5

Table 10.13 The age distribution of AIDS cases (based on total reported cases of 9695 as of November 2018)

	Number of cases		
Age (years)	M	F	T
0–14	165	34	199
15–29	1675	581	2256
30–44	2015	336	2351
>45	247	121	368
Total (%)	78.5%	21.5%	100%

Table 10.14 HIV prevalence levels in 2001 in selected states

	Prevalence (%)			
State/city	STD	ANC[a]	IVDU	CSW
Andhra Pradesh	30.0	2.60	–	–
Karnataka	12.8	1.68	4.23	–
Maharashtra (excluding Mumbai)	18.4	1.12	–	–
Mumbai	33.4	2.0	23.7	58.7
Tamil Nadu	16.8	1.0	26.7	–
Pondicherry	4.1	0.25	–	–

[a]*ANC* antenatal clinics

Table 10.15 Distribution of HIV positives

Mode	TM1
Neurological	30
Neurosurgical	02
Psychiatric	05
Tuberculosis (SD sanitarium)	17
Infected blood in donors	01
Voluntary testing	02
Others	43

A large-scale behavioral survey on AIDS awareness in India undertaken by NACO during March–August 2001 with a total of 84,473 respondents in equal proportions of males/females and urbanites/ruralites (www.naco.nic.in.com)

Table 10.16 Overview of HIV prevalence

State/city	Prevalence (%)			
	STD	ANC*	IVDU	CSW
TM1	77.8	64.6	84.6	67.1
TM2	77.6	64.9	84.6	67.2
TM3	79.1	65.9	86.3	68.3
TM4	71.2	63.1	79.7	63.4
Total	82.4	70.0	89.4	72.3

revealed that the awareness is higher among males as compared to females and similarly among urbanites as compared to ruralites (Table 10.16).

10.69 Summary

The stochastic simulation modelling techniques of HIV/AIDS are flexible enough to capture a wider variety of epidemic patterns than the classic formulation. However, the fitted models for estimating it converge more slowly than for the traditional model (e.g., back calculation, double-event model, etc.), as the flexible model contains a greater number of model parameters to estimate. Model fitting speed tends to be slowest in countries with extensive time series data in large numbers of HIV-affected sites or ART. Additionally, constrains on prevalence in the pre-surveillance period and constraints on the change of geometric progression of HIV as described in flexible specification for the infection rate have sometimes been used to eliminate unrealistic patterns of prevalence and incidence in the stochastic model. Those parameters are set based on local expert and physician knowledge, but must be set with cautions, because if they are set too aggressively, it may result in a prevalence trajectory that does not match HIV data sets.

References

Brown T, Grassly NC, Garnett G et al (2006) Improving projections at the country level: the UNAIDS estimation and projection package 2005. Sex Transm Infect 82(Suppl 3):34–40

Brown T, Salomon JA, Alkema L et al (2008) Progress and challenges in modelling country-level HIV/AIDS epidemics: the UNAIDS estimation and projection package 2007. Sex Transm Infect 84(Suppl 1):5–10

Brown T, Bao L, Raftery AE et al (2010) EPP 2009: bringing the UNAIDS estimation and projection package into the ART era. Sex Transm Infect 86(Suppl 2):3–10

Garcia-Calleja JM, Gouws E, Ghys PD (2006) National population based prevalence surveys in sub-Saharan Africa: results and implications for HIV and AIDS estimates. Sex Transm Infect 82 (Suppl 3):64–70

Ghys PD, Walker N, McFarland W et al (2008) Improved data, methods and tools for the 2007 HIV and AIDS estimates and projections. Sex Transm Infect 84(Suppl 1):1–4

Gouws E, Mishra V, Fowler TB (2008) Comparison of adult HIV prevalence from national population-based surveys and antenatal clinic surveillance in countries with generalised epidemics: implications for calibrating surveillance data. Sex Transm Infect 84(Suppl 1):17–23

Hogan DR, Zaslavsky A, Hammitt J et al (2010) Flexible epidemiological model for estimates and short-term projections in generalised HIV/AIDS epidemics. Sex Transm Infect 86(Suppl 1):84–92

Stover J et al (2004) Projecting the demographic consequences of adult HIV prevalence trends: the Spectrum projection package. Sex Transm Infect 80(Suppl 1):14–18

Stover J, Walker N, Grassly NC et al (2006) Projecting the demographic impact of AIDS and the number of people in need of treatment: updates to the Spectrum projection package. Sex Transm Infect 82(Suppl 3):45–50

Stover J, Johnson P, Zaba B et al (2008) The Spectrum projection package: improvements in estimating mortality, ART needs, PMTCT impact and uncertainty bounds. Sex Transm Infect 84 (Suppl 1):24–30

Stover J, Johnson P, Hallett T et al (2010a) The Spectrum projection package: improvements in estimating incidence by age and sex, mother-to-child transmission, HIV progression in children and double orphans. Sex Transm Infect 86(Suppl 2):16–20

Stover J, McKinnon R, Winfrey B (2010b) Spectrum: a model platform for linking maternal and child survival interventions with AIDS, family planning and demographic projections. Int J Epidemiol 39:7–10

Meta Analysis of Genetic Variants of HIV Mother to Child Transmission

11

11.1 Introduction

Nearly 80 million people have been infected by HIV, primarily through sexual aquition and 35 million have died from HIV –I and associated diseases. HIV infect infants through MTCT and adult through blood born or sexual transmission discussed in Chap. 1. The epidemic has affected sub population in heterozygous fashions, with rates varying by age, sex, predominant mode of exposure and geographic locations. The overall risks of transmission of HIV is thought to be low, roughly to 0.18% per sex act, but varies considerably from 0.02% to 1.6% in previous published mata analysis findings. Similarly, level of viremia during acute HIV infection, set point VL rate of CD4 T-cell depletion, and eventual rates of progression to AIDS all vary widely. For example, while some individuals have been observed to develop profound CD4 T cells lymphopenia and AIDS within 2 years, others remain AIDS free for up to 15 years following HIV seroconversion (Gray et al. 2009; Guay et al. 1999; Guevara et al. 2002). Since the sequencing of the human genome in large scale genetic and genomic studies have played an increasingly important role in delineating the pathogensis of human disease. Understanding the variable risk and course of HIV infection in vivo by studying host genetics has been instrumental to understanding the immunopathogensis of HIV. Moreover, it has complemented the invitro understanding of the biology of HIV infection and replication that led to development of ARV drugs, which are cornerstone of HIV prevention and therapy. Studies of host genetic correlates have reflected the wide ranging nature of possible HIV outcome measures over the course of HIV infection, beginning with acquition through disease progression and development of OIs and AIDS (Guindon & Gascuel 2003). Similarly, the studies reflects the heterogeneity in population affected by HIV. Hundreds of studies have been conducted into the genetic determinants of HIV aquition and disease progression. Previous studies, referred to as candidate gene studies were locus or gene centric, while larger recent studies have searched for correlates across the genome using genome wide genotypic or whole exome/genome sequencing is an unbiased "agnostic" manner. In total, 5 genome wide association studies of HIV acquisition and the 11 of markers of HIV disease

D. M. Basavarajaiah, B. Narasimha Murthy, *HIV Transmission*,
https://doi.org/10.1007/978-981-15-0151-7_11

course have been reported at global level (Johnson et al. 2003). Asper the literature survey GWAS have also been instrumental in generating estimates of the relative contribution of the host and viral genetic variation in HIV. Accordingly, the present study reviewed the relevant literature briefly, and then turns attention to the two well validated genetic correlates of HIV aquition and HIV disease outcome. We specifically highlight questions or hypothesis, which, in our view remain unanswered with regard to the mechanism of HLA effects in HIV (Katoh et al. 2005). We anticipate further progress in these areas and discuss additional future prospects in this mata analysis study intervention. Further, the biological mechanisms involved in HIV type –I &II transmission will remain largely unclear. A genetic compactability and bottleneck has been routinely monitored in both horizontal and vertical transmission at global level, although the research findings on various characteristics or attributes of these transmitted viruses are still conflicting and may depend on the mode of geometric progression or sub type of the infecting virus (Keele et al. 2008). Owing to this larg research gap many scientist to know the variants and extrapolate the reasons for growth of progression, in the essence of the availability of matched donor –recipient pairs and the relatively well defined timing of transmission, MTCT of HIV type I is tractable settings in which to study this bottle neck and determine the viral characteristics and or immune responses associated with transmission, with the potential to suggest mechanisms. The correlation between HIV I transmission, variable loop length and number of putative n linked glycosylation (PNG) sites encoded in the HIV *env* gene have been reported in some studies but in others. In horizontal transmission, acutely infected subjects were found to have shorter variable loops and fewer PNG sites encoded in env compared to subject with chronic HIV-I infection for sub type A and C, but not sub type B (Kimura 1980). In vertical transmission, one study of an HIV-I sub type CRFAE infected cohort found no difference in sequence length or PNG sites in transmitted viruses. Shorter variable loops and fewer PNG sites have separately been shown to correlate with increased viral fitness and greater neutralizing antibody sensitivity. One study suggested that HIV-1C viruses newly transmitted from MTCT were more fit, had significantly fewer PNG sites and were more resistant to autologus maternal serum than non transmitted viruses. For studies that analyzed vertical transmission stratified by timing, viral populations have been reported to have different properties if transmitted inutero (IU) or intrapartum (IP). There is no consensus on the neutralizing antibodies may play in MTCT (Kittinunvorakoon et al. 2009). Animal studies have demonstrated that neutralizing antibodies elicited by simian immunodeficiency virus (SIV) vaccine can at least slow disease progression. Ehile direct administration of antibodies matched to the challenge virus can block transmission. Studies of natural MTCT have yielded conflicting results a, although possibly for identifiable reasons. The breadth of the neutralizing antibody response may depend on the sub type of HIV-1 being studied and neutralizing antibody levels may be associated with the timing of transmission. A comprehensive picture of the effect of neutralizing antibodies on MTCT is difficult to obtain because of small sample sizes and different sub types accounting for transmission timing are needed to better understand the transmission mechanisms. There is also uncertainty about the role of antibodies in super infection (Kosakovsky et al. 2006). In the present chapter we analyzed and formulated the statistical model for describing the HIV sub type C env genes from 25 mothers –infant pairs: 15 transmitting IU and

10 transmitting IP data sets accrued from the meta analysis conducted at global level, and also correlate strong genetic bottle neck associated with vertical transmission. Compared to the maternal viral population, viruses' transmitted IP tended to have shorter variable loops and fewer PNG sites than viruses transmitted IU however, the present study also formulate env growth models approach to psuedo typed viruses from transmitted infants variants and maternal variants (Kuhn et al. 2007). The recently characterize chemokine receptor gen CCR_5 and its most frequent mutation have become the objects of intense interest since their roles in the entry of HIV-I in to target cells were identified. This mata analysis reports the estimation of genotypes distribution of the deletion in children born to HIV I infected mothers, the genotype distribution are in Hardy Weinberg equilibrium HW law suggesting the absence of deleterious genotypes. The δ32 allilic frequency in this populations. Homozygosity for a 32 bp deleted allele in CCR5 gene protects adults from HIV-I infection following blood or sexual exposure. So, it is possible that this mutated allele also has a protective effect in children born to HIV –I seropositive mothers (Kuiken et al. 2009). The present study not evidence may partial resistance to HIV I infection among heterozygous children. Many research cited that, the heterozygous adults are discordant Dean et al., Huang et al., and Zimmeraman et al. found no protective effect, where as, Samsn et al. and Micheal et al. suggested that, the existence of a protective effect as they reported a frequency of the heterozyogous state that was lower in those whose were infected than in the general population of naïve group. A major strength of prospective cohorts of children born to HIV I seropositive mothers is that infected and uninfected patients can be compared within single group rather than using reference group comparison. Considerations of the predictive biological factors for the disease in children have mostly addressed the risk of early and severe forms, which are associated with advanced maternal disease and viral replication in utero. Genetic factors have previously been suggested in HIV I infected children, namely the HLA genotype and complement system genotype, but only in analyses of small subgroup population (Kwiek et al. 2006). Those concerning HLA remain controversial due to low sensitivity and specificity.

11.2 Variation of Host and Viral Genetics in HIV

Classically, twin and family studies have been used to infer the host genetic contribution to disease risk. Such studies have been exceedingly challenging to perform in HIV either with regard to HIV acquition or disease progression due to poor sample size, although one very enlightening sibling study has been reported by Indian context, emphasizing the importance of the major histocomatibilty complex (MHC) in disease course. A second important determinant of disease course, unique to disease caused by a polymorphic pathogen, is the relative important of pathogenic variation (Kwiek et al. 2008a; 2008b). While estimates of the host relatives contribution to HIV aquition have not been reported, estimates of the genetic contribution to HIV control after infection suggest that around one third of the variance in septic viremia can be attributed to viral variation. Modern approaches that estimates the host polygenic heritability using genome wide range genotypic data have recently been reported in HIV. In a meta analysis of 6315 individuals for whom set point viremia was attributable to common host genetic variation outside of these could be explained by variation in the HLA or CCR5 loci leaving around 5.50% of variance attributable to variation outside of these two regions. Moreover, Btahrath et al. demonstrated this study, where, VL and host genetic were both available, that almost all of the effect of the HLA region on step point viremia is mediated through its pressure on viral genetic variation, and that human variants only in the HLA region and not else where in the genome are associated with specific VL mutations. VL in vivo taken together, these studies are striking on demonstrating that the CCR5 and HLA loci explain the majority of the host genetic effects on VL naive (Lathey et al. 1999). Larger studies may yet yield additional rare variants that alter disease, but more extensive coverage through whole genome studies has not yet yielded now insight effects may be identified, as is suggested by early GWAS in Asian populations, for e.g. the genetic mapping of HIV is amongst the most complete of any complex disease, as there are few other disease where the majority of the variance in genetically mediated modification of disease course has been mapped and attributed to specific genes. Efforts in HIV genetic research have therefore focused on delineating the nature of CCR5 or HLA mediated protection and finding therapeutic opportunities to exploit this.

11.3 Selected Host Factors Influencing MTCT of HIV Type I

11.3.1 Genetic Factor

The HIV epidemic continues to be a major world wide health and human problem as reflected in AIDS epidemic updates form the WHO (Li et al. 2006; Liu et al. 2005; Liu et al. 2008a; Liu et al. 2008b). HARRT has improved health management, especially in developed countries, such it was first introduced in the mid 1990s. However, access to ART in developing countries has been developed. Developing an effective vaccine as an ongoing mission, the success of which depends on understanding key aspects of the immune response to HIV. The existence of genetic factors that modulate immune response to infectious disease was described more than 10 years ago. Genetic factors may classified in to the followings

1. Fetal gender and HLA type
2. Maternal fetal HLA concordance
3. SNPs for chemokines/chemokines receptor/innate immune factors

Many authors recommend various recent and extensive review, that have focuses on the immunobiology of HIV infection, the immune response to HIV specifically the innate response. Innate and adaptive immune responses play a decisive role during the initial stages of HIV infection and will also affect the progression of the disease. Definitive evidence that host genetics plays a role in the immune response to HIV is the fact that HIV I infection doesn't always progress to AIDS. A small percentage (<0.20%) of HIV-I seropositive patients is able to control the infection, meaning that they can maintain a VL of fewer than 50 copies of HIV -1 RNA per ml over 10 years.these patients have been given different names viz HIV controller, HIV elite controller, long term non progressives (LTNPs) or natural virus suppressor. Further histopathological perspective is important parameters to know the association between the genetic variants. HLA disease association studies and HIV infection, the first review of HLA association with disease are from the late 1970s (Luo et al. 2005; Meddows et al. 2006) and early 1980s followed by other studies on HLA susceptibility to HIV infection (Mummidi et al. 2001). HLA genes exhibits linkage disequilibrium, meaning that they are found together on the same chromosomes at a higher frequency than expected according to their recombination distance.they are defined as a so called extended haplotype or combination of alleles that are transmitted together as a unit. As with any gene frequently found in linkage disequilibrium with others, it is difficult to identify the specific HLA gene that is responsible for a given association observed in a population. Studies of HLA association with infectious diseases must separate HLA effects from confounding factors, which are other factors that independently affect the risk of developing the disease. If the prevalence of these other factors differs between the groups being compared, they will distort the observed association, In the case of HLA/HIV associations, confounding detected and the resolution of the typing methods used. HLA association are considered to be consistent when a similar or equivalent association is observed across different ethnic groups. HIV association and ancestral haplotypes initial association analyses focused on ancestral haplotypes. An increases frequency of C4 null alleles was found in HIV infected individuals, which could in fact reflects an indirect association with discrete numbers of ancestral haplotypes. At that time a series of studies focused on the A1-B8-DR3-DQ2 haplotype, also known as the 8.1 ancestral haplotype, which has been implicated in disease susceptibility. In addition, the HLA-B27 allele was found to be related to slow HIV disease progression. Closer analysis of ancestral haplotype points to a direct role of HLA-B35 in rapid HIV progression, and this allele is thought to be associated with disease susceptibility.

Maternal or Infants Co Infection

Several maternal or infant factors will precursor variables to transmit the infection from infected mother to her child viz.

1. Chorioamnionitis
2. STIs: Genital ulcer disease including HSV2 and syphilis
3. Malaria
4. TB
5. Mastitis/breast abscess
6. Oral candidiasis

Several coexisting infections in the HIV-I mother (or, less frequently, in her infant) have been shown to increase MTCT risk. We summarize the evidence for the most important ones below.

11.3.2 Chorioamnionitis (Infection of the Fetal Membranes)

It has been associated with an increased risk of MTCT of HIV-I in several studies (Pedersen et al. 2007). Results are mixed, however, and not all studies have concluded MTCT. Chorioamnionitis is strongly associated with preterm labor and premature rupture of the membranes, both of which are associated with increased MMTCT. Contributing factors increasing the risk of a premature infant are the immaturity of the skin and mucosal membranes and reduced immnocompetence, resulting in higher permeability to HIV-I. The perforated mechanism through which the risk of infant HIV-I infection increased is through infection of the placenta, leading to disruption of the integrity of the placental barrier, with maternal white blood cells infected with HIV-I entering the amniotic fluid. Several organism are associated bacteria *N. gonorrhoeae, C.trachomatis, Trichomonas vaginalis* and group *B streptococcus*. Among 250 mother infant pairs in Kenyan Study, chorioamnionitis was an independent risk factor for perinatal MTCT, while controlling for viral shedding in the genital tract and maternal VL. The present mata analysis estimated that, the average MTCT rate was 12.80% attributed to choriomnionitis, assuming a casual relationship between choriomnionitis and MTCT.

11.3.3 Sexual Transmitted Infections

Due to shared acquisition risk factor and synergistic relationship between HIV-I and other sexually transmitted infections (STIs) are common among HIV-I infected women. It is well established that both ulcerative and non nuccreative STIs increase sexual HIV-I transmission. However, whether STIs are independent risk factors for increased HIV-I transmission or the result of increased HIV-I viral load is not clear. Further, the role of STIs in MTCT of HIV-I has not been fully characterized. Many studies have assessed the prevalence of any STI among HIV-I infected pregnant women, making it difficult to elucidate the relationship that specific STIs have on MTCT of HIV –I. Inflammation of the maternal genital tract mucosa, as occur in genital ulcer disease has been shown to increase MTCT independently of maternal Plasma HIV-I load. Syphilis and HSV-2 are both associated with genital lesions which increase local inflammation and genital shedding of HIV-I.

11.3.4 Malaria

Malaria infects the placenta and leads to adverse pregnancy outcomes.this is especially true in primi gravida women, among whom malaria tends to be more sever there are conflicting reports on the effect of malaria during pregnancy on MTCT OF hiv-I. Several earlier studies have failed to reveal an interaction between malaria and MTCT. However more recent data sets indicate that malaria increase HIV-I VL and treatment of malaria reduces HIV –I VL. A few recent studies have suggested an increased risk of MTCT of HIV –I in pregnant women with malaria, yet others have not shown a significantly increased risk. A study in global level of women who were infected with HIV-I and malaria found that higher parasitemia levels (>100,000 parasites/ml of blood) were associated with an increased risk of MTCT of HIV-I compared to lower levels of parasitemia. Inconsistencies in study results may be due, at least in part, to differences in epidemiology of malaria in different settings, which could affect maternal immunity. Further research is needed to characterize the association between malaria and MTCT.

11.3.5 Tuberculosis (TB)

TB is a leading cause of morbidity and mortality world wide and is of particular concern those infected with HIV-I, as PLHIV are 20–30 times more likely to develop TB. In 2009 there were as estimated 1.10 million incident cases of TB occur during the reproductive years (15–49 years old). Rates of TB in HIV in HIV-I infected women in study in South Africa ten times those in HIV-I uninfected pregnant women. Active TB infection increases HIV-I VL, which is a recognized risk factor for MTCT. Given the high rates of TB among HIV-I infected women, particularly those of reproductive age, a concern is whether TB increases the risk of MTCT of HIV-I independently or through increased HIV-I VL. To date, however, there have been few studies that have investigated TB infection as an independent risk factor for MTCT of HIV-I. In a south African meta analysis study, 42 HIV–I infected pregnant with active TB disease, a 19% inutero HIV-I transmission rate was observed. This was in comparison to a 5–10% overall rate of in utero HIV-I transmission in resource limited countries at that time. Overall, the MTCT rate for the duration of study follow up was 40%. The study did not have a naive group, nor was there statistically adjustment for confounders such as VL. A recent study in India found that maternal TB was associated with a 2.50-fold increase in the odds of MTCT of HIV-I, after adjusting for maternal and infant factors. This study support that TB is an independent risk factor for MTCT of HIV-I, however given the limited data available additional studies are warranted (Pohlmann et al. 2001).

11.3.6 Behavioral Factors

There are several mechanism by which behavioral factor could affect MTCT of HIV-I. So many Meta analysis report was opined that, approximately 15–20% behavioral factor will influenced MTC, asper our stuy we are enlisted the following factors responsible for MTCT.

1. Illicit drug use during pregnancy
2. Frequency of sexual intercourse during pregnancy
3. Number of sex partner during pregnancy
4. Infant feeding practices viz breast feeding, mixed feeding and food premedication

First, drug use during pregnancy can increase the risk of preterm birth which is associated with increased MTCT. Indeed, prenatal cocaine and amphetamine exposure have been associated with preterm birth. Secondly, and drug use may be associated with increased HIV-I VL or failure to suppress VL in the presence of HAART. Cocaine, heroin and amphetamine use have been shown independently increase HIVI plasma VL, despite the use of HAART.Additionally, several studies have also demonstrated that drug use is associated with lower adherence to HAART regimens, which is in turn associated with reduced VL suppression other mechanism by which illicit drugs may affect MTCT include drug interaction with ARV medication and placental injury. Cocaine exposure during pregnancy has been associated with increased risk of placental abruption.

11.3.7 Maternal Nutritional Status

The general state of health of the mothers is an important predictor of MTCT risk. Mothers with higher HIV-I VL, lower CD4 T cell count and more advanced disease stage are at increased risk of transmitting HIV-I to their infant, which is a result of the higher peripheral blood VL, increased shedding in the tract and decreased maternal immune responses to contain the virus.in addition, advanced AIDS is associated with a poorer nutritional status and a catabolic state, and is also a predictor of increased MTCT risk. We have enlisted the followings for nutritional deficiency.

1. Advanced maternal disease with immunosupression and malnutrition
2. Vitamin A deficiency
3. Other micro nutrient deficiencies

11.4 Methods

Meta analysis was done for extraction of HIV sub type C env genes from 25 mothers – infant pairs: 15 transmitting IU and 10 transmitting IP data sets, the methodological assumptions were assumed for accepting for the creation of the model set (data base); poly genetic analysis the sequences were manually edited seaview and the boundaries of the V1–V5 region were determined from the protein alignment in the HIV sequence DBT, GOI global compendium. A neighbor joining tree, including sequences from all pairs was constructed to confirm epidemiological linkage between the pairs and the absence of cross sample contamination. Matched maternal and infant sequences were most closely related to each other. All sequences were aligned by using standard operating protocol and suitable method. The model of evolution was determined by Finmodel for each pair, with GTR plus gamma often being the best fit and MLE's phylogenic tree was constructed without gap stripping using the mobile plat form for the PHYML program. Trees were re sampled 100–200 times and boot trap values greater than 70 were considered significant. Unrelated sub type C out group were used to root each tree (Tables 11.1 and 11.2) (Figs. 11.1 and 11.2).

Many scientific reports have reported that, the HLA polymorphism have an impact of MTCT HLA class (i) and (ii) alleles are the most polymorphism genes

Table 11.1 Associations between child DC-SIGN haplotypes and intrauterine (IU), intrapartum (IP) and postpartum (PP) HIV-1 transmission

Child DC-SIGN haplotyp	IU infection (cases)	IP infection(cases)
H1		
Absent	19	22
Present	05	03
H2		
Absent	17	18
Present	08	07
H3		
Absent	20	23
Present	05	02
H4		
Absent	21	22
Present	04	03

(a) Haplotypes found at a frequency above 5% in the study population. (b) Absent (referent category for all analyses) vs homozygote + heterozygote (present) for each haplotypes. (c) P-value as determined by Fisher's exact test

Table 11.2 Associations of risk factors of MTCT

	RF	Strength of association	Impact
(i)	Maternal		
	RNA VL	Strong	Large
	AIDS	Strong	Small to medium
	Immune deficiency	Strong	Medium
	Genetics	Weak	Small
	STI's	Medium	Small to medium
	Chorioamnionitis	Medium	Small
	VA deficiency	Medium	Small
(ii)	Obesterics		
	Mode of delivery	Strong	Large
	Duration of membranal rupture	Strong	Large
	RNA in vagina	Medium	Medium
	Invasive procedure	Strong	Small
(iii)	Paediatrics		
	Prematurity	Strong	Medium
	Breast feeding (BF)	Strong	Large
	Breast health	Strong	Small
	Genetics	Weak	Small

CI Confidence interval, *htSNPs* haplotype-tagged single nucleotide polymorphisms n, number, *NA* non applicable, *OR* odds ratio. (a) Wild-type (referent category for all analyses) vs homozygote + heterozygote for each htSNPs. (b) P-value as determined by Fisher's exact test. (c) Adjusted for the maternal viral load in logistic regression analysis

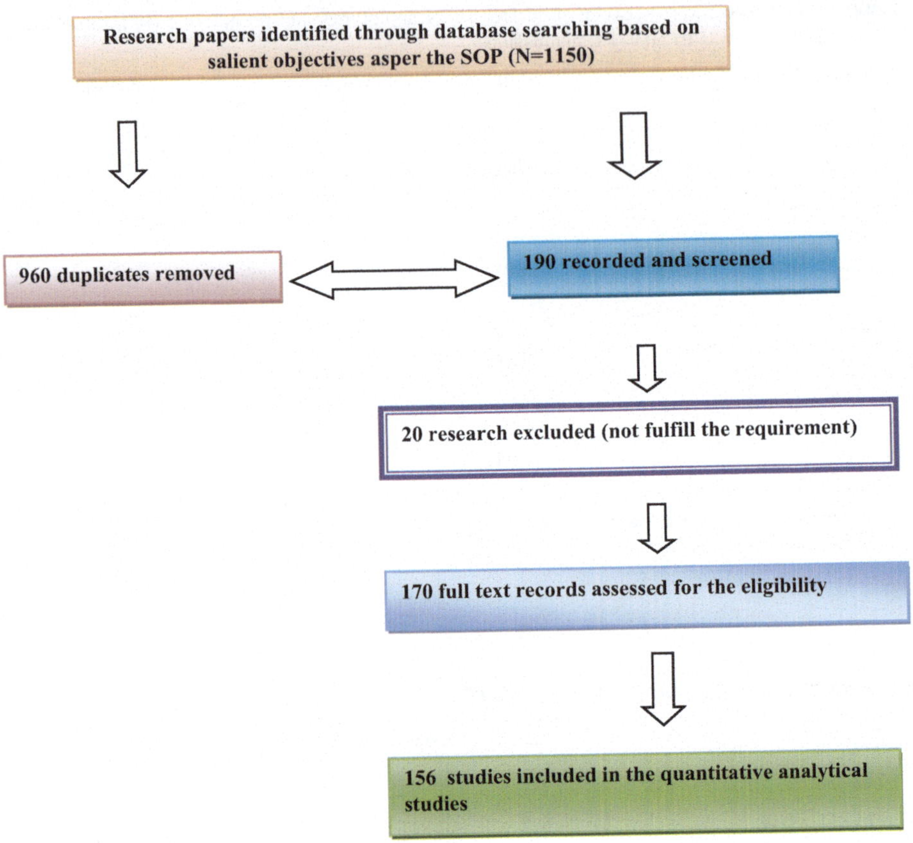

Fig. 11.1 Flow diagram of meta analysis conducted

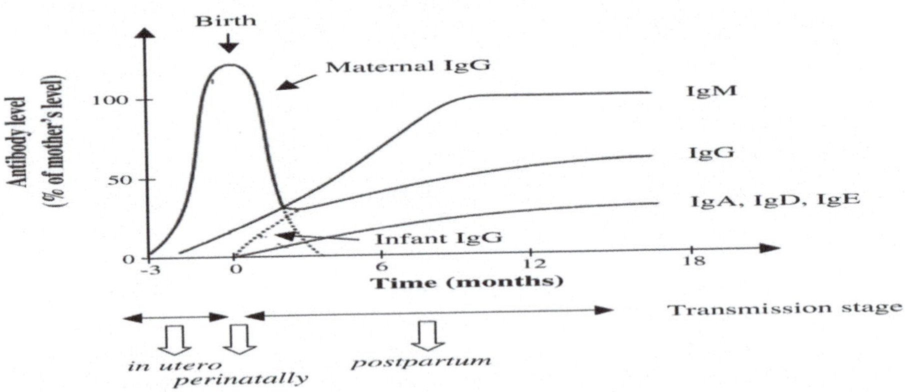

Fig. 11.2 Transmission stage of HIV

in human, they are currently 15,251 HLA and related alleles, more than 250 genes of diverse function including highly polymorphic antigen presenting protein. HLA genes are among the first genetic markers found to alter the risk of becoming infected with HIV-I genes are among the first genetic markers found to alter the risk of becoming infected with HIVI and the rate of disease progression. A class I is the most studies between the two classes, mainly due to his implication in the mechanism of HIV-1 infection. HLAB18 may protect breastfed infants against both early and late HIV-I acquition in Indian perinatal cohort also HLAB may be associated with the resistance to HIV infection upon mother to child exposure found in UK population as well a more specific genotype have shown that among infants the super type is associated with an estimated sevenfold protective effect from perinatal HIV-I transmission. In contrary HLA class (i) concordance between a mother and her infant and the homozygosity of the maternal HLA is associated with increased of overall risk, while HLA discordance decrease the risk of MTCT. The 14 bp insertion in HLA –G was associated with protection from utero and intrapartum of HIV. Mother child HLAG concordance was found not to be associated with increased perinatal HIV transmission. Genome wide association studies, interrogating 0.5–1 milllion SNP's has not confirmed the HLA system as the main contributor to HIV class ii genes with HIV –MTCT are scarce. A study conducted on African population showed that DRB genotype concordance between mother and child increased risk of perinatal HIV transmission, whereas, DPA1, DPB1 and DQB1 concordance between mother and child had no significant influence on perinatal HIV transmission. In addition to that, the summing of the findings showed that, the overall DRB1 discordance between mother and child provided fivefold protection. However, the protective effect of DRB discordance was diminished if and only one of the cases babay carried the DRB1. DRB3 positive phenotype children were less likely to be infected perinatally (Sing et al. 2008; Stephens et al. 2001). However; there was a fourfold increase in risk of being infected at birth if DB3 positive children were born to DRB1 as compared with other intervention.

11.5 Effect of Viral Genotype for MTCT

Viral genotype and inter sub type recombination may influence the rate and or timing of mother to child HIV-I transmission that is why it is important to know whether selective pressure influence the transmission of HIVI from mother to child.inter sub type recombinant genomes, and especially recombination within the LTR, might render HIV-I more fit for transmission via breast milk in comparision with non recombinant subtype A, C, and D. A significant difference in the distribution of transmission time according to sub type and a higher proportion of HIV-I with sub type C *env* transmitted in utero than HIV-I with sub type A env, sub type D env or both combined was reported by Renjifo et al. found that MTCT appears to be more common among mothers infected with sub type D compared with sub type A. A study 2009 supports these data in non B sub types virus infection, here the Abrahams et al. (2009) and Dieltjens et al. (2009) demonstrate that in five Uganda mother child pairs x4 and R5X45 viruses were transmitted before, during or shortly after delivery, and thus establish vertical transmission as an important source of CXCR4 using viruses in infants. But a contrary study have reported that polygenetic tree typologies argue selection process as the major mechanism driving mother to child transmission but support the hypothesis that virus variability is mainly driven by the in columns level and or exposure time. Another study did not find any association between clades A and D either frequency or mode of vertical transmission. The first studies comparing the genetic sequences of viruses from mother and child showed that the maternal viral populations is more heterogeneous than that of the child.if only a limited number variants are originally transmitted and or initially replicating in the child is still a matter of discussion. On the one hand it was shown that a minor viral variant of the mother constituted the dominant variants in the child, on the other hand that a major maternal variant could be detected in vertically infected children. On the other hand it was shown that selection may occur in relation to different transmission route, in utero versus intra partum. Indeed, a major maternal virus variant as well as sub type C variant compared to A and D were associated with in utero transmission. As shown, some studies share the hypothesis that the genetic variation of the HIV1 can drive the MTCT and some are against, but it was noted that in most of the studies the number of mother child pairs was small and information concerning the infection time of the infants was lacking, these limitation was a population size studied; inclusion of small number of mother pairs with incomplete sets of relevant data, limits the power to detect the effects of a common and rare genetic variants. There is need to consider both genetic profile of the mother as well as those of exposed children to avoid distortion between the population parameters for genetic polymorphism and susceptibility to HIV-I MTCT. There is also need to look at the effect of co infection when studying these polymorphism in the case of sub sharan countries. For future research, the recommendation is to study a larger population size, different ethnicities, looking at the effect of all described AIDS related genes (altogether) including those involved in innate immunity, using appropriate control groups and including other factors such as the presence of co infection, the age of the mother, the anti retroviral drugs administered and so on. These studies will benefit the development of a vaccine suitable for all population ground (Table 11.3).

11.6 Discussion

The present study showed bird eye view of genetic variants for MTCT, the results supported by expression assay in placenta, suggest the involvement of CCR5, CD4 and SDF1 in MTCT of HIV-I.Homozygosity for the haplotype H1 and H2 was associated with IU transmission in the Brownian stochastic mode and it was more converges geometric progression. However, the association disappeared after analysis was made for the maternal factors presumably because of the small number of G1 homozygote infants analysed in each sub groups (Subgroup analysis) (Boily et al. 2007). H1 and H2 were the most frequent haplotyes observed in the meta analysis and share a cluster of mutation. Grouping haplotype H1 and H2 increased the power of the study and permitted the identification of specific gene mutation associated with fourfold increased risk of IU

Table 11.3 Gene expression of MTCT (genetic polymorphisms of HIV-1 receptors and ligands on HIV-1 mother-to-child transmission and pediatric disease progression)

Gene	Polymorphism	MTCT	Disease progression
CCR5	Δ32	Decreased	Delayed
CCR5	59029A	Augmented	Accelerated
CCR2	64I	Contracting regularly	Delayed
CD4	1249	No effect	Accelerated
CX3CR1	C868T	Augmented, when heterogeneously expressed in children	Unknown
DC sign	P336C and P201A	Augmented, when expressed in children	Unknown
DC sign	Exon 4:R198Q, E241D, R221Q, and L242v	Augmented, when expressed in children	Unknown
DC SisnR	H1 and H3	Augmented	Unknown
CCL3	Copy number variation	Augmented, when presented in children	Unknown
SDF1	3UTR801A	Augmented, when presented in children	Accelerated

and sixfold increased risk of IP after adjustment for maternal factors. Although P201A and p198A variants was associated with IU transmission, the association disappeared after adjustment was made for the maternal VL. Neverthless, many study showed that this mutation reduces DC sign R transcriptional activity invitro and produces lower level of DC Sign R transcript in placental tissue in combination with the int2 180A variant. Since int2-180A is always transmitted with P 198a on the MTCT associated combined haplotype H1/H3, where as p198 a on the MTCT associated combined haplotypes, we can speculate that the P198A mutation alone may have a minor effect in vivo where as in combination with the int2 180 A variants, they both act to reduce the level of placental DC SIGNR expression resulting in an increased risk of MTCT (Li et al. 2006; Kuiken et al. 2009; Stephens et al. 2001).

The majority of IU transmission occurs during the last trimester of pregnancy. The full term placenta samples were not available for the current study and the expression assays were performed on first term placental tissues. A previous study looking at DC Sign R placental informs repertoire in full term placenta samples demonstrated similar diversity of DC Sign R transcripts as in the first term placental tissues studied herin. However, since levels of DC SIGN R expression have never been compared between the different terms of pregnancy, it is not known whether DC SIGN R expression varies during the course of pregnancy, Nevertheless, it is reasonable to assume that the inter-individual differences in both DC SIGN R isoform repertoire and transcript levels observed between the H_1 and H_2 homozygous infants would be reflected throughout the pregnancy.

11.7 Summary

In this study, we have reviewed 1190 research articles published globally with H factor, eigne value >2.0. Asper the resulted findings and demonstrated results presented in various published articles, summing of the results concludes that, the potential functional impact of CCR5, CD4 and SDF1 mutation on its expression in the placenta and in vertical transmission of HIVI. Many scientists believed that the presence of DC SIGN R at the placental endothelial cell surface may protect infants from HIV I infection by capturing virus and promoting its degeneration. However, in placenta containing low levels of DC SIGN R, HIV I would be preferentially binds CCR5 on endothelial cells resulting in a loss of placental barrier integrity and enhanced passage of maternal HIV I infected cells in a foetal circulation triggered to MTCT of HIV I. This mechanism may also apply to other vertically transmitted pathogens known to interact with DC SIGNR such as HIV2.

References

Abrahams MR et al (2009) Quantitating the multiplicity of infection with human immunodeficiency virus type 1 subtype C reveals a non-poisson distribution of transmitted variants. J Virol 83:3556–3553

Bashirova AA, Geijtenbeek TB, van Duijnhoven GC, van Vliet SJ, Eilering JB et al (2001) A dendritic cell-specific intercellular adhesion molecule 3-grabbing nonintegrin (DC-SIGN)-related protein is highly expressed on human liver sinusoidal endothelial cells and promotes HIV-1 infection. J Exp Med 193:671–678

Boily LG, Zijenah LS, Mbizvo M, Ward BJ, Roger M (2007) DC-SIGN and DC-SIGNR genetic diversity among different ethnic populations: potential implications for pathogen recognition and disease susceptibility. Hum Immunol 68:523–530

Dieltjens T et al (2009) Evolution of antibody landscape and viral envelope escape in an HIV-1 CRF02_AG-infected patient with 4E10-like antibodies. Retrovirology. 2009 6:113

Gray ES et al (2009) Antibody specificities associated with neutralization breadth in plasma from human immunodeficiency virus type 1 subtype C-infected blood donors. J Virol 83:8925–8937

Guay LA et al (1999) Intrapartum and neonatal single-dose nevirapine compared with zidovudine for prevention of mother-to-child transmission of HIV-1 in Kampala, Uganda: HIVNET 012 randomised trial. Lancet. 1999 354:795–802

Guevara H et al (2002) Maternal HIV-1 antibody and vertical transmission in subtype C virus infection. J Acquir Immune Defic Syndr. 2002 29:435–440

Guindon S, Gascuel O (2003) A simple, fast, and accurate algorithm to estimate large phylogenies by maximum likelihood. Syst Biol 52:696–704

Johnson WE et al (2003) Assorted mutations in the envelope gene of simian immunodeficiency virus lead to loss of neutralization resistance against antibodies representing a broad spectrum of specificities. J Virol 77:9993–10003

Katoh K, Kuma K, Toh H, Miyata T (2005) MAFFT version 5: improvement in accuracy of multiple sequence alignment. Nucleic Acids Res 33:511–518

Keele BF et al (2008) Identification and characterization of transmitted and early founder virus envelopes in primary HIV-1 infection. Proc Natl Acad Sci USA 105:7552–7557

Kimura M (1980) A simple method for estimating evolutionary rates of base substitutions through comparative studies of nucleotide sequences. J Mol Evol 16:111–120

Kittinunvorakoon C et al (2009) Mother-to-child transmission of HIV-1 in a Thai population: role of virus characteristics and maternal humoral immune response. Culture 778:768–778

Kosakovsky Pond SL, Posada D, Gravenor MB, Woelk CH, Frost SD (2006) Automated phylogenetic detection of recombination using a genetic algorithm. Mol Biol Evol 23:1891–1901

Kuhn L, Schramm DB, Donninger S, Meddows-Taylor S, Coovadia AH et al (2007) African infants' CCL3 gene copies influence perinatal HIV transmission in the absence of maternal nevirapine. AIDS 21:1753–1761

Kuiken C et al. (n.d.) HIV sequence compendium 2009. Theoretical Biology and Biophysics Group T-6, Los Alamos, NM

Kwiek JJ et al (2006) Maternal-fetal microtransfusions and HIV-1 mother-to-child transmission in Malawi. PLoS Med 3:e10

Kwiek JJ et al (2008a) The molecular epidemiology of HIV-1 envelope diversity during HIV-1 subtype C vertical transmission in Malawian mother-infant pairs. AIDS 22:863–871

Kwiek JJ, Arney LA, Harawa V, Pedersen B, Mwapasa V et al (2008b) Maternal-fetal DNA admixture is associated with intrapartum mother-to-child transmission of HIV-1 in Blantyre, Malawi. J Infect Dis 197:1378–1381

Lathey JL et al (1999) Lack of autologous neutralizing antibody to human immunodeficiency virus type 1 (HIV-1) and macrophage tropism are associated with mother-to-infant transmission. J Infect Dis 180:344–350

Li M et al (2006) Genetic and neutralization properties of subtype C human immunodeficiency virus type 1 molecular env clones from acute and early heterosexually acquired infections in Southern Africa. J Virol 80:11776–11790

Liu H, Hladik F, Andrus T, Sakchalathorn P, Lentz GM et al (2005) Most DC-SIGNR transcripts at mucosal HIV transmission sites are alternatively spliced isoforms. Eur J Hum Genet 13:707–715

Liu S et al (2008a) Analysis of putative N-linked glycosylation sites and variable region of envelope HIV-1 CRF07_BC recombinant in intravenous drug users in Xinjiang Autonomous Region, China. AIDS Res Hum Retrovir 24:521–527

Liu Y et al (2008b) Env length and N-linked glycosylation following transmission of human immunodeficiency virus type 1 subtype B viruses. Virology 374:229–233

Luo W, Yang H, Rathbun K, Pau CP, Ou CY et al (2005) Detection of human immunodeficiency virus type 1 DNA in dried blood spots by a duplex real-time PCR assay. J Clin Microbiol 43:1851–1857

Meddows-Taylor S, Donninger SL, Paximadis M, Schramm DB, Anthony FS et al (2006) Reduced ability of newborns to produce CCL3 is associated with increased susceptibility to perinatal human immunodeficiency virus 1 transmission. J Gen Virol 87:2055–2065

Mummidi S, Catano G, Lam L, Hoefle A, Telles V et al (2001) Extensive repertoire of membrane-bound and soluble dendritic cell-specific ICAM-3-grabbing nonintegrin 1 (DC-SIGN1) and DC-SIGN2 isoforms. Inter-individual variation in expression of DC-SIGN transcripts. J Biol Chem 276:33196–33212

Pedersen BR, Kamwendo D, Blood M, Mwapasa V, Molyneux M et al (2007) CCR5 haplotypes and mother-to-child HIV transmission in Malawi. PLoS One 2:e838

Pohlmann S, Soilleux EJ, Baribaud F, Leslie GJ, Morris LS et al (2001) DC-SIGNR, a DC-SIGN homologue expressed in endothelial cells, binds to human and simian immunodeficiency viruses and activates infection in trans. Proc Natl Acad Sci USA 98:2670–2675

Singh KK, Hughes MD, Chen J, Phiri K, Rousseau C et al (2008) Associations of chemokine receptor polymorphisms with HIV-1 mother-to-child transmission in sub-Saharan Africa: possible modulation of genetic effects by antiretrovirals. J Acquir Immune Defic Syndr 49:259–265

Stephens M, Smith NJ, Donnelly P (2001) A new statistical method for haplotype reconstruction from population data. Am J Hum Genet 68:978–989

12 Statistical Perspective Approach to Selection of Sample

12.1 Statistical Dealing with Success of Good Research

This note monologue, at a prior level, extensive postulates that apply to many different disciplines of research (Medical, Agriculture, Biological and Veterinary Sciences). Anyone that has a research degree/empathy should be aware of them, whether or not they arise in their own research process. They give, also, pointers that may help in getting a clear view of where the researcher's project headed. Many researchers have successfully venture to the research cascade itself and in the salient examples. They are several reasons why researchers should take an interest in broad ranging multiple issues at the time of research planning and hypothesis concord. Many assumed hypothesis have been precluded that the following key points will narrate the story of research. The immediate research project may take twists and turns that are different from those for which earlier has been a preparation (Cady et al. 2000; Cohen 1984). This is especially likely for highly applied research projects, which typically demand a range of diverse skills and other variants affected during the study period. Those who acquire a wide range of research skills and knowledge are thereby better placed, after objective finalization to turn their hand to tasks different from those for which their immediate research training has equipped them. As broad based research skills will best equip to nurture for the researchers to respond to changing the subject area, as they move from one task to another. The designing and planning of research is very important tool or indicator the instrument panel of a research on large questioner domains may appear like a multifaceted problem arise. It can be really emphasize the critical and questioning role of scientific ways of thinking is the best solution for obtaining trust worthy results. It does not much matter where you start practicing scientific thinking and project implementation etc. Because it's explanatory power is so great deal to maintain open pedagogy, once you get the hang of scientific reasoning you are bound to start applying it everywhere during the course of action (Fisher 1935).

Finally, the scientific criticism and questioning are in tension with the openness to imaginative insight that is equally important to the research continuum process. Data

D. M. Basavarajaiah, B. Narasimha Murthy, *HIV Transmission*,
https://doi.org/10.1007/978-981-15-0151-7_12

may be in tension with the theoretical and practical insight that generates their collection. Robert Langkjaer fellow of Royal statistical Society, UK has quoted that "data are not just numbers without meaning or context. The issue of evidence is central there must be an assessment of the evidence in the literature that is the starting points for the research. There must be a research strategy that will bring together data sets that blissfully address the research questions and hypothesis.Statistical analysis will plausibly extract from the real data evidence must be integrated into the body of the earlier knowledge, creating a coherent account that will assimilation of a research project/articles/thesis and monographs etc.

12.2 Research Perspectives in New Horizon

According to research prospective and ethical issues, there is an inherent frankness to new ideas and the ruthless criticism to which the scientific research process insists on extrapolating new idea. As well as research ethical issues, principles and methodological aspects to specify or describe the particular disciplines, there are general statistical principles and methodologies, though avoiding any attempt at rigid prescription of a acceptable scientific procedure. In order to criticize or address the research planning we would establish a frame work that is broad enough for the most of the research projects. The plan should include examination of existing knowledge, a decision on a research question or hypothesis a plan to follow in seeking answers, an analysis of the research data sets and an eventual report formulation (Fig. 12.1).

There are two key components to any research activity. Firstly, there must be generation of new ideas that may be worth investigation. This requires openness to new ideas. Secondly, there must be critical scrutiny of all ideas, whether they are an accepted part of knowledge or new. There will be an eventual rejection of ideas that cannot withstand criticism. These two components are in anxiety. Failure in either may spell doom for the scientific innovation and new ideas. If criticism comes on too strongly at too early a stage, good ideas may be squashed (Kirby et al. 2002; Basavarajaiah 2017). If it appears too late, there may be a huge waste of time from pursuit of unfruitful paths. When ideas that have not received adequate critical evaluation become accepted knowledge, nonsense readily masquerades as science. Different types of study call for different approaches. Unduly rigid prescription is undesirable. Any adequate account of scientific method must allow room for the exercise of imaginative insight. It must also pay regard to checks on the unconstrained use of the imagination. Unconstrained exercise of imagination leads to myth, fiction and to imaginative fiction that presents itself as science. It has led, at worst, to supposed science that has been little more than a vehicle for individual and cultural prejudices. Yet without productive forms of imaginative insight, science would stultify. Ideas may come in many ways, from working out the implications of existing theory, in reverie, from one's reading, from brainstorming sessions, from dreams, as a byproduct of the process of critical scrutiny and testing, and so on. What works for one person or for one research project may not work for another (Basavarajaiah 2017). The origins of creativity are a deep mystery, part of the mystery of our humanness. The study of creativity is itself a scientific study, one

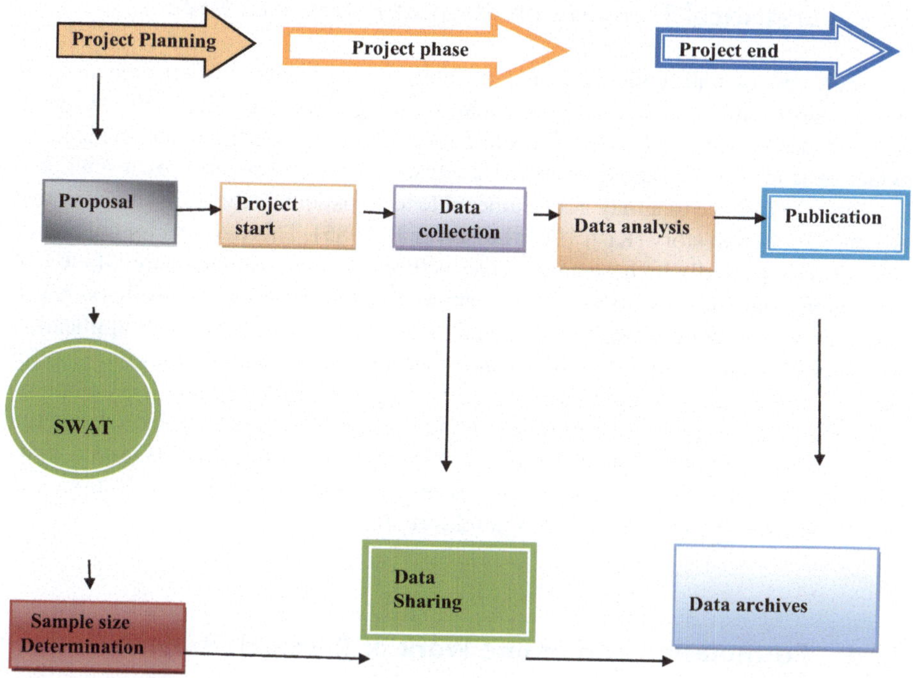

Fig. 12.1 Schematic diagram of research project flow

that has not yet advanced to the point where it can offer deep insights. Creativity has its best chance when the research enterprise has captured the imagination (Basavarajaiah 2017). Researchers who find their task boring and uninspiring are unlikely to be very creative. A sense of wonder is important. Generation of ideas is less the problem than the generation of ideas that has a good chance of withstanding scientific community. Ideas from these sources have been singularly unhelpful to the progress of science. When ideas appear, there must be mechanisms for deciding which are worth pursuing (Basavarajaiah 2017; Fisher 1935). The Juxtapose of any project will begins with SWAT analysis

1. Strength

   The ability to widely distributed project information to vast audience
2. Weakness

   Lack of Knowledge technical information which can lead to misinformation being disseminated, the exposure of information before formal announcement are made
3. Opportunities

   Promote communication and engagement through various types of media source
4. Threats

   Disgruntled environmentalists contracting the media

12.3 Statistical Thinking on Thematic Research Area

In the design of data collection, and in interpreting results, subject area insights should mesh with statistical and data analysis insights in ways that will vary from study to study. The researcher's challenge is to put together all the evidence – evidence from the literature, from the analysis of the researcher's own data, and less formal evidence that may not be amenable to statistical analysis, in a manner that presents a coherent story (Kish 1965; Larsen et al. 1985). This demand for coherence will appear repeatedly in these notes. This section is written from the point of view of a practicing statistician who has often been involved in the research of others. A key emphasis is that there must be a correlation of statistical insights with application area insights. There must be shoe leather as well as statistical analysis. Careful planning will greatly increase the chances that, when your data analysis is complete, there will be a compelling story to tell. It is a fortunate researcher whose data tell a story that is as compelling as R A Fisher (1935) and Basavarajaiah (2017) data, or as John Snow's data. Good planning of the project, and of the data collection, can greatly increase the chances of such good fortune.

12.4 Formulation and Frame Work of Research Project

The aim of the new research project is to develop a framework that will be helpful in the later discussion of research projects. Since, it is fragile to get started at all unless there is a research question, or at least the beginnings of a research questions. It will be convenient to group the different components of a research project under the following headings:

1. Define the state variables -Assessment of the state of existing knowledge
2. Implicit and explicit questions to presume your null hypothesis (Generation and honing of ideas)
3. Formulate proper design of experiment and execution of research that will explore or test specific ideas (Statistical methods for data analysis)
4. Analysis, interpretation and presentation of the resulting data sets

While statistical ideas may not have much role in idea generation, they are certainly important viz assessing existing knowledge, designing, executing research and data analysis and interpretation etc. In case of Veterinary and Medical Science Research emphasis on the review of existing knowledge, an area where the insights of experienced statisticians are sorely needed for guiding the research projects and Interim analysis work. An assessments of how effectively earlier workers have designed their study, and of how compelling their results are, may rely heavily on statistical insights or fore thoughts. Even if the study design seems to stand up to critical scrutiny, the funding agency will ask whether the data interpretation is correct. Mistakes in the statistical analysis or in the interpretation of the analysis may lead to quite wrong conclusions, as in some of the examples that we give later. Sound statistical tool will curb the error of sample or population (Nelder 1999).

12.5 Sample Size Determination

Perhaps the most frequently asked question concerning sampling is, "What size sample do I need?" The answer to this question is influenced by a number of factors, including the purpose of the study, population size, the risk of selecting a "bad" sample, and the allowable sampling error. This section reviews criteria for specifying a sample size and presents several strategies for determining the sample size etc.In very important criteria for sample size determination is level of precision, level of confidence or risk and the degree of variability in the attributes being measured. Usually sample size determination has been followed five basic approaches

1. Arbitrary approach –Rules of thumb (10% of the population)
2. Conventional approach-Average of similar studies (what others have done)
3. Cost basis approach –Availability of resources
4. Statistical approach-Statistical consideration (adequate for sub group analysis)
5. Confidence Interval approach-Concept of variability, sampling decision and SE (x) (allows us to predetermine how precise our estimates are)

Different approaches of Sample size (Fig. 12.2)

12.6 The Level of Precision

The level of precision, sometimes called sampling error (se), is the range in which the true likelihood values of the population is estimated to be. This range is often expressed in percentage numerals (e.g. ±5, ±10 percent), in the same way that results for survey on QOL are reported by the Basavarajaiah et al. Opined that 60% of the farmers who are rearing animal husbandry have adopted a recommended scientific practices with precision rate of ±5%, then he can concludes that between 55% and 65% of farmers in the population have adopted the practice (Basavarajaiah 2017).

12.7 The Confidence Level

Central Limit Theorem clearly states that, any state variables (quantitative/qualitative) can be normally distributed with parameters μ and common varianceσ^2. If the variable not normally distributed the confidence boundary as lead to be skewness (positive/negative). However, the researcher addressed the issues of variable of interest. Asper the theorem the key idea encompassed in the Central Limit Theorem is that, when a large population is repeatedly sampled with large entries, the average value of the attributed data obtained by those samples is equal to the true population

Fig. 12.2 Flow chart shows sample size determination wrt population and sample

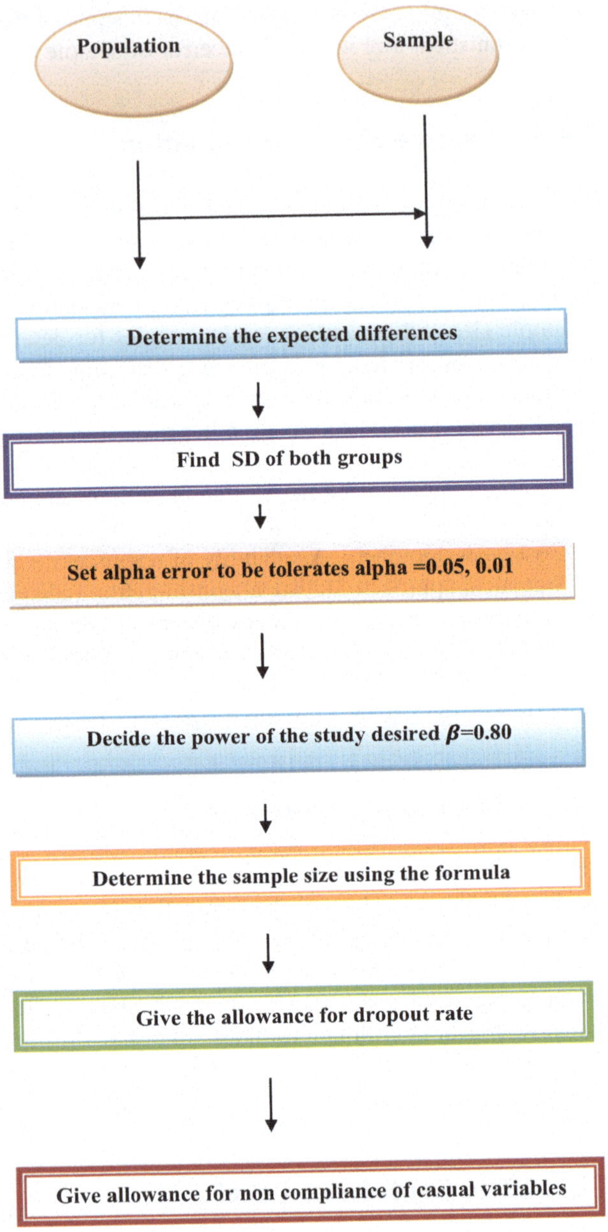

mean value μ. Furthermore, μ values were obtained by these samples are distributed normally $N(\mu, \sigma^2)$ about the true value, with some samples having a higher value and some obtaining a lower score than the true population value is accord. In a normal distribution approximation, approximately 95% of the sample values are within two standard deviations of the true population value (e.g. mean). In other words, this means that, if a 95% confidence level is selected, 95 out of 100 samples will have the true population value within the range of precision specified earlier (repetitions of the experimental value). There is always a chance that the sample you obtain does not represent the true population value. This risk is reduced for 99% confidence levels and increased for 90% (or lower) confidence levels.

$$\text{CI } 95\% = \overline{\mu} + Z_{\alpha\ 1/2} < \text{ND} < \overline{\mu} - Z_{\alpha\ 1/2}$$

12.7.1 Using a Sample Size of a Similar Study

Another salient approach is to use the sample size as those of studies similar to the one you plan. Without reviewing the procedures employed in these studies you may run the risk of repeating errors that were made in determine the sample size for another study. However, a review of the literature in your discipline can provide guidance about typical sample sizes which are used in the experimentation.

12.7.2 Degree of Variability

The important third criteria, the degree of variability in the attributes being measured refers to the distribution of attributes in the population, The more heterogeneous a population, the larger the sample size is required to obtain a given level of precision. The less variable (more homogeneous) a population, the smaller the sample size. The point to be noted that, the proportion of 50% indicates a greater level of variability than either 20% or 80% this is because 20% and 80% indicate that a larger majority do not or do, respectively, have the attribute of interest (Prakesh et al. 2010). Because a proportion of population is necessary. The research study indicates the maximum variability in a population; it is often used in determining a more conservative sample size *ie* the sample size may be larger than if the true variability of the population attributes were used.

12.7.3 Using Published Tables

A third way to determine sample size is to rely on published tables which provide the sample size for a given set of criteria. The sample size would be necessary for given combinations of precision, the confidence level and variability have been considered for determination of sample size it was presented in (Tables 12.1 and 12.2) The following note has been inclusion for sample size reflect viz., the number of obtained responses and not necessarily the number of surveys mailed or interview planned (this number is often increased to compensate for non responsive). Second, the sample sizes in (Table 12.1) presume that the attributes being measured in various characteristics and also measurements are distributed normally or nearly so. If these assumptions can't be met, then the entire population may need to be surveyed with cost minimization.

Table 12.1 Matrix shows various formulas to determine sample size

Types	Sample	Population
Proportion	$n = \frac{Z_\alpha{}^2 p\, q}{e^2}$	$n = \frac{n_0}{1+\frac{n_0-1}{N}}$
	$Z_\alpha =$ Table value for ND	$n =$ sample size
	$p =$ Estimated proportion of sample	$n_0 =$ slected population small in size
	$q = (1 - p)$	$N =$ population
	$e =$ precision of the experiment(0.05)	
Mean	$n = \frac{Z_\alpha{}^2 \sigma^2}{e^2}$	$n = \frac{Z_\alpha{}^2 \mu_\sigma{}^2}{\mathrm{Me}^2}$
	$Z_\alpha =$ Table value for ND	$Z_\alpha =$ Table value for ND
	$\sigma =$ SD of the sample	$\mu_\sigma =$ SD of the population
	$e =$ precision of the experiment(0.05)	$\mathrm{Me}^2 =$ Marginal error
	$\mathrm{ME} = Z_\alpha \sqrt{\frac{P(1-P)}{n}}$	
	$\mathrm{ME} = 1.96\sqrt{\frac{P(1-P)}{n}}$	
	Formula based on t score	
	$\mathrm{ME} = t\left(\frac{\sigma}{\sqrt{n}}\right)$	
	$n = \left(\frac{\sigma t}{\mathrm{ME}}\right)^2$	
	$N = \frac{N}{1+\mathrm{Ne}^2}$	
	$n =$ the sample size, $N =$ the Population size, $e =$ the acceptable SE	
	$n = \frac{\left(\frac{\mathrm{Range}}{2}\right)^2}{\left(\frac{\text{Accuracy level}}{\text{Confidence level}}\right)^2}$,	
	$\text{size} = \frac{\chi^2 \mathrm{np}(1-p)}{d^2(n-1)+\chi^2 p(1-p)}$	
	Where $\chi^2 =$ table value of chisquare	
	$N =$ population size	
	$P =$ population proportion	
	$d =$ degree of accuracy (expression as proportion)	
	Pocock sample size formula	
	$n = \frac{[P_1(1-P_1)+P_2(1-P_2)](Z_\alpha+Z_\beta)^2}{(P_1-P_2)/2}$	
	$n =$ required sample	
	$P_1 =$ estimated proportion of study outcome in the exposed group	
	$P_2 =$ estimated proportion of study outcome in the un exposed group	
	$Z_\alpha =$ represents the desired level of significance 0.05	
	$Z_\beta =$ represents the desired power 0.84	
	Calculating sample size for independent t test	
	$n = \frac{(M_1-M_2)-(\mu_1-\mu_2)}{(\mu_1-\mu_2)^2}$	
	$n = \frac{N\sum N_h S_h{}^2}{N^2 D^2+\sum N_h S_h{}^2}\ D = \frac{e^2}{t^2}$	
	$n =$ sample size	
	$N_h =$ Number of respondents in acceible population	
	$S_h =$ SD of each stratum	
	$D^2 =$ Desired variance	
	$e =$ Permitted error	
	$t =$ table t value	

Kish 1965. Survey Sampling

Table 12.2 Sample size for ±5%, ±7% and ±10% precision levels where confidence level is 95% and $P = 0.05$

Size of the population	±5%	±7%	±10%
100	81	67	51
125	66	78	56
150	110	86	61
175	122	94	64
200	134	101	67
225	144	107	70
250	154	112	72
275	163	117	74
300	172	121	76
325	180	125	77
350	187	129	78
375	194	132	80
400	201	135	81
425	207	138	82
450	212	140	82

12.7.4 Using a Census for Small Populations

One approach is to use the entire population as the sample. Although cost considerations make this impossible for large populations a census is attractive for small populations (e.g. 200 or less respondents) (Sudman 1976). A census eliminates sampling error and provides data on all the individuals in the population in addition some costs such as questionnaires design and developing the sampling frame are fixed. They will be the same for samples of 50 or 200. Finally, virtually the entire population would have to be sampled in small populations to achieve a desirable level of precision of the experiments or research etc (Tables 12.3, 12.4, and 12.5).

12.8 Merits of Sample Size Determination

1. Low cost of sampling –Cost minimization (Reduced cost)
2. Less consuming in Sampling –Consistency result
3. Scope of sampling is high (Error of sample is very less)
4. Maintain good accuracy and precision of the experiment
5. Suitable in very limited resources *wrt* geographical location
6. Better rapport of research insight

12.9 Demerits of Sample Size Determination

1. Chance of bias at induction or end of the experiment

Table 12.3 Sample size for ±3%, ±5%, ±7% and ±10% precision levels where confidence level is 95% and $P = 0.05$

	Sample size for precision 'e'			
Size of the population	±3%	±5%	±7%	±10%
500	A	222	145	83
600	A	240	152	86
700	A	255	158	88
800	A	267	163	89
900	A	277	166	90
1000	A	286	169	91
2000	714	333	185	95
3000	811	353	191	97
4000	870	364	194	98
5000	909	370	196	98
6000	938	375	197	98
7000	959	378	198	99
8000	976	381	199	99
9000	989	383	200	99
10,000	1000	385	200	99
15,000	1034	390	201	99
20,000	1053	392	204	100
25,000	1064	394	204	100
50,000	1087	397	204	100
1,000,000	1099	398	204	100
>1,000,000	1111	400	204	100

a assumption of ND is poor (Yamane 1967). The entire population should be sampled Source data: University of Florida press 1992 fact sheet report, Medical Science -single arm and dual arm study, the table is available in (Larsen et al. 1985)

Table 12.4 Comparison of independent sample groups based power (group I and II)

	Percent of group I									
Percentage of group II	0	10	20	30	40	50	60	70	80	90
10	74									
20	34	199								
30	21	62	293							
40	15	32	81	356						
50	11	20	39	93	387					
60	8	13	23	42	97	387				
70	6	10	14	23	42	93	356			
80	5	7	10	15	23	39	81	293		
90	4	5	7	10	14	20	32	62	19	
100	2	4	5	6	8	11	15	21	34	74

$\alpha = 0.05, \beta = 0.80$

Table 12.5 Matrix for medical/veterinary study for sample size determination

	CI-95%									
Population	10	20	30	40	50	60	70	80	90	95
60	37									
70	41	18								
80	44	19	19							
90	47	19	18	16						
100	49	20	20	17	16					
110	52	20	20	17	16	15				
120	54	20	20	17	16	14	14			
130	55	20	20	17	16	14	14	13		
140	57	21	20	17	16	14	14	12	10	
150	59	20	20	17	18	14	14	12	10	9
160	60	21	20	17	18	14	14	12	10	9
170	62	21	20	18	18	14	14	12	10	9
180	63	21	20	18	19	14	13	12	10	9
190	64	21	20	18	19	13	12	12	10	9
200	65	22	20	18	19	14	12	12	10	9
210	66	22	20	18	19	14	12	12	10	9
220	67	22	21	19	19	12	12	12	10	9
234	68	22	21	19	20	13	12	12	10	9
240	69	22	21	19	20	12	12	12	10	10
250	70	22	21	19	20	12	12	12	10	10
>250	71	24	22	19	20	12	12	12	10	11

2. Difficulties in selecting random true representative samples during the study period
3. Need for subject expertization
4. Changeability of sampling unit due to intrinsic and extrinsic factors
5. Plausible changes of sampling unit due to accidental causes (bottle neck effect)

12.10 Discussion

As per the previous studies, sample size is very important domain for drawing correct decision about the population and solves the real world problems at larger extent, the insight of study will describe the characteristics of parameters tested (Cady et al. 2000). Too small a sample size is more likely to generate inconclusive, incorrect or spurious results. This is because a smaller sample size will generate estimates which have higher variation. These estimates will then be less useful in modelling and understanding the real underlying hypothesis of interest. Secondly, studies which more likely to fail due to inadequate sample size are considered unethical (Yamane 1967; Basavarajaiah 2017; Nelder 1999). This is because exposing human subjects or lab animal/patients recruitment for the study to the possible risks associated with research is only justifiable if there is a realistic chance that the study will yield useful information. Additionally, a study which is too large faces the same ethical problem and will also waste scarce resources such as money, subjects and time. When conducting research, quality sampling may be characterized by the number and selection of subjects or observations. Obtaining sample size that is appropriate in both regards is critical for many reasons. Most importantly, a large sample size is more representative of the population, limiting the influence of outliers or extreme observations. A sufficiently large sample size is also necessary to introduce results among variables that are significantly different. For qualitative studies, where the goal is to reduce the chances of discovery failure. a large sample size broadens the range of possible data and forms a better picture for analysis. Sample size is also very important for economic, physical, psychological and ethical reasons (Nelder 1999). As Rususell Lenth from the University of lowa explains "An under sized study can be a waste of resources for not having the capability to produce useful results, while an oversized one uses more resources than necessary. In an experiment involving human or animal subjects, sample size is a pivotal issue for ethical reasons. An undersized experiment exposes the subject to potentially harmful treatments without advancing knowledge. In an oversized experiment, an unnecessary number of subjects are exposed to a potentially harmful the experiments or research of interest.

12.11 Conclusion

In designing experiments or study, sample size calculation is very important for methodological, ethical reasons, as well as for reasons for human and animal intervention and also financial resources. When conducting a research, the researcher should be alert to ascertain that, the study is subjected to sample size determination. In the absence of the sample size determination, the findings of the study should be interpreted with serious caution and elucidate with probable realistic threat. An appropriate sample size renders the research more efficient, data generated are reliable, and resource investment is as limited as possible, while conforming to ethical and research perspectives. The use of sample size determination directly influences the research intuition and findings. Researcher would have confine to validate the samples at inception of research study, as a result, eliminate the biasness and hypothetical errors.

12.12 Summary

Any research starts with the selection of a problem. Many characteristics or attributes may look for their problems of research viz novelty, interesting, importance, feasibility availability of data and hypothesis testing etc.In the essence of biological research we should make a formulated hypothesis at greater accuracy and precise level of significance $'\alpha'$. The research hypothesis is a presumptive statement of a proportion or a reasonable guess based upon the available evidences or attributes, which the researcher seeks to prove through his course of study. It is also driven from deductive reasoning from a scientific theory. The researcher may begin his study by selecting the sample size is very important dogma in his own area of interest. After selecting the particular theory, the researcher proceeds to derive the hypothesis from his theory. The required sample numerals (size of the sample) are very much concern for success of the research pedagogy and also how much data will require making a correct decision about the population parameters. If we have accurate sampled data sets, then our decision will be more accurate and there will be less standard error of the parameters estimates of research concern. In this accord the present research paper address the basic principles adopted for sample size determination *with respect* to biological field.

References

Basavarajaiah DM (2017) Recent statistical techniques in clinical research. Educreation, Inc, India

Cady RK, Sheftell F, Lipton RB, O'Quinn S, Jones M, Putnam G et al (2000) Effect of early intervention with sumatriptan on migraine pain: retrospective analyses of data from three clinical trials. Clin Ther 22:1035–1048

Cohen IB (1984) Florence nightingale. Sci Am 250:98–107

Fisher RA (1935) The design of experiments. Oliver and Boyd, Edinburgh

Kirby A, Gebski V, Keech AC (2002) Determining the sample size in a clinical trial. Med J Aust 177:256–257

Kish L (1965) Survey sampling. Wiley, New York

Larsen S, Osnes M, Eidsaunet W, Sandvik L (1985) Factors influencing the sample size, exemplified by studies on gastroduodenal tolerability of drugs. Scand J Gastroenterol 20:395–400

Nelder JA (1999) From statistics to statistical science. J R Stat Soc Ser D 48:257–267

Prakesh B, Babu SR, Sureshkumar K (2010) Response of Ayurvedic therapy in the treatment of migraine without aura. Int J Ayurveda Res 1:29–35

Sudman S (1976) Applied sampling. Academic, New York

Yamane T (1967) Statistics, an introductory analysis, 2nd edn. Harper and Row, New York

Summary and Implications for Future Study 13

13.1 Introduction

HIV is a scourge; more than 2.5 million of the infected populations die every year. For control of non-curable diseases, there is a need for implementation of new innovative public health programs. Till date, HIV infection continues to have a significant impact, especially on children. In the year 2012, approximately 2.10 million children were living with HIV worldwide. In Indian context national adult HIV prevalence was 0.27% in 2011. Of these, women constituted 39% of all people living with HIV (PLHIVs), while children less than 15 years of age constituted 7% of all infections. As of March 2015, 0.10 million HIV-positive children had been registered under the antiretroviral therapy (ART) program, and 38,579 are receiving free ART. There has been a significant scale-up of HIV counseling and testing, prevention of parent-to-child transmission (PPTCT), and ART services across the country over the last 5 years (Kuhn et al. 2005a, b; Kuhn et al. 2008; Kumwenda et al. 2008; Lallemant et al. 2004; Lanjewar et al. 1996; Li N Sando et al. 2015; Lihing et al. 2009; Lounes et al. 1986; Low-beer et al 1997; Madhi et al. 2000a; 2000b; Marais et al. 2006; Marazzi et al. 2011; Marcenko et al. 2008; Martelli et al. 2002; Martin et al. 2010; May et al. 1998; Menzies et al. 2009). It is a great economic burden on National GDP and public health. AIDS also poses a threat to economic growth in many countries already in distress. The World Bank estimates an annual slowing in growth of income per capita by an average of 0.6% per country in ten worst affected countries. The negative impact of AIDS on households, productive enterprises, and countries seems to be partly from the high cost of treatment, which diverts resources from productive investments. Modelling is an essential tool for understanding disease progression and its relationships with social, biological, and environmental mechanisms that influence the spread of HIV/AIDS (Mermin et al. 2008; Ministry of Health Uganda 2006; Mofenson et al. 2012; Moges et al. 2011; Moges et al. 2014; Mohammed et al. 2012; Mustapha et al. 2010; Nagelkerke et al. 1995; NACO 2006; Nduati et al. 2000; Nelson et al. 2001; Nguena et al. 2014; Nico et al. 2002; Obimbo et al. 2004; Onyango-Makumbi et al. 2010; Palme et al. 2002;

D. M. Basavarajaiah, B. Narasimha Murthy, *HIV Transmission*,
https://doi.org/10.1007/978-981-15-0151-7_13

Pinkerton et al. 2012; Ramharter et al. 2004; Raminez et al. 2006; Ramos et al. 2010; Rauner et al. 2005; Read et al. 2003; Rollins et al. 2004, 2008; Ross 1993; Selekman et al. 2006; Shankar et al. 2005; Shapiro et al. 2010; Sharma et al 2005; Sperling et al. 1996; Spira et al. 1999; Springer et al. 2004; Srinivasrao 2009; Stark et al. 2003; Stover et al. 2000; Sun et al. 2012; 2009; Swaminathan et al. 2004; Taha et al. 2002; 2016; Thamattor et al. 2015; Thior et al. 2006; Thomas et al. 2002; Thomas et al 2007; Towne et al. 2007; Uganda Bureau of Statistics 2007; Ugochukwu et al. 2006; UNAIDS 2007; 2008). Due to paucity of research work on modeling, the policymakers are unable to implement the new innovative programs at national level. The entitled book *HIV Transmission: Statistical Modelling* is an outcome of a series of analyses carried out by developing and applying mathematical and statistical models on a body of real-life data compiled in Karnataka State AIDS Control Societies to know the rate of HIV transmission from mother to child in Bangalore city. Several researchers developed mathematical and statistical models to analyze and test the HIV disease progression rate of mother-to-child transmission (MTCT). However, there are practical issues on which mathematical and statistical models are developed and applied and should be addressed to arrive at reasonable analytical reasoning on HIV transmission from mother to child. In that context, examination of practical issues related to building of mathematical modeling of HIV MTCT large data sets for reduction of high-dimensional HIV data sets is necessary. The methodology attempted in the present thesis is at three levels. First is to build the model on real-life HIV mother-to-child transmission large data sets to know the disease epidemic and endemic equilibrium with varied parameters. The validity of the developed model is examined through the estimation of proportion of babies who got HIV infected through defined risk factors. Second, two common practical issues, viz., the statistical criteria in terms of reduction of large high-dimensional HIV data sets on the basis of theoretical model and intervention with numerical simulation for the estimation of defined risk parameters of HIV MTCT, are considered. Third, sometimes it may not be feasible to build the desired and efficient models for the estimation of HIV mother-to-child transmission. In such a situation, if the researcher or statistician estimates the progression rate effectively by the way of building or developing mathematical models through different analytical procedures, it will be useful for nurturing HIV epidemic at population level. There are several data sets generated from HIV clients, viz., drug reaction, HIV TB co-infection, HIV-associated neurological disorders, ophthalmological complications, etc., for describing clinical complications. HIV itself is a life-threatening deadly disease, and many real-life data sets are generated from the lifelong treatment and their follow-up records. Over the past era, statisticians, researchers, and policymakers have put a great amount of efforts in developing and comparing suitable mathematical and statistical models on HIV data sets (UNAIDS/WHO 2005; Vajpayee et al. 2001; Vieira et al. 2002; Vieira 2003; Waema et al. 2005; Walker et al. 2002; Wallers et al. 2008; WHO, 2000; 2006; WHO collaborative study team, 2000; Wishart 1928; Yui et al. 2001; Zaba et al. 2003; Zar et al. 2000). These fitted models must be general and broad enough to allow for building theoretical and predictive models. The consistency of findings of the fitted models suggests that the quality of estimation is good, taking into consideration of the practical, analytical, and statistical issues and the efficient quality of estimation of parameters with varied socioeconomic, behavioral, and risk factors.

13.2 Objectives

The specific objectives of the book are:

(i) To provide a brief introduction and background about mathematical and statistical model building, review of the relevant literature on estimation of HIV transmission from mother to child by considering the various risk factors and HIV biomarkers. To discuss certain issues related to the development of modeling
(ii) To describe the real-life data sets including flowchart of HIV transmission risk factors, procedure of model building, and estimation of factors associated for HIV MTCT
(iii) To examine the developed model by relevant diagnosis (Runge and Kutta method and MLEs) and illustrate the fitted model with HIV MTCT real-life data sets
(iv) To examine the suitability of well-known predictive models approach to HIV transmission from mother to child and HIV TB co-infection ascertained with lower CD4 count at the time of inception of HAART and high RNA plasma viral load
(v) To attempt various analytical methods adopted for model building and examine whether it is feasible to identify optimal analytical procedure for estimation of HIV MTCT
(vi) To summarize the thesis, provide recommendations, and discuss implications for future line of research work

13.3 HIV MTCT Data Sets and Methodology

The relevant information for this thesis was compiled from the data obtained from Karnataka State AIDS Control Societies (SACs) program with written permission during 2009–2013. The data pertaining to demographic features of ANCs, viz., risk factors of HIV mother-to-child transmission; gravida status; clinical parameters like type of regimen, WHO staging, opportunistic infections (OIs), etc.; laboratory parameters, CD_4 cell count(micro/dL) and viral load(micro/dL); transmission rate, timing of transmission, and mechanisms and risk factors of transmission; breastfeeding types and methods of feeding; duration of feeding; secondary prevention strategies; tertiary strategies; HAART type of therapy (I line or II line); duration of therapy; drug toxicity; WHO clinical stages; and different modes of delivery, were considered for the study. The collected data was analyzed by using Matlab-10.50

and SPSS-16.50 version software. Different statistical, mathematical, and epidemiological models were fitted to test the significance of certain risk factors.

13.4 Salient Findings

The present study developed simulation mathematical model. Theoretically model was simplified and formulated on the basis of higher order differential equations. Positivity of the solution, stability analysis, and equilibrium point of the model (diseases endemic and epidemic equilibrium) was obtained from the basis of reproduction number Ro. Model forward bifurcation was proved by Castillo-Chavez and Song theorem. Model suggested that due to absence of ARVs, prolonged breastfeeding, lower CD4 count, and high plasma viral load of infected mother were directly proportional to increase HIV transmission from mother to child. Fitted model could undergo further mathematical and algebraic treatment easily with varied population size and parameters. Considering the issue on the reduction of large matrix of high-dimensional data sets fitted, random walk-free probability and entropy model become orthogonal symmetric and followed Gaussian of complex valued $N \times K$ matrix, where K is the number of transmitting children, while "N" is the same for receiving from mother side, which was simplified by the way of random walk-free probability with weak topology. The model clearly suggest that, the newborn child will undergo HIV testing at different interval of time, the probability values were expected to meet P(n, m). This model is more useful for reduction of large data coverage and high-dimensional HIV data set. It was demonstrated that statistical modeling is more useful for the estimation of HIV mother-to-child transmission rate and construction of appropriate design. It could be useful to validate the findings from the empirical analytical results for real-life data. The present study fitted different statistical and mathematical models for understanding disease progression in HIV mother-to-child transmission. As per the fitted model, mother-to-child HIV cumulative transmission rate was 23.84%. Prolonged breast feeding, lower CD4 count at inception of HAART, high plasma viral load, low body weight, and no use of ARV prophylaxis at the time of onset of birth are considered as the predictors of HIV mother-to-child transmission. The disease transmission susceptible mathematical model, genetic, random walk, and probability models were found to be best models for the analysis of HIV large data set and can also achieve a local asymptotically stabilization and globally disease-free equilibrium (reproduction $R_0>1$ & $R_0<1$). The present study helps policymakers, researchers, mathematicians, statisticians, and clinicians for the implementation of innovative program for preventing HIV MTCT.

13.5 Significance of the Study

The outcome of this study will help the government and NGOs to establish policies, programs, and optimal plan for control of the disease by taking into account the aspect of treatment and vertical transmission. It will help the society in general to have an understanding on how the disease can be controlled through treatment of infective with ARV. Also, it will add more knowledge to the existing literature on HIV/AIDS and help researchers to do more research on this disease. Lastly, this study will help educationists to develop educational seminars, workshops, or training programs to educate people on the impact of treatment and vertical transmission in creeping down the HIV/AIDS epidemic.

13.6 Study Limitation

This study comprised data from a series of cross-sectional surveys rather than a randomized controlled trail design and without suitable control groups. Hence, it is not possible to rule out that the results may have occurred independently out of the intervention, personal privacy and confidentiality is respected at all times.

13.7 Implication for Future Research

The possibility of identification of various components of different mathematical and statistical model building for estimation of HIV MTCT rate and developing analytical and predictive models assume significance, when there exist large computerized data sets. With advanced statistical theory and by developing mathematical and statistical methods in future, the HIV transmission can be split into many folds by considering risk factors and their associated parameters. It needs further research to look for the suitability of the models to account for estimation of diseases progression rate. Baseline parameters of HIV transmission may be studied in the future. Survival analysis is yet another important procedure to look for the effectiveness of the HAART treatment program; Cox proportional hazards and Kaplan-Meier model are the statistical tool employed for this purpose. It may be worthwhile, as future activity to look for the coding of independent variable in Cox proportional hazard model and logistic regression model for treatment outcomes with a real-life data of time to the event in HIV lifelong treatment. In HIV diseases progression estimation, the desired mathematical and statistical models may not be met its full bloom or may be inadequate. In such a situation, our fitted model may be explored to examine the accurate estimation of HIV progression rate with desired level of significance. However, this model needs to be applied with real-life HIV data set, globally. This thesis provides an opportunity to look into various forces that act upon while analyzing HIV high-dimensional data sets.

13.8 Challenges

Challenge is striking the right balance between prevention and treatment initiatives. Since the epidemic is still concentrated, the interventions need to be target-oriented and location-specific. The decentralization planning and intervention strategies will greatly help to achieve this objective. Considering the size and magnitude of the country, the resources required to meet the programmatic demands are substantial and call for sustained partnerships at all levels. In this context, a more accurate estimate of the HIV burden will help in strategic evidence-based planning and designing for more elective programs at national, state, and district levels. In addition, this approach will also strengthen the decentralized target-oriented interventions in selected locations. Accordingly, the present NACP IV program at national level will have to invest more in public and PPP sector, service delivery mechanisms, and infrastructure; capacity building of public sector, civil society, and private sector; and a robust strategic information management system. To achieve this complex set of objectives and the overall goal of halting and reversing the HIV MTCT epidemic, the national program will have to strengthen partnerships with donors, civil society, and the private sector at micro level.

References

Kuhn L, Kasonde P, Sinkala M et al (2005a) Does severity of HIV disease in HIV infected mothers affect mortality and morbidity among their uninfected infants? Clin Infect Dis 41:1654–1661

Kuhn L, Kasonde P, Sinkala M et al (2005b) Prolonged breast-feeding and mortality up to two years postpartum among HIV-positive women in Zambia. AIDS 19:1677–1681

Kuhn L, Aldrovand GM, Sinkala M, Zambia Exclusive Breast feeding Study et al (2008) Effects of early, abrupt weaning on HIV-free survival of children in Zambia. N Engl J Med 359:130–141

Kumwenda NI, Hoover DR, Mofenson LM et al (2008) Extended antiretroviral prophylaxis to reduce breast-milk HIV-1 transmission. N Engl J Med 359:119–129

Lallemant M, Jourdain G, Le Coeur S (2004) Single-dose perinatal nevirapine plus standard zidovudine to prevent mother to child transmission of HIV, Thailand. N Engl J Med 351 (3):217–228

Lanjewar DN, Rodrigues C, Saple DG, Hira SK, Dupont (1996) Cryptosporidium, isospora and strongyloides in AIDS. Natl Med J India 9:17–19

Li N Sando MM, Chalamilla G, Spiegelman D, Hertzmark WFE (2015) Antiretroviral therapy in relation to birth outcomes among HIV-infected women: a cohort study. J Infect Dis Adv 1–7

Lih-ing W, Feng RZ, Castillo-Chavez C (2009) Modelling TB and HIV co-infections. Math Biosci Eng 6(4):815–837

Lounes R, Arazoza HD, Sanchez A et al (1986) Epidemiology of HIV in Cuba, modelling detection with temporally varying parameters. Int J Math 4(1):107–117

Low-beer D, Stone Burner RL et al (1997) An age–and sex structured HIV epidemiological model; features and applications. Bull World Health Organ 75:312–316

Madhi SA, Huebner RE, Doeders L, Aduc T, Wesley D, Cooper PA (2000a) HIV-1 co-infection in children hospitalized with TB in South Africa. Int J Tuberc Lung Dis 4:448–454

Madhi SA, Huebner RE, Doeders L, Aduc T, Wesley D, Cooper PA (2000b) HIV-1 co-infection in children hospitalized with TB in South Africa. Int J Tuberc Lung Dis 4:448–454

Marais BJ, Graham SM, Cotton MF, Beyer N (2006) Diagnostic and management challenges of childhood TB in the era of HIV. J Infect Dis 196:576–585

Marazzi MC, Palombi L, Nielsen-Saines K et al (2011) Extended antenatal use of triple antiretroviral therapy for prevention of mother-to-child transmission of HIV-1 correlates with favorable pregnancy outcomes. AIDS 25:1611–1618

Marcenko V, Pasture L (2008) Distribution of some sets of random matrices, Mat.Sb. J Comput Res 1:507–536

Martelli TCM et al (2002) Mother to child transmission of HIV: risk factors and missed opportunities for prevention among pregnant women attending health services in Brazil 23. J Infect Dis 10:1028–1032

Martin DJ, Sim JG, Sole GJ, Rymer L, Shalekoff S, Van Niekerk AB et al (2010) CD4 lymphocyte count in African patients co-infected with HIV and TB. J Acquir Immune Defic Syndr Hum Retrovirol 8:386–391

May RM, Anderson RM et al (1998) Transmission dynamic of human immunodeficiency virus (HIV). Phil Trans R Soc A 321:565–607

Menzies N, Homsy J, Chang Pitter JY et al (2009) The cost-effectiveness of routine rapid HIV antibody testing before DNA-PCR testing for early infant HIV diagnosis in resource-limited settings. Pediatr Infect Dis J 28:819–825

Mermin J, Were W, Ekwaru JP et al (2008) Mortality in HIV-infected Ugandan adults receiving antiretroviral treatment and survival of their HIV-uninfected children: a prospective cohort study. Lancet 371:752–759

Ministry of Health Uganda, AIDS Control Programme (n.d.) National guidelines for the prevention of mother to child HIV transmission. Revised ed. August 2006

Ministry of Health Uganda and ORC Macro (2006) Uganda HIV/AIDS sero-behavioral survey. Uganda Ministry of Health and ORC Macro, Kampala

Mofenson LM et al (2010) Protecting the next generation eliminating perinatal HIV-1 infection (editorial). N Engl J Med 362(24):2316–2318

Mofenson L et al (2012) Antiretroviral prophylaxis to reduce breast milk transmission of HIV type 1: new data but still questions. J AIDS 48:237–240

Moges H, Carla J, Chibwesha MD, Mark J et al (2011) Optimal time on HAART for prevention of MTCT of HIV. J AID 58(2):224–228

Moges H, Fentaw WA, Sahu O et al (2014) Statistical modelling and analysis of mother-to-child transmission of HIV: a case study in referral hospital and health center of Hawassa Town, south nation nationality people, Ethiopia. Int J Data Envelopment Anal Oper Res 1(3):49–52

Mohammed I, Seidu DB et al (2012) Modelling the effect of irresponsible infective immigrants on the transmission dynamics of HIV/AIDS. Adv Appl Math Biosci 3(1):31–40

Mustapha MG, Rabasa AI, Ashir MG, Usman AB, Mohammed SY et al (2010) Management of childhood tuberculosis: the experience in a tertiary health re-facility in Nigeria. Niger Med Pract 57:5–6

Nagelkerke NJ et al (1995) The duration of breastfeeding of HIV-1 infected mothers in developing countries: balancing benefits and risks. AIDS 8:176–181

NationalAIDS ControlOrganization(NACO) (2006) Annual report http://www.nacoonline.org

Nduati R, John G, Mbori-Ngacha D et al (2000) Effect of breastfeeding and formula feeding on transmission of HIV-1: randomized clinical trial. JAMA 283(9):1167–1174

Nduati R, Richardson BA, John G et al (2001) Effect of breast feeding on mortality among HIV-1 infected women: a randomized trial. Lancet 357:1651–1655

Nelson P, Mittler J, Perelson A et al (2001) Effect of drug efficacy and the eclipse phase of the viral life cycle on estimates of HIV-1 viral dynamic parameters'. AIDS 26:405

Nguena HL, Nguefack H, Gwet M, Téjiokem P et al (2014) Estimating mother-to-child HIV transmission rate in Cameroon: a computer simulation approach. AIDS 24th International conference Melbourne http://pag.aids2014.org/Abstracts.aspx?AID=7582

Nico JD, Nagelkerke James F, Blanchard, Jha P et al (2002) Modelling HIV/AIDS epidemics in Botswana and India: impact of interventions to prevent transmission. Bull World Health Organ 80(2):89–96. http://www.who.int/bulletin/archives/80(2) 89.pdf

Obimbo EM, Mbori-ngacha DA, Ochieng JO et al (2004) Predictors of yearly mortality in a cohort of human immunodeficiency virus type1-infected African children. Pediatr Infect Dis J 23:536–543

Onyango-Makumbi C, Bagenda D, Mwatha A et al (2010) Early weaning of HIV-exposed uninfected infants and risk of serious gastroenteritis: findings from two perinatal HIV prevention trials in Kampala, Uganda. J Acquir Immune Defic Syndr 53:20–27

Palme IB, Gudetta B, Bruchfeld J, Muhe L, Giesecke J et al (2002) Impact of human immunodeficiency virus infection on clinical presentation, treatment, outcome and survival in a cohort of Ethiopian children with tuberculosis. Paediatr Infect Dis J 21:1053–1061

Pinkerton SD et al (2012) HIV transmission rate modelling: a primer, review, and extension. AIDS Behav 16(4):791–796

Ramharter M et al (2004) Shared breastfeeding in Central Africa. AIDS 18(13):1847–1849

Raminez-cardich ME, Kawai V, Oberhelman RA, Bautista CT et al (2006) Clinical correlates of TB co-infection in HIV infected hospitalized in Peru. Int J Infect Dis 10:278–281

Ramos JM, Reyes F, Tesfamariam A et al (2010) Childhood and adult tuberculosis in a rural hospital in Southeast Ethiopia: a ten-year retrospective study. BMC Public Health:215–219

Rauner MS, Brailsford SC, Flessa S et al (2005) Use of discrete-event simulation to evaluate strategies for the prevention of mother-to-child transmission of HIV in developing countries. J Oper Res Soc 56:222–233

Read JS et al (2003) Human milk, breastfeeding, and transmission of human immunodeficiency virus type 1 in the United States. Am Acad Pediatr Comm Pediatr AIDS Pediatr 112 (5):1196–1205

Rollins N et al (2004) Preventing postnatal transmission of HIV-1 through breast-feeding: modifying infant feeding practices. J Acquir Immune Defic Syndr 35(2):188–195

Rollins NC, Becquet R, Bland RM et al (2008) Infant feeding, HIV transmission and mortality at 18 months: the need for appropriate choices by mothers and prioritization within programmes. AIDS 22:2349–2357

Ross SM (1993) Introduction to probability models. Academic, Boston

Selekman J et al (2006) Changes in the screening for tuberculosis in children. Pediatr Nurs 32:73–75

Shankar AV et al (2005) Making the choice: the translation of global HIV and infant feeding policy to local practice among mothers in Pune, India. J Nutr 135(4):960–965

Shapiro RL, Hughes MD, Ogwu A (2010) Antiretroviral regimens in pregnancy and breast-feeding in Botswana. N Engl J Med 362(24):2282–2294

Sharma SK, Mohan A, Kadhiraran T (2005) HIV-TB co-infection. Epidemiology, diagnosis and management. Indian J Med Res 11:5–10

Sperling RS, Shapiro DE, Coombs RW (1996) Maternal viral load, zidovudine treatment, and the risk of transmission of human immunodeficiency virus type 1 from mother to infant. N Engl J Med 335(22):16219

Spira R, Lepage P, Msellati P et al (1999) Natural history of human immunodeficiency virus type 1 infection in children: a five year prospective study in Rwanda. Pediatrics 104(5):56–62

Springer V, Castillo-Chavez C, Songe B (2004) Dynamical models of tuberculosis and their application. Math Biosci Eng 1:361404

Srinivasrao A (2009) Mathematical modelling on HIV. Ph.D thesis submitted to Bangalore University

Stark JR et al (2003) Pediatric tuberculosis: time for a new approach. Tuberculosis 83:208–212

Stover et al (2000) Influence of mathematical modelling of HIV and AIDS on policies and programs in the developing world. Sex Transm Dis 27(10):572–578

Sun Y, Gilbert PB (2012) Estimation of stratified mark-specific proportional hazards models with missing marks. Scand J Stat 39:34–52

Sun Y, Gilbert PB, Mckeague IW (2009) Proportional hazards models with continuous marks. Ann Stat 37:394–426

Swaminathan S et al (2004) Tuberculosis in HIV-infected children. Paediatr Respir Rev 5:225–230

Taha TE, Kumwenda NI, Hoover DR et al (2016) The impact of breast feeding on the health of HIV-positive mothers and their children in sub-Saharan Africa. Bull World Health Organ 84:546–554

Taha TE, Kumwenda J, Kafulafula G et al. (2002) Maternal highly active antiretroviral treatment (HAART): does it improve child survival? 5th IAS Conference on HIV Pathogenesis, Treatment and Prevention; July 19–22, Cape Town

Thamattor U, Thomas T, Banandur P et al (2015) Multilevel analysis of the predictors of HIV prevalence among pregnant women enrolled in annual HIV sentinel surveillance in four states in South India. PLoS One 10(7):1–11

Thior I, Lockman S, Smeaton LM, Mashi Study Team et al (2006) 20 breast feeding plus infant zidovudine prophylaxis for 6 months vs formula feeding plus infant zidovudine for 1 month to reduce mother-to-child HIV transmission in Botswana: a randomized trial: the Mashi study. JAMA 296:794–805

Thomas T, Masaba R, Ndivo R et al. (2002) Rates of diarrhea associated with early weaning among infants in Kisumu, Kenya. 14th Conference on Retroviruses and Opportunistic Infections; February25–28, Los Angeles

Thomas T, Masaba R, Ndivo R et al. (2007) Prevention of mother-to-child transmission of HIV-1 among breastfeeding mothers using HAART: the Kisumu Breastfeeding study, Kisumu, Kenya, 2003–2007. 15th Conference on Retroviruses and Opportunistic Infections; February3–6, Boston

Towne-gold B, Ekouevi DK, Viho I et al (2007) Antiretroviral treatment and prevention of peripartum and postnatal HIV transmission in West Africa: evaluation of a two-tiered approach. PLoS Med 4:1362–1373

Uganda Bureau of Statistics, Ministry of Health and Macro International Inc. (n.d.) USA Uganda demographic and health survey, 2006. August 2007, Kampala

Ugochukwu EF et al (2006) Clinical spectrum of pediatric HIV infection in Nnewi. West Afr J Med 25:10–14

UNAIDS (2007) Report of the global AIDS epidemic. Joint United Nations programme on HIV/AIDS

UNAIDS (2008) Report on the global AIDS epidemic, WHO Library Cataloguing-in- Publication Data: UNAIDS/08.25E/JC1510E. WHO, Geneva

UNAIDS/WHO (2005) Guidelines for measuring HIV prevalence in population-based surveys. UNAIDS/WHO Working Group on Global HIV/AIDS and STI Surveillance, Geneva

Vajpayee N, Kanswal S, Seth P, Wig N (2001) Spectrum of opportunistic infection and profile of cd4 counts among AIDS patients in north India. Infection 31:336–340

Vieira TI, Harper RP, Shahani AK, De senna V (2002) Mother to child transmission of HIV a simulation based approach for the evaluation of intervention strategies. J Oper Res Soc 54:713–722

Vieira TI, Harper RP, Shahani AK, De senna V (2003) Mother-to-child transmission of HIV: a simulation-based approach for the evaluation of intervention strategies. J Oper Res Soc 54 (7):713–722

Waema R, Olowofeso OE et al (2005) Mathematical modelling for human immunodeficiency virus (HIV) transmission using generating function approach. Kragujevac J Sci 27(115):130

Walker N, Schwartlander B, Bryce J et al (2002) Meeting international goals in child survival and HIV/AIDS. Lancet 360:284–289

Wallers E, Cotton MF, Rabie H, Schaaf HS, Wallers LO, Marais BJ (2008) Clinical presentation and outcome of tuberculosis in human immunodeficiency virus infected children on anti-retroviral therapy. BMC Paediatr 8:1–6

WHO (2000) Improving access to quality care in family planning: medical eligibility criteria for contraceptive use, 2nd ed. WHO/RHR/00.02WHO global strategy for infant and young child feeding. Geneva, World Health Organization 3(1):98–101

WHO (2006) Management of TB in the HIV-infected child. Int J Tuberc Lung Dis 10:1331–1336. WHO.HIV transmission through breast feeding review of available evidence

WHO Collaborative Study Team on the Role of Breastfeeding on the Prevention of Infant Mortality (2000) Effect of breastfeeding on infant and child mortality due to infectious diseases in less developed countries: a pooled analysis. Lancet 355:451–455

Wishart J (1928) Entropy and its application. J Biometricka 20:32–52

World Health Organization (2013) Treatment of children with HIV report. http://www.who.int/hiv/topics/paediatric/en/index.html 153–168

Yui LL, Chen RY et al (2001) Pregnancy outcomes and risk factors for low birth weight and preterm delivery among HIV-infected pregnant women in Guangxi, China. Chin Med J (Engl) 125:403–409

Zaba B, Whitworth J, Marston M et al (2003) HIV and mortality of mothers and children: evidence from cohort studies in Uganda, Tanzania, and Malawi. Epidemiology 16:275–280

Zar HJ, Tannenbaum E, Apolles P, Roux P, Hanslo D, Hussey G (2000) Sputum induction for the diagnosis of pulmonary tuberculosis in infants and young children in an urban setting in South Africa. Arch Dis Child 82:305–308

The manufacturer's authorised representative in the EU is Springer Nature Customer Service Centre GmbH, Europaplatz 3, 69115 Heidelberg, Germany. If you have any concerns regarding our products, please contact ProductSafety@springernature.com

Printed and bound by CPI Group (UK) Ltd, Croydon, CR0 4YY
23/09/2026
02221542-0012